AF615370

A Primate Model for the Study of Colitis and Colonic Carcinoma

The Cotton-Top Tamarin

Saguinus oedipus

Edited by
Neal K. Clapp, D.V.M., Ph.D.
Director
Marmoset Research Center
Oak Ridge, Tennessee

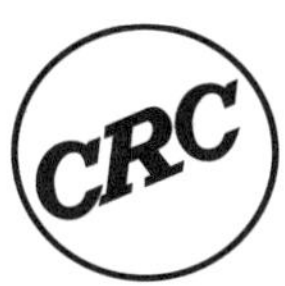

CRC Press
Boca Raton Ann Arbor London Tokyo

Library of Congress Cataloging-in-Publication Data

A Primate model for the study of colitis and colonic carcinoma : the cotton top tamarin (Saguinus oedipus) / edited by Neal K. Clapp.
p. cm.
Includes bibliographical references and index.
ISBN 0-8493-5363-7
1. Colitis--Animal models. 2. Colon (Anatomy)--Cancer--Animal models. 3. Saguinus oedipus--Diseases. I. Clapp, Neal K., 1928- .
[DNLM: 1. Colitis. 2. Colonic Neoplasms. 3. Disease Models, Animal. 4. Saguinus. WI 522 P952]
RC862.C6P75 1993
616.3′447--dc20
DNLM/DLC
for Library of Congress 92-48271
CIP

This book represents information obtained from authentic and highly regarded sources. Reprinted material is quoted with permission, and sources are indicated. A wide variety of references are listed. Every reasonable effort has been made to give reliable data and information, but the author and the publisher cannot assume responsibility for the validity of all materials or for the consequences of their use.

Direct all inquiries to CRC Press, Inc., 2000 Corporate Blvd., N.W., Boca Raton, Florida 33431.

International Standard Book Number 0-8493-5363-7

Library of Congress Card Number 92-48271

Printed in the United States of America 1 2 3 4 5 6 7 8 9 0

Printed on acid-free paper

PREFACE

Advances through medical research are frequently hampered by the absence of appropriate animal models for human disease. Animal models developed by induction or intervention, which offer the advantage of predictability in time of expression, can mimic human disease in some parameters, e.g., production of inflammatory mediators, but frequently deviate from typical human disease pathogenesis. Spontaneous animal models may also deviate from normal human pathogenesis but more commonly suffer from the problem of unpredictability in the time of disease expression. The cotton-top tamarin (CTT) has been proposed as an animal model of spontaneously occurring idiopathic colitis and colonic carcinoma which offers the further research advantage of predictable expression, in that colonic carcinoma is expressed in 35% of the adult CTT population found in 14 different colonies worldwide.

In this volume, researchers report results of studies involving three of the larger biomedical research CTT colonies in the world. Many of the studies represent just the beginning in defining the CTT as a model of colitis and of colon carcinoma. Several investigators, however, have identified similarities between colon disease expressions in CTTs and humans. Furthermore, both humans and animals potentially may benefit from knowledge gained from repetitive sampling possible only in the animal model.

A further advantage of the cotton-top tamarin model is the shortened chronology between onset of colitis and eventual progression to colon carcinoma. The opportunity is thus available, within a reasonable time frame and in a primate model, to assess therapeutic efficacy of both anti-colitic agents and anti-cancer protocols. Tumor biologists also have the possibility of evaluating expression of disease markers and designing approaches to alter the sequence of disease progression.

As indicated earlier, many of the studies reported in this book represent beginnings. Our colony also is experiencing a new beginning. The foresight of Oak Ridge Associated Universities' administration in establishing the cotton-top tamarin colony has been succeeded by the vision of The University of Tennessee Medical Center in maintaining and expanding the colony. The colony remains a fertile resource for investigators dedicated to the vision of improving the well-being of both animals and humans through biomedical research.

Neal K. Clapp

THE EDITOR

Neal K. Clapp, D.V.M., Ph.D., is the Director of UTMCK's Marmoset Research Center at Oak Ridge (UT/MARCOR) and is Professor of Pathology at The University of Tennessee Medical Center at Knoxville, TN.

Dr. Clapp received his B.S. degree from Purdue University in 1950, his D.V.M. from The Ohio State University in 1960, and his M.S. (Radiology) and Ph.D. from Colorado State University in 1962 and 1964, respectively. He was an NIH postdoctoral fellow at Colorado State University from 1961 to 1964. He was an experimental pathologist at the Biology Division of Oak Ridge National Laboratory from 1964 to 1981 and directed the Marmoset Research program in Oak Ridge Associated Universities from 1981 to 1992.

Dr. Clapp is a member of American Association for Cancer Research, American Veterinary Medical Association, Inflammation Research Association, American and International Primatology Associations, Radiation Research Society, and American Society of Laboratory Animal Practitioners.

Dr. Clapp has been the recipient of research grants from the National Institutes of Health and several pharmaceutical company research programs. He has presented seminars internationally at universities, in the private sector, and at numerous international meetings. He has published more than 100 research papers. His current research interests include the pathogenesis, diagnosis, and therapeutic efficacy of treatment in colonic diseases.

CONTRIBUTORS

Linus J. Adams, M.D.
Chief, Director of Gastroenterology and Nutrition
Department of Medicine
University of Tennessee Medical Center at Knoxville
Graduate School of Medicine
Knoxville, Tennessee

Garth Anderson, Ph.D.
Department of Molecular and Cellular Biology
Roswell Park Cancer Institute
Buffalo, New York

Richard B. Andrews, B.S.
Senior Research Assistant
Department of Medical Biology
University of Tennessee Medical Center
Knoxville, Tennessee

Dennis Barnard, M.S.
Nutritionist
Veterinary Resources Program
National Center for Research Resources
National Institutes of Health
Bethesda, Maryland

C. Richard Boland, M.D.
Associate Professor
Internal Medicine
University of Michigan
Ann Arbor, Michigan

David A. Brian, D.V.M., Ph.D.
Professor
Department of Microbiology
College of Veterinary Medicine
University of Tennessee
Knoxville, Tennessee

Robert L. Carson
Marmoset Nurse
Marmoset Research Center
University of Tennessee Medical Center
Oak Ridge, Tennessee

Sreeniwas Chintalapani, M.B., B.S.
Internal Medicine
Wayne State University
Detroit, Michigan

Neal K. Clapp, D.V.M., Ph.D.
Director, Marmoset Research Center
Professor of Pathology
Graduate School of Medicine
University of Tennessee Medical Center at Knoxville
Oak Ridge, Tennessee

Bertram I. Cohen, Ph.D.
Assistant Director
Surgical Research Lab
Beth Israel Medical Center
New York, New York

James E. Crook, M.D., Ph.D.
Consultant
MARCOR
Oak Ridge, Tennessee

Joseph E. Fuhr, Ph.D.
Professor
Medical Biology and Pathology
University of Tennessee Medical Center
Knoxville, Tennessee

Robert M. Hansard, B.A., B.S.
Research Associate
Marmoset Research Center
Oak Ridge Associated Universities
Oak Ridge, Tennessee

Lemuel Herrera, M.D.
Surgical Oncology
Medical Center of Delaware
Wilmington, Delaware

Marsha A. Henke, M.S.
Research Associate
Marmoset Research Center
Oak Ridge Associated Universities
Oak Ridge, Tennessee

Lorna D. Johnson, M.D.
Lecturer
Obstetrics, Gynecology, and
Reproductive Biology
Harvard Medical School
Boston Massachusetts

Norval W. King, D.V.M.
Associate Director for Research
New England Regional Primate
Research Center
Harvard Medical School
Southborough, Massachusetts

Karel Kithier, M.D., Ph.D.
Associate Professor
Pathology
Wayne State University of Medicine
Detroit, Michigan

Joseph J. Knapka, Ph.D.
Staff Nutritionist
Veterinary Resources Program
National Center for Research
Resources
National Institutes of Health
Bethesda, Maryland

Norman L. Letvin, M.D.
Associate Professor
Department of Medicine
New England Regional Primate
Research Center
Southborough, Massachusetts

Gordon D. Luk, M.D.
Patterson Professor
Internal Medicine
VA Medical Center
University of Texas
Southwestern Medical Center
Dallas, Texas

Kenneth Manley, Ph.D.
Department of Molecular and
Cellular Biology
Roswell Park Cancer Institute
Buffalo, New York

Roderic B. Mast
Conservation International
Washington, D.C.

Stuart Van Meter, M.D.
Assistant Professor
Department of Pathology
University of Tennessee Medical
Center
Knoxville, Tennessee

Russell A. Mittermeier
Conservation International
Washington, D.C.

Erwin H. Mosbach, Ph.D.
Director
Surgical Research Laboratory
Beth Israel Medical Center
New York, New York

Gloria M. Petersen, Ph.D.
Assistant Professor
Department of Epidemiology
The Johns Hopkins University
School of Hygiene and Public Health
Baltimore, Maryland

Nicholas J. Petrelli, M.D.
Chief
Surgical Oncology
Roswell Park Cancer Institute
Buffalo, New York

Daniel K. Podolsky, M.D.
Chief
Gastrointestinal Unit
Massachusetts General Hospital
Boston, Massachusetts

José Vicente Rodriguez
Santafé de Bogotá
Colombia, South America

Marie-Paule Roth, M.D.
Research Scientist
CRPG du CNRS
Toulouse Cedex, France

Prabhat K. Sehgal, B.V.Sc.
Assistant Professor of Pathology
Division of Primate Resources
New England Regional Primate Research Center
Harvard Medical School
Southborough, Massachusetts

Linda J. Shockley, M.S.
Lieutenant Colonel
Chemical Corps
United States Army
Alexandria, Virginia

Suzette D. Tardif, Ph.D.
Research Assistant Professor
Department of Anthropology
University of Tennessee
Knoxville, Tennessee

Martin Tobi, M.D., Ch.B.
Assistant Professor
Department of Medicine
Wayne State University
Detroit, Michigan

Kaila Vijaya, M.B.B.S.,
Resident Internal Medicine
Wayne State University
Detroit, Michigan

Bryan F. Warren, M.D., Ch.B.
Department of Pathology and Microbiology
University of Bristol
Bristol, United Kingdom

David I. Watkins, Ph.D.
Assistant Professor
Department of Pathology and Regional Primate Research Center
University of Wisconsin
Madison, Wisconsin

ACKNOWLEDGMENTS

To management and staff of Oak Ridge Associated Universities and The University of Tennessee Medical Center at Knoxville, who had the vision and commitment to support and encourage the research and merit of the Marmoset Colony through many years.

To many collaborators and co-workers who have encouraged and labored with us in seeking knowledge to understand the animal model and its value in studying both animal and human diseases.

DEDICATION

To my family who have offered support and encouragement for many years: my wife, Dot, our children, Cheryl, Mark, and Steve, their spouses, and our grandchildren. Thanks.

TABLE OF CONTENTS

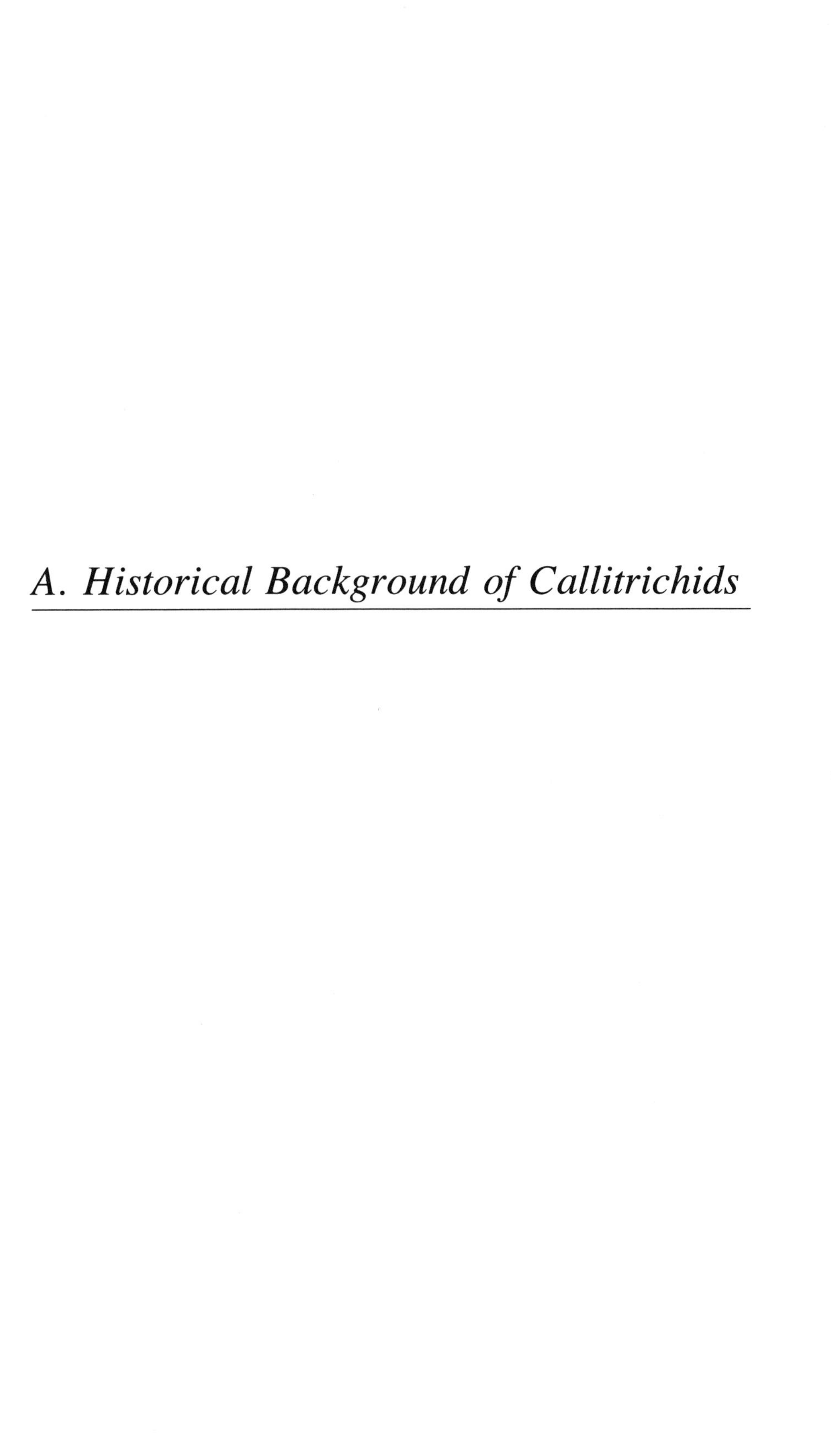

A. Historical Background of Callitrichids

Chapter 1

THE COLOMBIAN COTTON-TOP TAMARIN IN THE WILD

Roderic B. Mast, José Vicente Rodriguez, and Russell A. Mittermeier

TABLE OF CONTENTS

0-8493-5363-7/93/$0.00 + $.50

I. INTRODUCTION

Due to its unique natural history and physiology, the cotton-top tamarin is one of the most important primate models for biomedical research, and has been used for laboratory research on numerous maladies, from Epstein-Barr virus to colitis and colon cancer. As will be discussed throughout this volume, the cotton-top tamarin is indispensable for the study of colitis and colon carcinogenesis, as it is the only primate model which, like humans, spontaneously develops colitis preceding and often accompanying the onset of colon cancer.[1-4]

Although the cotton-top is found abundantly in both zoological and research colonies throughout the world,[5-7] it is considered highly endangered in its wild habitat. The cotton-top's entire distribution is in a small area of northwestern Colombia, South America; there, its native forests have been substantially reduced, and free-ranging monkeys have been threatened by live capture for local and international pet markets and the biomedical industry.[8]

The cotton-top tamarin is just one endangered resident of these high diversity forests but is noteworthy because of its beauty and charisma, as well as its economic and utilitarian importance as a tool to catalyze a more rapid cure for colon cancer, one of the leading causes of death, second only to lung cancer[1] in Europe, North America, Australia, and New Zealand. As such, the cotton-top is an ideal flagship species to draw attention to the plight of its tropical forest habitat, and hence should be used (through education and awareness campaigns) both to rally public support and to muster financial resources for conservation in Colombia.

This paper discusses the taxonomy, distribution, and conservation of the cotton-top tamarin in the wild and the authors recommend actions to ensure the long-term survival of the species and the integrity of its natural habitat, as well as a rationale and general guidelines for ways in which biomedical researchers can play a greater role in conserving the natural habitats of cotton-tops and other primate species used in biomedical research.

II. TAXONOMY

A. THE FAMILY CALLITRICHIDAE

The Callitrichidae make up the most diverse family of New World monkeys, with 32 species in all. Apart from the 16 marmoset species within the genera *Callithrix* (15) and *Cebuella* (1),[9] there are four lion tamarin species within the genus *Leontopithecus*,[10] and 12 tamarin species within the genus *Saguinus*.[9,11] Snowdon and Soini[12] have divided the tamarins into two groups, the Hylaen (or Amazonian) and the extra-Amazonian. The latter group of trans-Andean tamarins comprises three taxa (*S. geoffroyi, S. oedipus,* and *S. leucopus*), all of which are found in Colombia.

Overall, the callitrichids are the smallest of the New World monkeys, have nonprehensile tails, possess claws instead of nails, and move quadrupedally.[13,14] The callitrichids are the size of, and move in a similar fashion to, squirrels; Kavanagh[15] has aptly referred to the Callitrichidae as the "little squirrel-like monkeys with claws." In addition, all monkeys of the family Callitrichidae lack a set of paired molars that are typical of the other families of New World primates. The four callitrichid genera can be further distinguished on the basis of dentition. The "short-tusked" lower anterior dentition characteristic of the genera *Callithrix* and *Cebuella* is a physiological adaptation allowing these taxa to perforate tree bark and induce the flow of exudates (gum and sap), which are important food sources. In contrast, the genera *Saguinus* and *Leontopithecus* possess the "long-tusked" dental configuration in which the canines are much longer than the incisors.

B. THE COTTON-TOP AND ITS CONGENERS

Of Colombia's 26 primate species (12 genera and 45 taxa, see Table 1),[17] three are endemic; these include one species of douroucouli or owl monkey (*Aotus brumbacki*), and two congeneric callitrichids, *Saguinus leucopus* (the white-footed tamarin) and the subject of this chapter, *S. oedipus* (the cotton-top tamarin, Figures 1A and 1B). A large mane of cottony white fur on its head gives the cotton-top tamarin its most appropriate name. This notable feature makes the animal one of the world's most striking primates and is also the source of its other vernacular name, used mostly in Germany, the "Franz Liszt" monkey, for the Hungarian piano virtuoso and composer (1811–1886) also known for his ashen pompadour. First described by Linnaeus in 1758, the cotton-top tamarin is often mistakenly referred to in the literature as the cotton-top "marmoset." In Colombia it is called *tití, titis,* or *tití pielroja* in the northern portion of its range, plus *bichichi* in the southwestern portion (where it is confused with *Saguinus geoffroyi,* called by the same common name, see Figure 2).[18]

It is noteworthy to mention that Hershkovitz[13] describes both the cotton-top and Panamanian (or Geoffroy's) tamarins as subspecies of *Saguinus oedipus (S. o. oedipus* and *S. o. geoffroyi,* respectively), and Hernández Camacho and Defler[19,20] have also suggested that these two taxa fall beneath a single superspecies.[21] We have chosen to utilize herein the more widely accepted view that both of these taxa are full species.[9,22]

The debate regarding the taxonomy of the three extra-Amazonian tamarins results largely from a severe lack of data on wild distribution and ecology. The Panamanian tamarin (*S. geoffroyi*) is found in extreme eastern Panama and northwestern Colombia roughly to the west of the Atrato River (see maps, Figures 3A and B); a few sightings of the Panamanian tamarin have been made to the east of the Atrato, in the vicinity of Quibdo.[18] The cotton-top's other closely related congener, the white-footed tamarin (*S. leucopus,* see Figure 4), ranges to the south and east of the cotton-top's distribution; its range is roughly bounded to the north and west by the Cauca River and the Magdalena River, respectively. The distribution and ecology of the white-footed tamarin is the most poorly known of the three extra-Amazonian callitrichids especially in the eastern and southern portions of its range.[23]

TABLE 1
Primates of Colombia

Present in Colombia	Spanish common name	English common name	Conservation status CITES, IUCN, Authors**
Cebuella pygmaea pygmaea[1]	tití, leoncito, pielroja, chichico	pygmy marmoset	2, N, V
Saguinus fuscicollis fuscicollis[2]	tití	saddle-back tamarin	2, N, S
Saguinus nigricollis nigricollis	bebeleche	black-mantled tamarin	2, E, A
*Saguinus nigricollis hernandezi**	bebeleche	" " "	2, N, U
Saguinus graellsi[3]	tití	Graells' black-mantled tamarin	2, N, U
Saguinus inustus	gueviblanco, mico diablito	mottle-faced tamarin	2, N, U
Saguinus geoffroyi	tití, bichichi	Panamanian tamarin	1, N, V
*Saguinus oedipus**	tití, tistis, tití pielroja, tití cabeciblanco	cotton-top tamarin	1, E, A
*Saguinus leucopus**	tistis, tití gris	white-footed tamarin	1, E, A
Callimico goeldii	chichico diablo	goeldi's marmoset	1, R, A
Aotus lemurinus zonalis	marteja, marta, micodenoche, tutamono	Douroucouli or owl monkey	2, N, A
Aotus lemurinus griseimembra	" " "	" " "	2, N, A
*Aotus lemurinus lemurinus**	" " "	" " "	2, N, A
*Aotus brumbacki**	" " "	" " "	2, N, V
Aotus vociferans	" " "	" " "	2, N, V
Aotus nancymai	" " "	" " "	2, N, V
Callicebus cupreus discolor	zocai, zocayo, zogui-zogui	dusky titi	2, N, V
*Callicebus cupreus ornatus**	" " "	" " "	2, N, V
Callicebus torquatus lugens	viudita, macaco, zogui-zogui	collared titi	2, N, V
Callicebus torquatus lucifer	" "	" "	2, N, V

*Saimiri sciureus albigena**	tití vizcaino, tití frayle, fraylecito, macaco de cheiro	squirrel monkey	2, N, S
Saimiri sciureus macrodon	" " "	" "	2, N, S
Saimiri sciureus casiquiarensis	" " "	" "	2, N, S
*Pithecia monachus milleri**	mico volador, huapo negro, huarpo negro	saki monkey	2, N, V
Pithecia monachus monachus	" " "	" "	2, N, V
Cacajao melanocephalus ouakary	chucuto, rabón	black-headed uakari	2, V, V
Cebus capucinus capucinus	cariblanco, mico negro, maicero, machín	white-faced capuchin	2, N, V
*Cebus capucinus curtus**	" " "	Gorgona Island capuchin	2, N, S
*Cebus albifrons malitiosus**	mico tanque, coruptela de takke, (nombre en Andoque), machín, yurac-machín, yana-machín (Quechua), cairara	white-fronted capuchin	2, N, V
Cebus albifrons cesarae	" " "	" " "	2, N, A
Cebus albifrons versicolor[4]	" " "	" " "	2, N, V
*Cebus albifrons albifrons**	" " "	" " "	2, N, V
Cebus albifrons unicolor	" " "	" " "	2, N, V
Cebus albifrons yuracus	" " "	" " "	2, N, V
Cebus apella apella	cachón, cachudo, macaco prego	tufted capuchin	2, N, S
Alouatta seniculus seniculus	aullador, guariba, cotumono, mono cotudo, araguato, arauato, mono colorado, bramador	red howler monkey	2, N, S
Alouatta seniculus stramineus	" " "	" " "	2, N, V
Alouatta palliata aequatorialis	gueviblanco, chongón, aullador negro	mantled howler monkey	1, N, V

TABLE 1 (continued)
Primates of Colombia

Present in Colombia	Spanish common name	English common name	Conservation status CITES, IUCN, Authors**
Lagothrix lagotricha lagotricha	barrigudo, churuco, choyo	wooly monkey	2, V, A
Lagothrix lagotricha lugens	" " "	" "	2, V, A
Ateles belzebuth belzebuth	mica, coatá, mona marimba, marimonda chomba, braceador, maquisapa	black spider monkey	2, V, A
Ateles belzebuth hybridus	" " "	" " "	2, V, A
*Ateles belzebuth brunneus**	" " "	" " "	2, V, A
Ateles fusciceps rufiventris	" " "	brown headed spider monkey	2, V, A
Ateles fusciceps grisescens	" " "	" " "	2, V, A
Possibly present in Colombia			
Saguinus labiatus thomasi[5]	tití	Thomas' moustached tamarin	2, N, U
Aotus nigriceps[6]	marta, marteja	Dourucouli or owl monkey	2, N, U
Pithecia aequatorialis[7]	mico volador		2, N, U
Chiropotes satanas chiropotes[8]	?	bearded saki	2, E, U
Cacajao calvus rubicundus[9]	uakari, mico inglés, macaco inglés, huapo, huarpo rojo	red uakari	2, V, U
Cebus nigrivitattus[10]	maicero, machín	Weper capuchin monkey	2, N, U
Ateles fusciceps fusciceps	marimonda	brown-headed spider monkey	2, V, U

Undescribed primate taxa from Colombia			
Saguinus sp.[11]	tití cardonero	?	?, ?, V
Aotus sp.[12]	marteja, marta, micoden-oche, tuta mono	?	?, ?, A

Note: * = endemic to Colombia; **: CITES: 1 = Appendix I; 2 = Appendix 2. IUCN: N = not listed; E = endangered; R = rare; V = vulnerable. Authors: V = vulnerable; S = satisfactory; A = endangered; U = insufficient data.

1 This subspecies name is derived from the supposition that *Cebuella pygmaea niveiventer* should be a valid subspecies, based on revision of specimens from Brazil.

2 Recent information pemits the supposition that the resident population in the Trapezio of the Colombian Amazon should be referred to as a new subspecies.

3 Hershkovitz considers this a subspecies of *Saguinus nigricollis.*

4 This includes *C. c. leucocephalus, C. c. adustus,* and *C. c pleei.*

5 This taxon is found north of the Solimões River and the headwaters of the Putumayo River.

6 Individuals of this taxon may have been introduced from Perú.

7 This taxon may be found in the Trapezio of the Colombian Amazon.

8 A dubious report of this animal has been recorded near the Orinoco River.

9 This taxon may be found in the Trapezio of the Colombian Amazon.

10 This species is synonymous with *C. olivaceus* and is possibly found in Colombia, in the Departments of Guainia and Amazonas.

11 Numerous visual records of an undescribed species bearing the local name ''tití cardonero'' have been made by Hershkovitz and others from: the watershed of the Guachaca River, near Pueblito, Department of Magdalena; the watershed of the River Ariguani, near Carcolicito and near Bosconia, Department of Cesar; and from the Tarra River, town of San Calixto, Department of Norte de Santander. Recently at La Gabarra, near the Catatumbo River in the Norte de Santander Department, captive individuals were also reported by Gerardo Viña. Hershkovitz has indicated that this animal could be a species of *Callimico*.

12 This species is in the process of description, with type locality from the upper Cusiana River, Department of Boyacá.

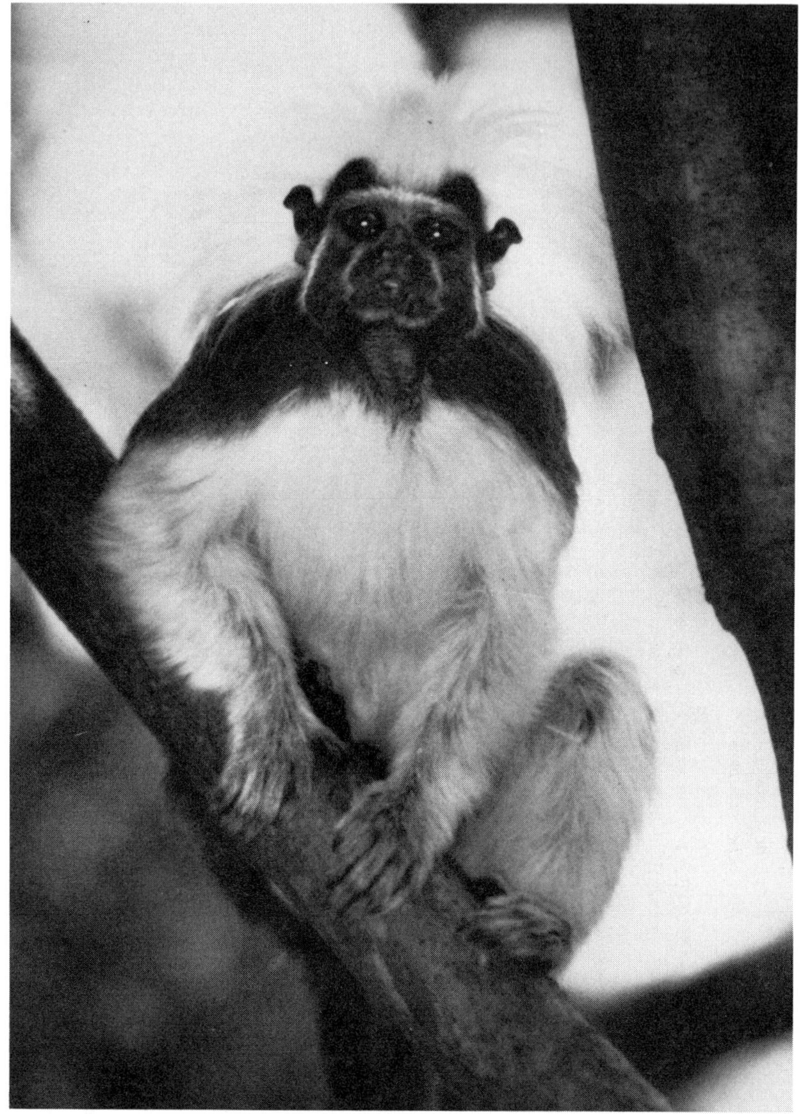

FIGURE 1A. The cotton-top tamarin (*Saguinus oedipus*) is well represented in captive zoological and research colonies in the U.S. and Europe, but is highly endangered in its native tropical forest habitat in northwestern Colombia. (Photo by Roderic Mast.)

The biological species concept assumes that if two taxa can interbreed and produce viable offspring in the wild, they cannot be considered separate species. Often, the ability of two taxa to interbreed can be tested in captivity and Benirschke has indicated that hybrids would likely occur within all the callitrichid genera if the animals were given the opportunity to interbreed.[24]

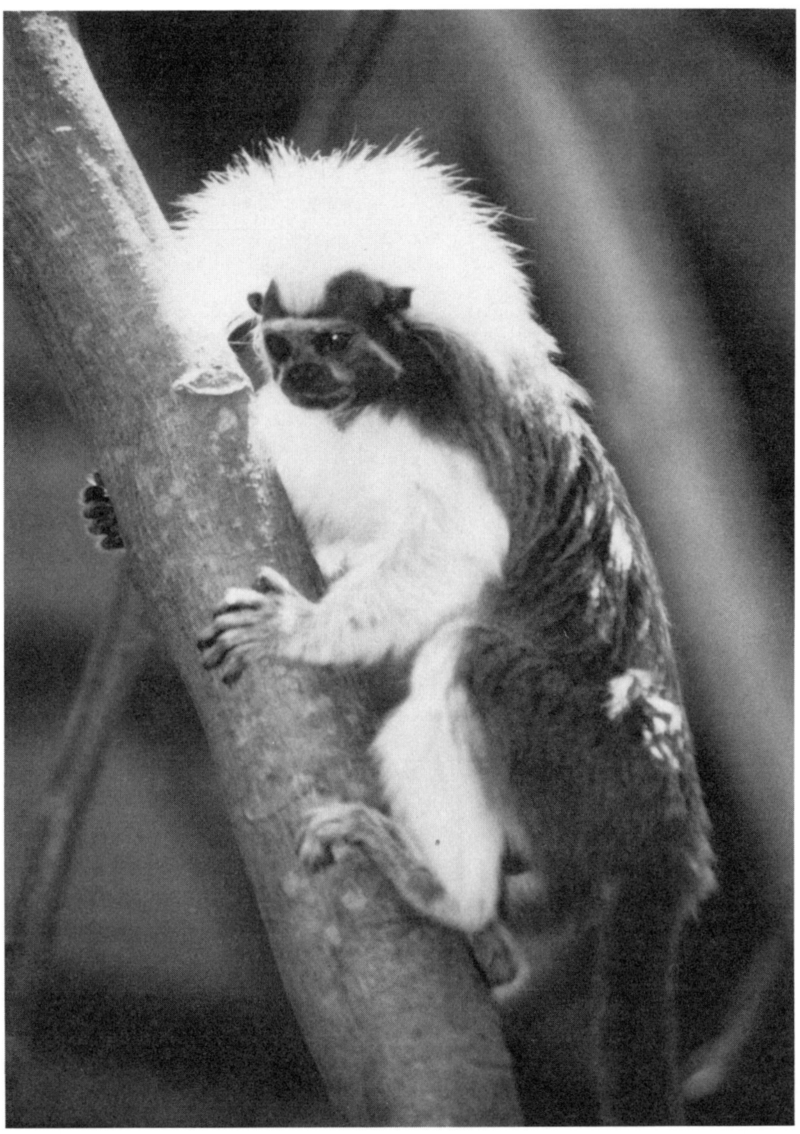

FIGURE 1B.

Interestingly, there seem to be many hybrids produced by *Saguinus* species,[13] though there are no confirmed reports of such offspring being fertile. Epple,[25] for example, reports a specific case of hybridization between *Saguinus oedipus* and *S. geoffroyi,* although it is unknown if the two litters produced were fertile. Hybrid offspring have also been produced between *S. oedipus* and *S. midas*.[25]

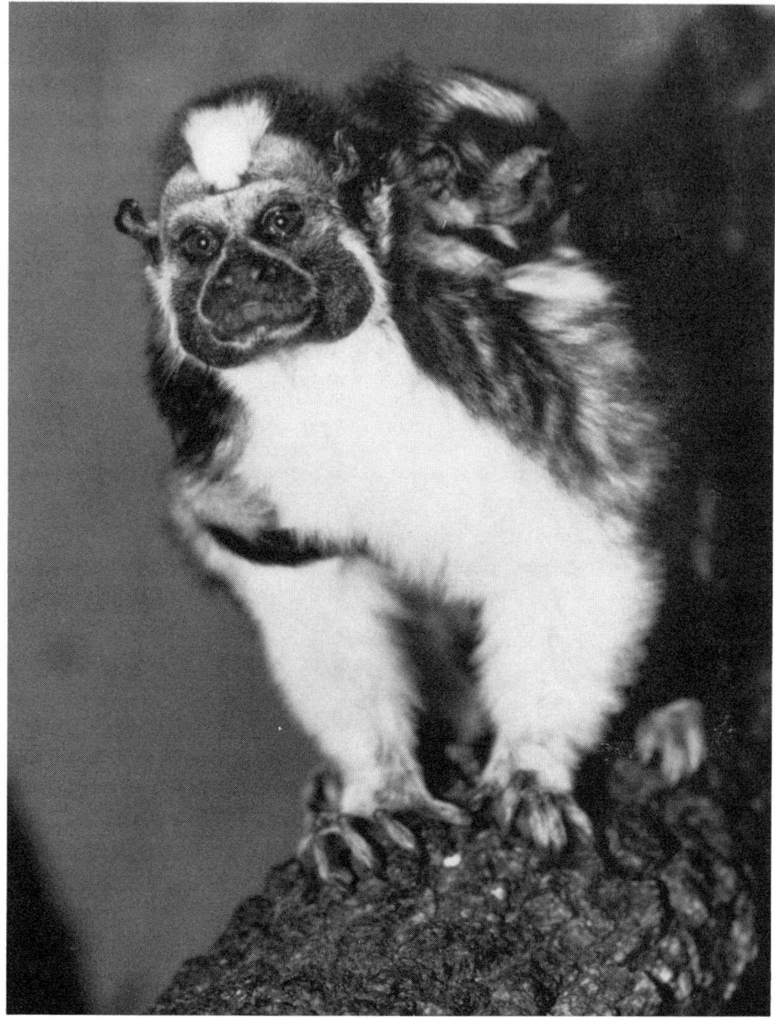

FIGURE 2. The Panamanian tamarin (*Saguinus geoffroyi*). (Photo by Russell Mittermeier.)

When the geographic distribution and ecology of closely related varieties is as poorly known as is the case with the three aforementioned tamarin species, the biological species concept is difficult to apply; Skinner[24] suggests that, in such cases, taxonomists must resort to other methods, such as morphological comparisons. Skinner compared morphological traits for 17 characteristics among *S. geoffroyi, S. leucopus,* and *S. oedipus*. She concluded that *S. leucopus* and *S. oedipus* were more closely related than either species

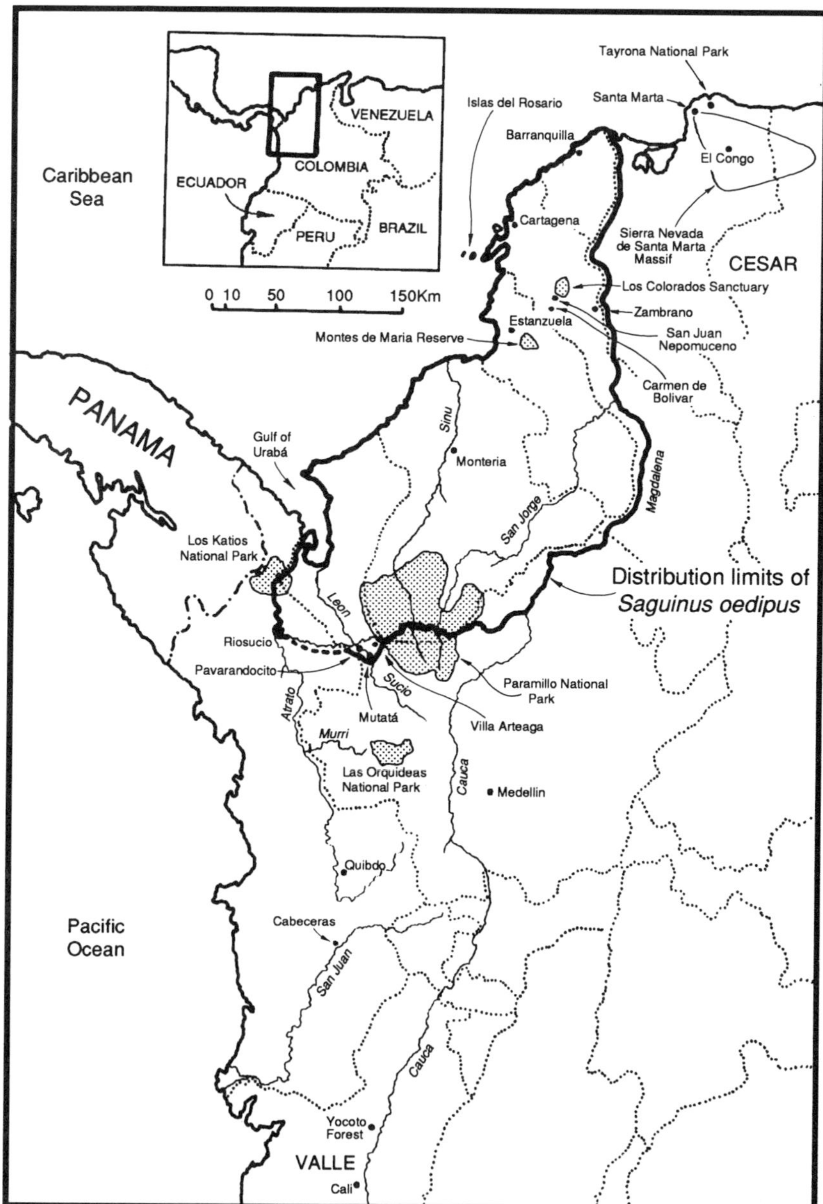

FIGURE 3A. Map of distribution limits for *Saguinus oedipus* showing parks and protected areas, major rivers, principal collection and study sites, and sites of introduced populations of cotton-tops outside the distribution.

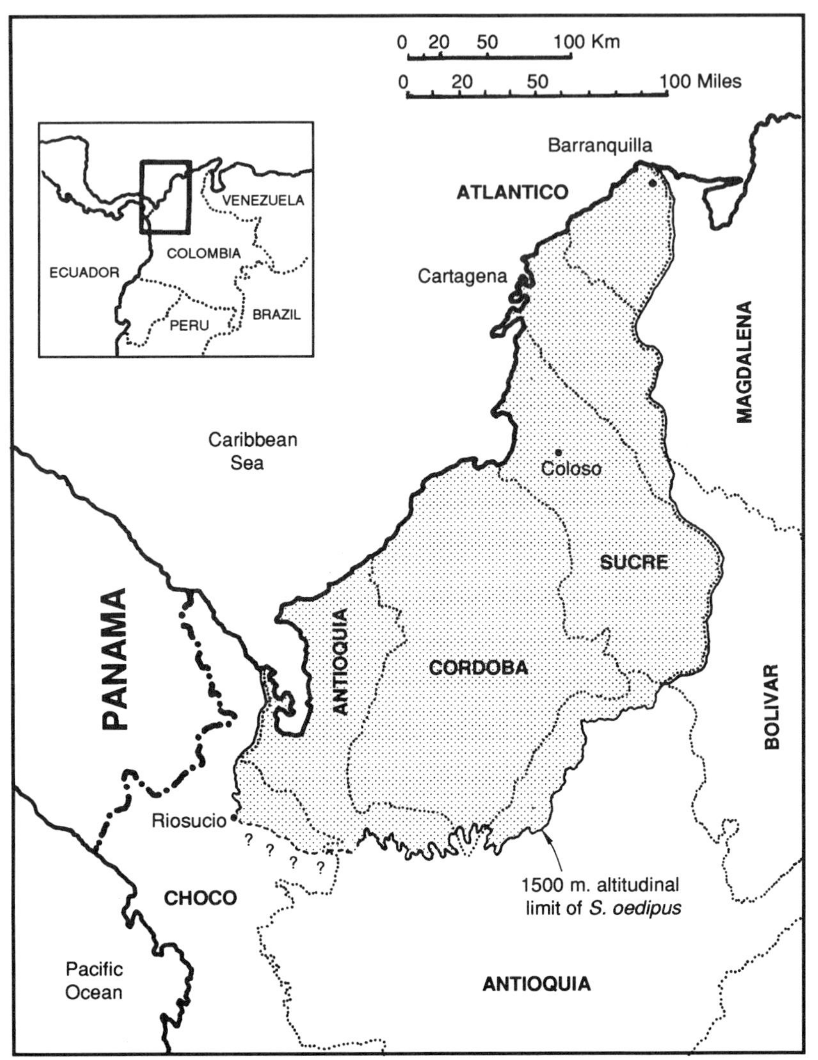

FIGURE 3B. Map of distribution limits for *Saguinus oedipus* showing political divisions and details of the southern extent based on a calculated altitudinal limit of 1500 m. Question marks indicate areas where further field data are necessary to clearly establish southern limits.

were to *S. geoffroyi;* on that basis alone she prefers to refer to the latter two as separate species. When considering the contrasts in morphology and physiology of *S. oedipus* and *S. geoffroyi* as evidence in favor of full-species status for each, it is noteworthy to mention also the fact that the latter does not develop colon cancer; indeed, to date the only species known to spontaneously develop colon cancer is *S. oedipus.*[1]

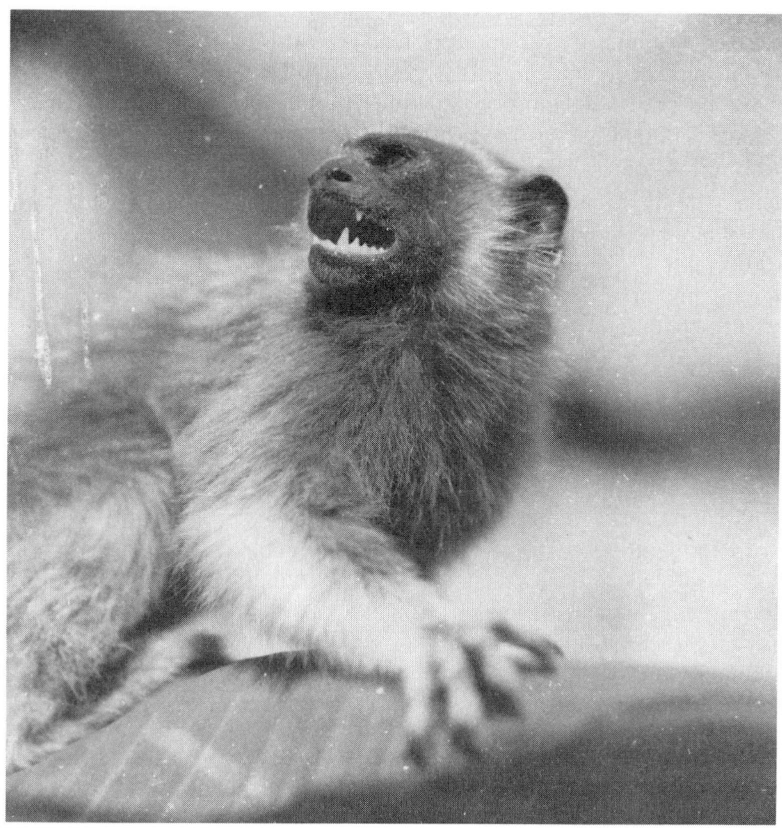

FIGURE 4. The white-footed tamarin (*Saguinus leucopus*). (Photo by Federico Medem.)

Nonetheless, the question remains as to whether the Panamanian and cotton-top tamarins have entirely allopatric distributions, and the answer will derive from additional field study. If their distributions are allopatric, then morphological distinctiveness is unquestionably sufficient to make them separate species. And even if these species do indeed interbreed in the wild, yet only produce hybrids within a narrow hybrid zone, full species status is likely warranted.

III. NATURAL HISTORY OF COTTON-TOP TAMARINS

An exceptional review of the genus *Saguinus,* including descriptions of the species, habitat, diet, population dynamics, social and reproductive behavior, expression and communication, locomotor and postural behavior, and learning and cognitive behavior is provided by Snowdon and Soini.[12]

In general, tamarins are considered primarily insectivore-frugivores with a tendency to omnivory. Cotton-tops feed on fruit, insects, frogs, lizards, and tree gums (especially the gum of the "caro" tree, *Enterolobium cyclocarpum*[26]), and live in extended family groups of 2 to 13 animals, though Barbosa et al.[18] have reported groups of up to 20 individuals. Average adult weight for a wild cotton-top is 410 g ($N = 21$) for males and 420 g ($N = 22$) for females.[27] Wild densities are dependent on available habitat and have been recorded at 78 individuals/km^2.[27] Cotton-top home range size varies from 7.8 to 10 hectares.[27] Cotton-tops generally breed in the wild from April to June, producing one offspring, though twins are also common and reports of triplets exist.[12] Sexual maturity in cotton-tops is reached in less than two years, and fathers and older sibling cotton-tops assist in caring for newborn offspring, which is one of the most characteristic behaviors of callitrichids in general.[12,13]

Cotton-tops and most other callitrichid species thrive in secondary forest where clearing has taken place. Some callitrichids survive well in small forest fragments,[12] and in general callitrichids prefer to utilize edge habitats to continuous forest.[28] In the case of the cotton-top, they have little choice, as most of the continuous forest is gone, but nonetheless Dawson's[29,30] work with *S. geoffroyi* indicates that this species actually avoids primary forest, preferring edge and degraded forest habitats. Cotton-tops live in both moist and dry forest formations up to 1500 m.[26] The ability of the species to prosper in secondary and degraded habitats could well have prevented its extinction.

IV. STATUS OF COTTON-TOP TAMARINS IN THE WILD

Members of the genus *Saguinus* range from Costa Rica to northern Bolivia.[16] The three extra-Amazonian (trans-Andean) species, *S. geoffroyi, S. oedipus,* and *S. leucopus,* reside in southeastern Panama and adjacent Costa Rica and northern Colombia, the latter two occurring exclusively in Colombia. The maps (Figures 3A and 3B) present the distribution limits for *S. oedipus,* showing parks and protected areas, major rivers, principal collection and study sites, political boundaries, and sites of introduced populations.

A. HABITAT CHARACTERISTICS

The major geographic features of this portion of northwestern Colombia are the northern termini of the western and central Andean cordilleras, separated by the Cauca River, and the eastern cordillera, lying to the west of the Magdalena River. An isolated massif, the Sierra Nevada de Santa Marta juts from the northern coast, rises from sea level to 5785 m (the highest point in Colombia) in just 42 horizontal km, and as such is the tallest coastal mountain on earth. The cool, moist Andes (2000 to 4000 mm annual rainfall) decline northward into the warm, dry, Caribbean coastal plain (less than 1000 mm annual rainfall), through which several major rivers drain into the Caribbean (such as the Rivers Sinú and the Magdalena River System with its tributaries including the San Jorge and the Cauca). To the west of the western cordillera and extending north into southern Panama (Province of Darién), lie the Chocoan forests, through which the Atrato River drains to the Atlantic. These are the wettest and most biologically diverse forests on earth, receiving up to 13,000 mm annual rainfall. The original vegetation types within the cotton-top's range are generally wet tropical forest in the west (Chocó), moist forest in the Andes and Sierra Nevada de Santa Marta, and dry thorn forest savannah in the northern coastal plane. Throughout the range, however, habitats have been moderately to severely altered by human activity.

B. COTTON-TOP DISTRIBUTION

In broad strokes, the distribution of the cotton-top tamarin extends from the eastern bank of the Atrato River to the western bank of the Cauca and lower Magdalena Rivers, bounded by the Colombian Caribbean coast to the north. To the south, the distributional range proposed in Figure 3B follows the 1500-m contour from east to west (based on calculated altitudinal limits reported by Hernandez Camacho and Defler[19,20] and Hershkovitz,[13] beginning at the Cauca River and crossing the Serranía de Ayapel and the Serranía de San Jerónimo.[34] The southwestern boundary of the cotton-top's range is also determined by collection records at Villa Arteaga on the Rio Sucio.[13]

Uncertainty regarding the southwestern limits of the range occurs where the altitude drops again below 1500 m on the western slope of the Andes, as indicated in Figure 3B by question marks; however, specimens have been collected in the vicinity of Mutatá and Pavarandocito.[18] Hershkovitz[13] states that "eventual dispersal south of the coastal Chocó is predictable on the basis of present conditions." It is reasonable to expect that the species occurs at least as far south as the Las Orquideas National Park,[26] although it appears to be completely replaced by *Saguinus geoffroyi* further south.[18]

At least four other sightings of wild *Saguinus oedipus* have been made well outside this range and are shown on Figure 3A: (1) by Velasco and Alberico in 1984 near the village of Cabeceras, along the San Juan River, Chocó Department;[18] (2) at the Yotoco forest, approximately 50 km north of Cali on the western bank of the Rio Cauca in the Department of Valle de Cauca, by Ramirez, Barbosa, and Santacruz in 1978;[18] (3) at "El Congo" in the valley of the Río Frio on the northern flank of the Sierra Nevada de Santa Marta in eastern Magdalena;[36] and (4) at Tayrona National Park, which lies on the Caribbean coast east of Santa Marta. These additional sites are shown on Figure 3B.

The first of these reports is considered to be a misidentification of *Saguinus geoffroyi,* based on field surveys and interviews conducted by Barbosa et al.;[18] they further postulate that the other two confirmed sightings at Yotoco and the Sierra Nevada represent introduced populations made up of, or founded by, ex-captive animals. The same is likely true for the apparently thriving group of cotton-tops at the Tayrona National Park. This is not an unreasonable hypothesis, given: (1) the proximity of these two small populations to urban centers where cotton-tops are frequently sold as pets (the cities of Cali and Buga in Valle de Cauca, and Santa Marta in Magdalena); (2) that primates kept as pets often escape and/or that pet-owners customarily tire of their charges and release them to the wild; and (3) these taxa are highly adaptable to survival in marginal habitats. Since the habitat at these sites is suitable for cotton-tops, they may thrive indefinitely. Similarly, disjunct populations of mona monkeys (*Cercopithecus mona*) have permanently established in Grenada; mona monkeys had been brought to that Caribbean island by slave ships in the 17th Century[37] and are still found living in the wild there. Based on interviews with local residents, Scott et al.[38] also report verbal accounts of what may be cotton-tops outside their known range to the east of the Magdalena (see section on Field Studies, following). An additional unconfirmed report of a small cotton-top tamarin population to the south of Panama City, Panama also begs further investigation.[39] Cotton-tops have also been reported to thrive on the Colombian Caribbean Rosario Islands. These latter reports may also be a result of the wide distribution of the animal by the pet trade.

It must be noted that while Figures 3A and 3B attempt to express the historic boundaries of the range of the cotton-top tamarin, the actual current range is limited to areas of suitable forest habitat within those boundaries. As mentioned earlier, habitats within the cotton-top tamarin's original range have been altered by anthropogenic forces, and parts of the range, such as the dry forest formations adjacent to the Caribbean coast, are among the most devastated ecosystems in Colombia (Figure 5).

The northern coastal plane was one of the first areas of Colombia to be colonized and has been the site of continuous human habitation for over 300 years. What little remains of the natural vegetation is isolated in forest fragments and strips of riverine forest, the remainder having been converted to pasture or farmland.

V. CONSERVATION

Colombia is one of the earth's most biologically diverse countries and is second only to Brazil in overall numbers of plant and animal species; given its size (one seventh that of Brazil), Colombia harbors greater concentrations of species per unit area than any other country on the planet. Not surprisingly, Colombia is one of the most important countries worldwide for primates, being home to approximately 10% of all extant primate species worldwide and approximately one third (26 of 87 species) of the primate species found in the Neotropical Realm.[40,41]

Colombian biodiversity in general and especially the country's tropical forests, in which the native primates are found, are under grave threat. Colombia is among the top ten countries worldwide in terms of deforestation (Figure 5) and is topped only by Brazil in the Western Hemisphere in terms of numbers of hectares deforested, both of them losing more than 4000 km^2

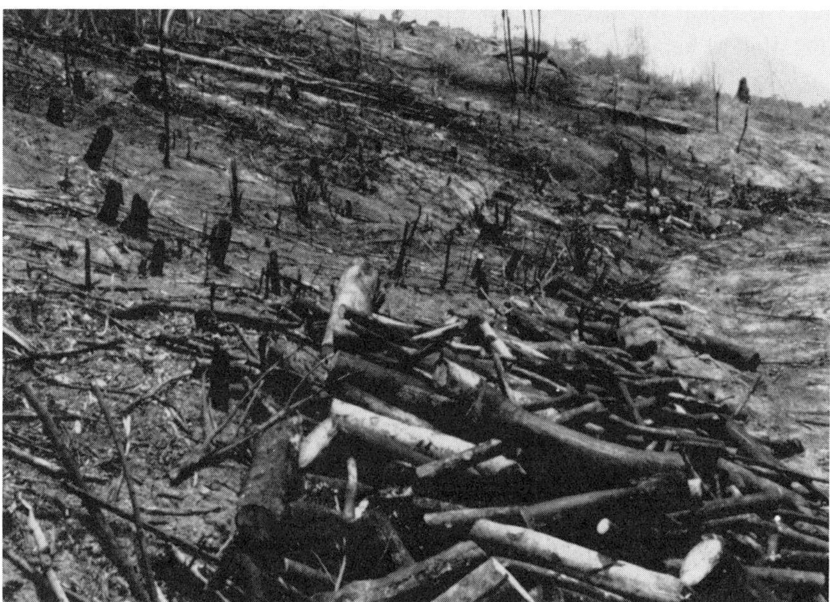

FIGURE 5. Deforestation and loss of habitat is the most severe threat to the cotton-top tamarin in the wild. Very little of northern Colombia's dry forest formations remain intact as a result of urban expansion and clearing for agriculture and pasture. (Photo by Roderic Mast.)

of forest annually.[42] As a result of these and similar figures for wetlands, dry forest, estuaries, and other major biomes, Colombia ranks among the world's most urgent and critical conservation priorities.

There are 12 Colombian primate taxa listed as either endangered, vulnerable, or rare by IUCN, The World Conservation Union.[43] Table 1 lists the 45 primate taxa known to be present in Colombia, the 7 taxa possibly present in Colombia, and the 2 currently undescribed taxa that may occur there; Spanish and English common names have also been provided in Table 1, along with a summary of conservation status for each taxa, including CITES rating (Convention on International Trade in Endangered Species of Flora and Fauna), IUCN rating, and a third status rating (*authors*) based upon the authors' knowledge of the current status of these animals in the wild.[44] In conservation terms, the most noteworthy are the white-footed and cotton-top tamarins, which have been given the highest rating of threat by the IUCN (Endangered), as well as being accorded the highest CITES rating. Coupled with the fact that these two species are endemic to limited ranges within Colombia, it is clear that they are of particular conservation concern.

A. THREATS TO WILD COTTON-TOP TAMARINS

The threats to wild cotton-top tamarins (and indeed to all primates) are many and can be characterized as direct pressures to the animals themselves (e.g., hunting and live capture) or threats which derive from the loss or alteration of habitat.[17]

1. Habitat Loss or Alteration

The most severe threat to primate populations worldwide is loss of tropical forest, where 90% or more of the world's primates reside, and the cotton-top tamarin is no exception.[17,45] According to Marsh et al.,[46] forest disturbance can be classified in six categories:

1. Removal of selected plant products by traditional means
2. Clearance or damage of the forest understorey
3. Changes in water regime
4. Shifting cultivation
5. Commercial selective logging
6. Large-scale clearance, usually for agriculture or ranching

In the northern part of the cotton-top's range (the Departments of Atlantico, Bolivar north of the Cauca, Sucre, northern Cordoba, and the Caribbean portion of Antioquia), category 6 (above) best describes the nature of habitat loss. While the present near-total absence of forest may have begun as removal of selected plant products, clearance of the understorey, or shifting cultivation, the final result is large-scale clearance and the remaining grasslands support agriculture (where soil fertility allows) and cattle pasture. The remaining forest patches in this part of the country generally lie atop agriculturally useless land (e.g., limestone outcroppings, seasonally flooded river margins).

It has been suggested by Marsh et al.[46] that understorey clearance might have an adverse effect on insectivorous primates that spend a great deal of time in the lower forest; this might well be the case for cotton-tops in parts of the northern range where forest patches still exist but where the understorey has been cleared for firewood. No research has been done on the effects of forest disturbance on arthropod density in these habitats; in such dry habitats, however, even minor fluctuations in food species abundance are likely to effect mortality rates, especially in the dry season.

The portions of the cotton-top's distribution that lie in the foothills of the northern termini of the western and central Andean cordilleras face fuelwood collection and small-scale agricultural encroachment threats of unknown intensity. However, the most damaging imminent threat comes from flooding of forest for hydroelectric projects (category 3 above, changes in water regime).

Colombia's electric power is approximately 70% hydroelectric, yet only about 6% of the country's hydroelectric potential has been exploited to date. Planned hydroelectric projects for Colombia, if completed, would flood thousands of hectares of the country's high-diversity ecosystems. One proposed hydroelectric project alone, URRA (comprised of two dams, URRA I and URRA II), could inundate over 60,000 ha in the upper Sinú river basin (within the cotton-top's range).[32] This area includes more than 54,000 ha of primary and secondary forest lying inside the Parramillo National Park (see Figure 3A) and its buffer zone, one of the last major strongholds for the cotton-top tamarin.[8,32,47]

Fortunately, Colombia's power sector has historically side-stepped any major negative environmental and social impacts resulting from hydroelectrics compared to other countries (such as Brazil). In recent years under the terms of the World Bank's power sector adjustment loan (loan 2889-CO) to that country, the Colombian central power agency (ISA) and its eight regional affiliates have undertaken a program to minimize the environmental impact of hydroelectric expansion under the National Power Expansion Plan. Efforts have been made to develop methodologies for more effectively prioritizing projects to minimize their adverse environmental and socioeconomic impacts, to provide environmental training for power sector staff, and to develop more stringent environmental standards for hydroelectric and thermal projects.[48]

As a result of these improvements, the Colombian power sector has committed itself to pursuing a "least cost expansion plan", which incorporates environmental and socioeconomic considerations. Among the hydroelectric projects that will be constructed under this plan are URRA I, Miel II, and Porce II. The more damaging URRA II project mentioned earlier, which would have flooded more than 50,000 ha of prime cotton-top tamarin habitat and displaced dozens of indigenous human communities, has not been approved for construction under the plan. Nonetheless, URRA II is still listed in the "feasibility study" stage;[49] hopefully, given the Colombian power sector's redoubled interest in minimizing environmental and social impacts, the URRA II project will be permanently cancelled as a result of these studies.

Of the three approved projects, URRA I is perhaps of greatest concern in terms of its overall environmental impact, especially when considering its impact on wild cotton-top tamarins. It will flood approximately 7000 ha of largely secondary forest and degraded habitats in the Department of Cordoba, where cotton-tops are known to reside. Optimistically, however, should the power sector authorities provide for adequate watershed protection and rehabilitation through empowering of local communities to undertake reforestation programs, as well as sanctuary or park establishment in collaboration with government authorities, the overall impact of URRA I could prove positive for the cotton-top tamarin and other native inhabitants within the zones around the proposed reservoir site. The Miel II hydroelectric project, which will flood a known *Saguinus leucopus* habitat, is already being approached responsibly by the power sector authorities at ISA, which is sponsoring endangered primate and other surveys in the area to be inundated.[23]

In the western and southwestern portions of the cotton-top's range, especially in the Chocó, commercial selective logging is also a threat to habitat. The forest of the Chocó biogeographic zone were considered until recent years to be among the most undisturbed on the planet, yet today they are being increasingly exploited for hardwood timber, both legally and illegally;

pulpwood extraction has also increased. The country as a whole shows a 63% increase in paper production since the period 1977 to 1979,[50] much of which comes from the Pacific region.

Overall, the threats posed by human expansion into forested areas exist throughout the cotton-top's range, and these threats are likely to increase. Colombia has already lost one third of its forest and the existing forests are depleted by 1.8% per annum,[50] the third highest rate in all of tropical South America. A trend toward continued forest loss in Colombia is largely driven by population growth (at 1.97% per annum),[50] especially in rural areas. The subsequent increased demand for agricultural and pasture lands, coupled with the continued construction of roads for logging or other commercial resource exploitation endeavors and access to coastal areas (e.g., the road being completed to Nuquí in the Department of Chocó), open up once remote areas to human encroachment. In addition, the forest-to-pasture conversion process is the preferred way to privatize publicly owned lands in Colombia, as government policies indirectly encourage deforestation through the titling of recently cleared lands and the provision of credit for cattle pasture establishment.[48]

2. Direct Threats: Hunting and Live Capture

Worldwide, hunting is the second most important threat to primate populations, behind habitat loss.[17,40,45,51] Primates are hunted throughout the world as food items, for medicinal purposes, as bait, as crop pests, for their skins and other body parts for ornamentation, as evil omens and for other quasi-religious purposes, and often simply for sport.[52] Generally, hunting pressure increases with the size of the species;[53] for larger animals, more meat, skin, bait, or other products can be derived, whereas a small animal will barely recompense the hunter for the cost of the bullet. As a result, hunting pressure does not greatly affect the survival of cotton-top or other tamarins. To the authors' knowledge, cotton-tops serve no medicinal function, nor are they notorious crop pests; their skins or body parts are not typically used for ornamentation and they are not considered evil or harbingers of bad luck.

Live capture, on the other hand, has historically caused a major decline in the numbers of wild cotton-tops. Live-trapped animals were sold internationally in great numbers for use in biomedical research institutions and as pets until the early 1970s.[19,20,28] The impact of these industries was great; between 1968 and 1972, as many as 14,000 cotton-tops were imported to the U.S., and between 30,000 and 40,000 cotton-tops were exported from Barranquilla, Colombia between 1960 and 1975 alone.[22] The actual numbers of cotton-tops extracted from the wild during this period is undoubtedly higher, given the inevitable mortality of animals between capture and export, which has been estimated by Thorington[54] for marmosets to be from 3 to 33%.

Colombia undertook a phased ban on the exportation of cotton-tops from 1969 to 1972 and the species was declared endangered, though appreciable numbers (2500 to 3500 animals) entered the U.S. during those three years; in 1972 all primate exportation was prohibited by Colombian authorities with

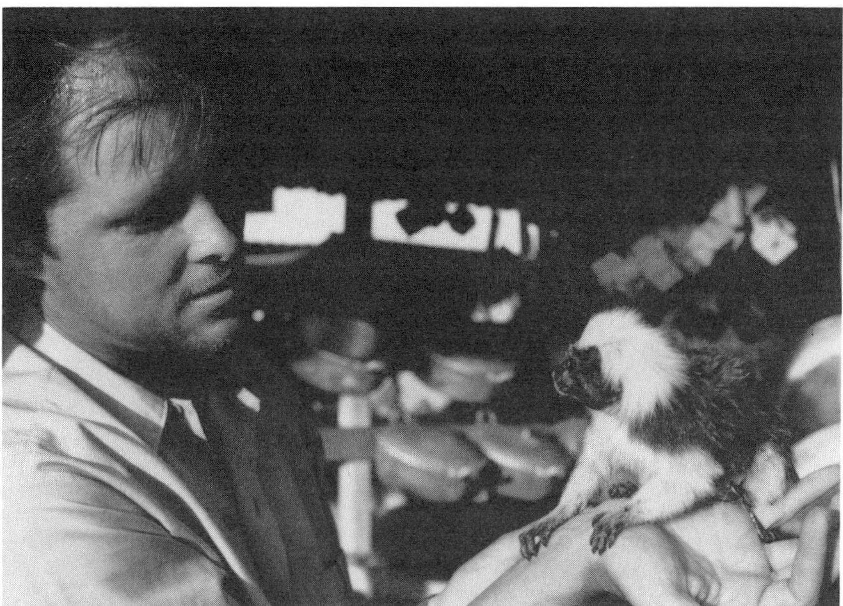

FIGURE 6. The principal author examines a cotton-top tamarin being sold as a pet at a market in Cartagena, Colombia. Though international trade in cotton-tops as pets is now curtailed, an active (albeit illegal) national market still exists. (Photo by Angela Mast.)

an exception for limited numbers used in biomedical research, and the following year even this exception was dropped. In 1975, the U.S. Public Health Service also prohibited the importation of primates for sale as pets, putting an end to this drain on wild cotton-tops. Despite the 1973 Colombian ban and the listing of *Saguinus oedipus* in Appendix I of the Convention on International Trade in Endangered Species of Wild Flora and Fauna (CITES) that same year, importation of cotton-tops to the U.S. continued in small numbers after 1973, mostly transshipped through countries like Panama.[28,55,56] Today, however, international trade in cotton-tops has been eliminated.

Nonetheless, an active local market still exists for cotton-tops within Colombia.[8,47] Indeed, all three extra-Amazonian (trans-Andean) callitrichids are popular pets in their countries of origin. Though no statistics are available, caged cotton-tops in homes and on farms, particularly in northern Colombia, are still a relatively common sight; and to find a cotton-top in the market is a simple task (Figure 6). Barbosa et al.[18] report that a wildlife dealer from Córdoba provided monkey traps to local people near the town of Chinulito, then paid 300 pesos (≈ $0.50 U.S.) per live monkey and resold the animals as pets in Barranquilla up until 1986. According to recent reports from field researcher Zorayda Calle,[57] the white-footed tamarin (*Saguinus leucopus*) is also greatly affected by the pet trade. Mittermeier and Coimbra-Filho[28] also

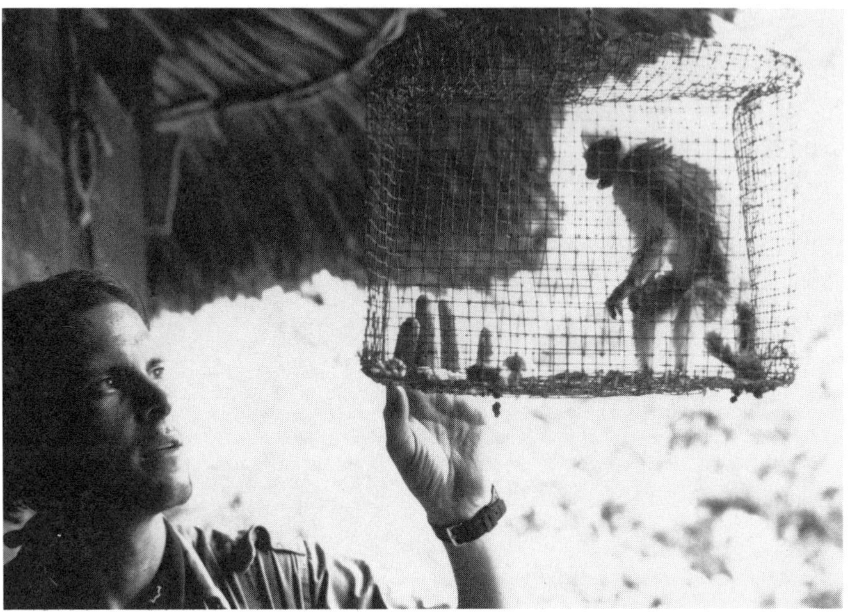

FIGURE 7. The principal author with a captive cotton-top tamarin in northern Colombia. This animal was kept by a rural family as a caller monkey or *llamador* for the purpose of live-trapping cotton-tops. (Photo by Anne Savage.)

indicate that the local pet trade has had an adverse affect on the Panamanian tamarin (*Saguinus geoffroyi*) in Panama, and that young animals were once commonly sold as pets in Panama City markets.

While these animals are apparently still captured in small numbers for the pet trade using a technique whereby the hunter merely trails the prey until it can be shaken from a tree or captured on the ground, a more effective method is through the use of a trap which employs a caller monkey or *llamador* (Figure 7). Such traps have numerous compartments with doors that can be shut by an observer hiding in a nearby blind. The vocalizations of the *llamador* attract other cotton-tops which, once nearby, are further lured into the compartments with bait of bananas or other fruit. Once inside, the compartment doors are lowered by the observer who loosens a string dropping the spring-operated door (Figure 8).

Another novel capture method used in the upper San Jorge river valley consists of habituating cotton-top tamarin troops to provisioning with bananas, then one day "spiking" the bananas with hot pepper sauce. The monkey is temporarily blinded or distracted by the burning in its mouth and nose, and is then easy prey for hand capture.[18]

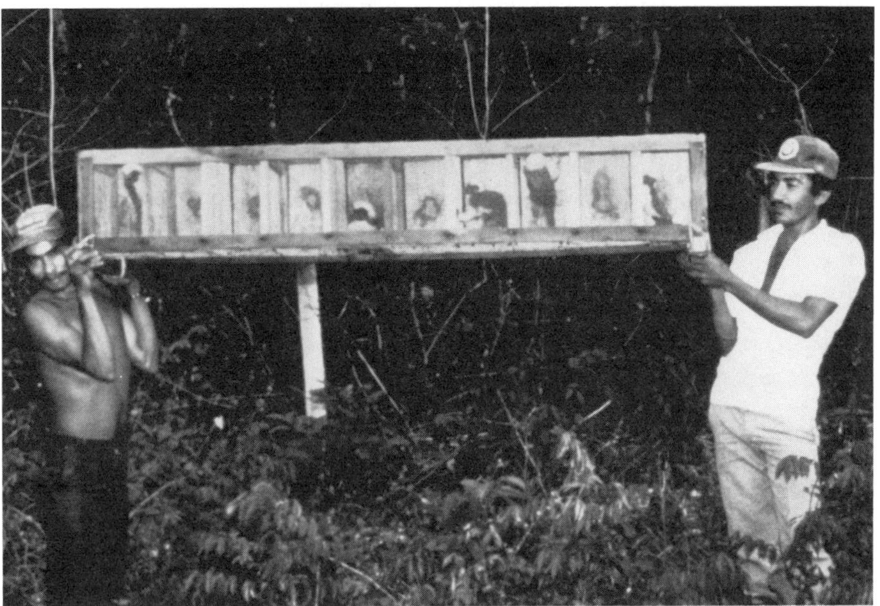

FIGURE 8. The typical design of a tamarin live trap consists of a number of separate compartments with doors that can be closed from a nearby blind. Tamarins are attracted by a caller monkey in the center compartment and food items within the compartments. (Photo by Anne Savage.)

B. COTTON-TOP TAMARINS IN CAPTIVITY

Cotton-tops are one of the best-represented primate species in captive collections, and one of the best studied by a number of disciplines. The combined effects of their popularity and availability in the 1960s and 1970s as biomedical research models, and the relative ease with which they reproduce in captivity, have resulted in numerous sizeable captive collections numbering in excess of 1700 animals in research institutes and zoos throughout North America and Europe.[5-7] Initially, cotton-tops were used as biomedical research models in a number of different types of research as they were readily available and inexpensive, but given their current endangered status, they are now used conservatively and seldom, if ever, are they sacrificed in terminal research.[56]

An *International Cotton-Top Tamarin Studbook* was established in 1987 and is now in its third edition;[7] the studbook maintains a record of individual animals and their genetic lineages and serves as a means by which captive population fluctuations can be monitored and captive genetic variability controlled. The most recent edition of the studbook reports that, among the studbook collaborators, there are 644 animals in zoo and private collections and another 1122 in research colonies; more than half of these 1766 animals are housed at 58 separate sites in the U.S. (53 zoo and private collections, 5 research colonies).[7]

Captive management techniques for these animals have improved as a result of the lessons learned from continued ethological and biomedical research over the past decade, and, given the attention paid to the proper genetic management of the taxa through the studbook and other efforts, it is likely that a vigorous captive population of the cotton-top tamarin can be maintained for years to come. An in-depth assessment of captive breeding is provided in Chapter 2.

C. PAST AND PRESENT FIELD CONSERVATION EFFORTS

Field work on the cotton-top tamarin prior to the 1970s centered primarily on the collection of animals for museums and on general descriptive studies of the animal's range, characteristics, and habitat. These early studies are well documented by Hershkovitz[13,58] and Hernandez-Camacho and Cooper;[22] it was not until the 1970s that conservation-oriented field work on the cotton-top tamarin began in Colombia.

Dr. Patricia Neyman conducted a field study of cotton-top tamarins from 1973 to 1975 which resulted in her doctoral dissertation, Ecology and Social Organization of the Cotton-Top Tamarin, in 1979.[59] This and other publications documenting Neyman's work remain among the most oft-cited literature on the species in the wild. Her research comprising over 2500 active field hours and approximately 750 hours of contact with marked and unmarked cotton-tops, took place at a forested site about 15 km to the northeast of Tolú, Department of Sucre, in the alluvial plain between the Caribbean coast and the San Jacinto hills (Estanzuela; see Figure 3A).[27,59] At that time, this was one of the larger forest fragments in the northern portion of the cotton-top's range. Her studies focused on ecology, population dispersion and characteristics, use of space, social organization, and reproduction.

In subsequent visits to Colombia, Neyman also provided some of the first concrete data regarding the endangerment of the cotton-top tamarin, documenting the widespread deforestation in the region, even in remote areas such as the upper Sinú River valley.[35] Neyman visited Colombia from June to September, 1977 with support from the New York Zoological Society for a survey of potential protected areas in the Departments of Sucre and Córdoba, and made recommendations for reserve establishment to INDERENA at that time. Neyman's work was of great importance in gathering the first long-term field data on the ecology of the species and in bringing the plight of the cotton-top tamarin to the attention of conservationists worldwide.

Two other noteworthy primate censuses which provided data on the cotton-top tamarin's conservation status were undertaken with support from the Pan American Health Organization in 1973 by Bernstein et al., and in 1974 by Dr. Norman Scott et al.; the results of these two studies are published together.[38] An initial aerial reconnaissance totalling 16.3 hours of flying time in northern Colombia (covering an area of approximately 160,000 km^2 over the Departments of Bolivar, Cordoba, Sucre, Magdalena, Guajira, Cesar, and northern Antioquia) was used to plan a two-month ground expedition to selected areas with both extensive forest or imminent deforestation threats. Foot and boat surveys were conducted to determine primate presence and abundance and interviews with area residents were undertaken.

Scott et al.[38] reported that the entire 160,000-km^2 study area was likely capable of supporting forest cover, but that only six discrete forest blocks remained in northern Colombia at that time, comprising 15% of the survey area (approximately 24,000 km^2). Moreover, the survey team pointed out that these six remnants were rapidly being cut. Cotton-tops were observed at only 1 of the 20 sites visited (at Estanzuela, Dr. Patricia Neyman's study site, Figure 3A), where 5 to 7 groups were seen. Interviews indicated the presence of cotton-tops at 4 other sites as well. Two of these latter sites were dry forest areas well outside the known range of *Saguinus oedipus* (to the south of the Sierra Nevada massif in the Department of Cesar); one was in dry forest in the southern portion of the San Jacinto hills, Department of Sucre, where farm workers indicated that the animals had been nearly trapped-out some four years earlier, and one was in wet forest in southern Cordoba where local Indians were familiar with cotton-tops but could not provide localities.

Aside from the confirmation that habitat destruction was severe in the region and a threat to primate populations, perhaps the most interesting aspects of the findings of Scott et al.[38] were the two reports of *Saguinus sp.* in northern Cesar, well outside the range of either *S. oedipus* or *S. leucopus* and a third report from Minca, western Department of Guajira, of a troop of "small, dark monkeys" determined to be of the genus *Saguinus* from verbal descriptions. Hershkovitz[13] also mentions reports from hunters of the existence of a black tamarin-like monkey in the Norte de Santander Department, upper Rio Catatumbo, which he did not see, but he postulated could be *Callimico*. It is conceivable that such far-removed populations could be the result of the wide distribution of these animals by the pet trade, as mentioned earlier. However, confirmation of these reports by qualified field primatologists should be attempted, as the existence of a native *Saguinus* species, especially *S. oedipus,* or even *Callimico* from this part of Colombia would substantially alter the currently accepted zoogeographic interpretations of the ranges of these genera.

Scott et al.[38] also made recommendations for habitat protection at three sites, both through stricter enforcement in existing parks, and by the creation of new parks. The three areas mentioned were the north flank of the Sierra Nevada de Santa Marta (a national park created in 1964 and expanded in 1977) and the adjacent coastal Tayrona National Park (also created in 1964); a 9000-km^2 area in and around the San Lucas hills, and an area of approximately 10,000 km^2 in the upper San Jorge and Sinú river valleys (partially protected within the Paramillo National Park, created in 1977). The latter is the only area of the three which lies within the known range of *Saguinus oedipus,* and indeed the Paramillo National Park remains the most important national park for the protection of the cotton-top and its habitat.

Another important refuge for the cotton-top was given protected status in October, 1984 (Ministry of Agriculture Resolution No. 204) at the Coraza Hills — Montes de Maria Protected Forest Reserve (Reserva Forestal Protectora Serranía de Coraza — Montes de Maria), lying in the southwestern San Jacinto hills. This zone was mentioned by Neyman,[27,35,59] Barbosa et al.,[18] and Scott et al.[38] as important for cotton-tops, the latter suggesting it as a suitable site for the development of a management plan for sustainable cropping of primates for biomedical research.

Largely as a result of the aforementioned field studies, the need for conservation measures to protect the cotton-top and its habitat was well known among Colombian conservationists by 1985, when Dr. Jairo Ramirez Cerquera of the Colombian National Institute of Health (Instituto Nacional de Salud) approached the authors.[60] Expressing his concern for the future of the cotton-top tamarin in light of the imminent habitat destruction that would have occurred had the proposed URRA I and URRA II hydroelectric projects been carried out, Dr. Ramirez Cerquera recommended the initiation of a long-term conservation effort to incude field studies, the creation of a captive breeding facility, public awareness and education campaigns, pressure on policy-makers to halt destructive development projects, and the establishment of additional protected areas for the cotton-top.[32,61]

With support from the World Wildlife Fund-U.S. Primate Program and INDERENA, the authors acted upon Dr. Ramirez Cerquera's suggestions and organized a detailed survey of the cotton-top's known range in an effort to provide baseline data upon which to build a multifaceted conservation program. Public awareness T-shirts and stickers were produced by artist Stephen Nash (Figure 9), and a team of Colombian field biologists was mustered.[47]

Ground surveys covering some 5000 km by four-wheel drive vehicle, boat, and foot were undertaken by the survey team from November 19, 1986 to February 27, 1987 in selected areas of the Departments of Sucre, Bolívar, Atlántico, Córdoba, and northwest Antioquia (the northern portion of the cotton-top's range). Additional surveys totalling 700 km were undertaken in the southern portion of the range (Departments of Valle, central and southern Chocó, western Antioquia, and the San Juan river) from November 16 to December 17, 1987. Transect sampling was carried out, botanical specimens were collected, and interviews were conducted with local residents throughout the survey area. The survey team provided detailed botanical descriptions of the forest types, as well as documented forest conditions and threats to the habitat throughout the range. Observations of cotton-top reproductive behavior, predation, food species, and the adverse effects of air pollution and pesticides on the species are also contained in an unpublished INDERENA report written by Barbosa et al.[18]

ESPECIE COLOMBIANA EN PELIGRO DE EXTINCION
Mono Tití Blanco
(Saguinus oedipus)
CONSERVATION
INTERNATIONAL

Mono Tití Blanco
en peligro de extinción
Ayúdanos a salvarlo
EL BOSQUE ES MI HOGAR
NO LO DESTRUYAS
CONSERVATION
INTERNATIONAL

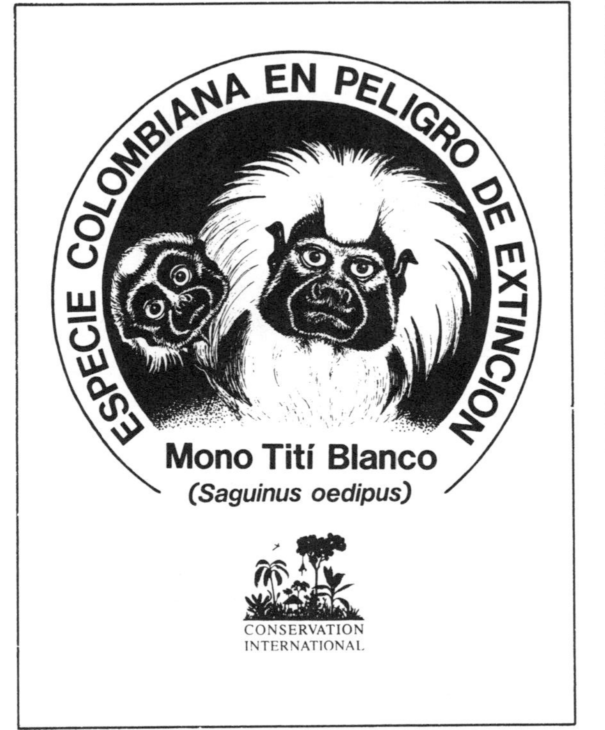

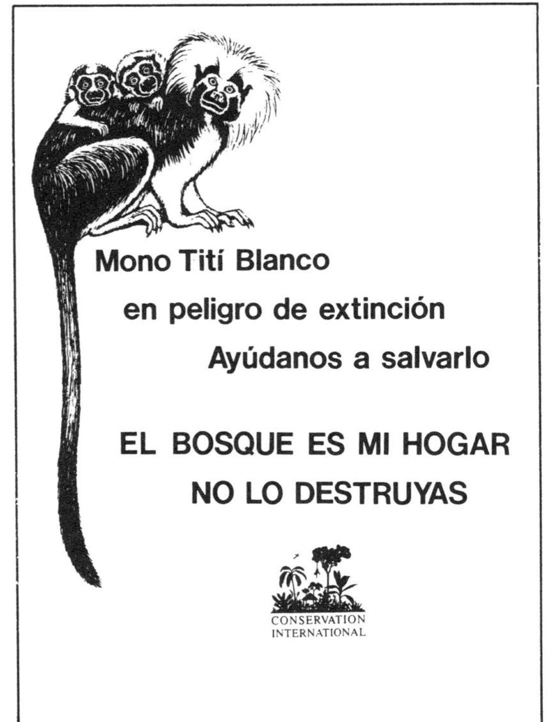

FIGURE 9. Designs used on T-shirts and posters as part of a public awareness campaign to draw attention to the plight of the cotton-top tamarin and its disappearing habitat in Colombia. The text reads (on left) ''Colombian Species in Danger of Extinction — Cotton-Top Tamarin,'' and (on right), ''The Cotton-Top Tamarin is in danger of extinction — help us to save it — the forest is my home — please do not destroy it.'' (Artwork by Stephen Nash.)

Barbosa et al.[18] reported that cotton-top populations were almost totally eliminated in the entire department of Atlántico, where they had not been seen for as much as 37 years in some areas. In Bolívar department, conditions for the cotton-top were much the same, though populations were found in secondary forest patches near Carmen de Bolivar, San Juan Nepomuceno, and Zambrano, and in the San Jacinto hills at the Los Colorados Sanctuary.

In the Department of Sucre, the researchers found noteworthy populations of cotton-tops in the Coraza Hills — Montes de Maria Protected Forest Reserve, at Estanzuela (Neyman's research site),[27,35,59] and at several forest fragments in the swamp vegetation of the Caribbean alluvial plain (in the municipalities of San Marcos, Sucre, Majagual, and Guaranda). They pointed out that the Montes de Maria Reserve was under great threat from uncontrolled clearing for agriculture and pasture land. Unlike a national park which is the property of the government, a protected forest reserve such as Montes de Maria can contain a combination of private and state-owned land. Much of the land within the reserve is still in the hands of private land-owners who have held titles for hundreds of years, hence regulation of forest clearing is a complex problem. Pressure to remove forest is also fueled by the fact that cleared land sells at twice the price of forested land. In addition, Barbosa et al.[18] mentioned that, based on Neyman's descriptions from 1977,[27,59] forests at Estanzuela had been degraded substantially in the ensuing ten years and a consequent decline in the numbers of cotton-tops was noted.

Barbosa et al.[18] reported the complete disappearance of the cotton-top in the coastal plains of the Department of Córdoba, but indicated that populations remained in good condition in the upper Sinu and San Jorge River valleys of that department, where colonization and deforestation had been slowed by the fear of local people to enter areas with active guerrilla activity. Similarly, social disorder in the countryside had also slowed colonization in Antioquia south of the Gulf of Urabá, where forest remained to the east of the León River. Their surveys identified the northern terminus of the Western Andean Cordillera, at the border between Córdoba and Antioquia, as an area of lightly disturbed forest where chances of conserving the cotton-top and its primary habitat remained good. To the contrary, however, they found the area of Antioquia near the border with Chocó to be highly altered by colonization except in the high altitudes. The Chocoan forests west of the border with Antioquia were also found to be largely unaltered and hence of conservation importance.

Regarding its overall conservation status, Barbosa et al.[18] place *Saguinus oedipus* clearly in danger of extinction in the wild. They note a direct relationship between forest condition and cotton-top abundance in the wild, and point out that given the high, continuous, and accelerating rate of deforestation in the cotton-top's range, the outlook for the future is bleak; indeed, in many areas the species had disappeared during the five years between 1972 and 1977.

In terms of conservation recommendations, Barbosa et al. felt that adding parks and protected areas to the existing network would not assure habitat preservation, unless on-the-ground enforcement of park boundaries could be achieved. They referred specifically to the fact that forest destruction was underway already in both the Los Colorados Sanctuary and the Montes de Maria Reserve. They encouraged the creation of private reserves and listed several potential sites, and further elaborated upon the need for public education as a means to preserve the species.

Since 1988, Dr. Anne Savage, Director of Research at the Roger Williams Park Zoo, Dr. Chuck Snowdon of the University of Wisconsin, and INDERENA have spearheaded a long-term field study of wild cotton-top tamarins centering on the Coraza Hills — Montes de Maria Protected Forest Reserve at the INDERENA field station (Estación Experimental de Fauna Silvestre de Colosó). Their research, which has been conducted through field monitoring of several radio tagged groups of cotton-tops and periodic capture of animals, has focused on determining such variables as general health[62] and physiological conditions of wild individuals, group composition and dynamics,[63] reproductive success and behavior,[64,67] home range size,[63] genetics,[64,66] and demographics.[63,64] The data emanating from this work represent the best available information on cotton-top tamarins in the wild and will serve to provide valuable insights for the design of conservation programs for the species.[65]

The initial conclusions of the aforementioned study highlighted the need for education programs to enlighten local Colombians to the need for forest conservation, and this prompted the Savage/Snowdon/INDERENA team to develop "Proyecto Tití" (tití is the local vernacular name for the cotton-top tamarin).[69,70] Proyecto Tití is a public awareness program which initially targetted the children of the small town of Colosó, near the cotton-top study site. Through school lectures (Figure 10), a small-scale tamarin reintroduction effort, and a field monitoring program involving 12 high school students, Proyecto Tití effectively raised local public awareness concerning the need for wildlife and forest conservation; the project continues to inspire young conservationists and foster local involvement.[68]

In recent years, Proyecto Tití has expanded beyond Colosó to involve other Colombian communities in collaboration with the Cali-based foundation, Fundación Herencia Verde (Green Inheritance Foundation), and even to the U.S., where the Colosó experience is serving as the basis of an international video exchange program between American and Colombian schools.[69] Proyecto Tití is a model for the types of public awareness activities that are critically necessary in Colombia and other tropical countries, as well as in the developed countries of the North, in order to bring about the paradigm shift in people's attitudes about their natural surroundings that will be necessary to maintain the world's biological diversity into the future.

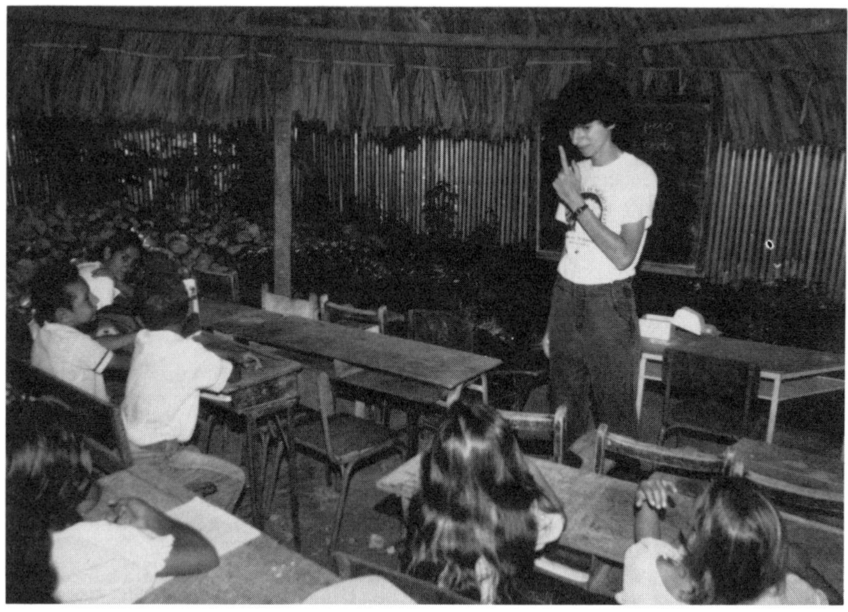

FIGURE 10. Dr. Anne Savage lectures to elementary school children about the value of natural resources in the municipality of Colosó, near the Coraza Hills — Montes de Maria Protected Forest Reserve, one of the last important refuges of the cotton-top tamarin. (Photo by Roderic Mast.)

D. CONSERVATION RECOMMENDATIONS

1. Additional Studies and Priority Setting

In order to clearly define the distribution of the cotton-top tamarin, additional field studies will be necessary in the southwestern portion of its range. Observations in this area will also be useful in clarifying the taxonomic relationship between the cotton-top, Panamanian, and white-footed tamarins (see Section II.B). Initially, such field surveys should focus on the region of the Rio Murrí and further south to the Las Orquideas National Park (Figure 3A),[18,26] the only zone where hybridization potentially occurs between *S. oedipus* and *S. geoffroyi*. Barbosa et al.[18] have indicated that they believe *Saguinus oedipus* and *S. geoffroyi* are found parapatrically in this zone. A rapid biological assessment of this area will be conducted during 1993 by Conservation International's RAP Team (Rapid Assessment Program), an international group of several top field scientists incuding botanists, mammalogists, ornithologists, and ecologists; this survey should shed additional light on the relationship between these taxa. Zorayda Calle's work with *S. leucopus* will also most certainly aid our understanding of the relationship between this taxon and its two northern Colombian congeners.[23] An effort should be made in these surveys to provide accurate estimates of the wild populations of these taxa.

These ground surveys should be preceded by a program of remote sensing to determine habitat extent and condition throughout the zone. Such an effort could be spearheaded by Colombia's Geographic Institute, IGAC (Instituto Geográfico Augustín Codazzi), which has access to remote sensing imagery, as well as local government authorities and private institutions in Colombia. An analysis of forest cover should be undertaken at regular intervals (perhaps annually) and comparative studies conducted in order to determine those sites of most rapid habitat loss for the purposes of prioritizing conservation efforts.

The aforementioned assessment of habitat extent and quality should also be augmented by land tenure studies to determine the ownership categories of lands within the cotton-top's distribution (e.g., private ownership, state ownership, protected areas, etc.).

With accurate data on cotton-top demography, biology, and remaining habitat, a Population and Habitat Viability Assessment (PHVA) workshop could be conducted as has been done with other endangered taxa, including the lion tamarins in Brazil's Atlantic forest.[71] Such assessments intensively review the biology and status of an endangered species or a protected area, assess the real risk of extinction, develop a stochastic simulation model of the population dynamics, and assist the formulation and testing of an adaptive management plan. About 30 of these PHVA workshops have brought together diverse and often conflicting interests to achieve a concensus on the risk of extinction and on needed management actions. PHVA workshops are catalyzed and carried out by the Captive Breeding Specialist Group (CBSG) of the World Conservation Union's Species Survival Commission (IUCN/SSC).[72]

From these types of surveys and priority setting activities, a detailed action plan for conserving the cotton-top and its habitat could be derived to include at least the activities listed below.

2. Conservation Actions

1. Provision of enhanced protection for the cotton-top and its habitat within the existing government conservation units inside its natural range (Paramillo National Park, Los Colorados Sanctuary, Coraza Hills — Montes de Maria Protected Forest Reserve, Los Katios National Park, Las Orquideas National Park, and others) through support for the activities of INDERENA and private Colombian conservation groups.
2. Encouragement of the establishment of new areas for protection of the cotton-top and its habitat (e.g., private reserves, new and expanded government protected areas). Key sites for consideration include:

   - The forest islands which dot the savannahs of the department of Bolivar
   - The wetland "la Mojana" zone of the upper San Jorge river valley near the town of San Marcos, Department of Córdoba

- The privately owned forest patches surrounding the Coraza Hills — Montes de Maria Protected Forest Reserve near Colosó, Department of Sucre
- The remaining forests in the Serranía la Coraza
- The fragments of riverine forest along the lower San Jorge River
- The forest patches on the savannahs north of Sincelejo and continuing northward to Cartagena
- The forest patches to the southwest of Carmen de Bolívar
- Most of the riverine forests of Magdalena Department
- The remaining dry forests between San Juan de Nepomuceno and the Magdalena river (including the forests around the Los Colorados Sanctuary)
- The Monterrey forestry project near Zambrano, Department of Bolivar, owned and operated by Pizano, S.A., which has from 5000 to 6000 ha of riparian and dry forest
- Maderas del Darién, a concession containing more than 25,000 ha of protected forests (23% riparian) south of the Golfo de Urabá, between the Atrato and León rivers

3. Support for expansion of conservation education efforts throughout the range of the cotton-top and beyond. The model ''Proyecto Tití'' program begun by Savage, Snowdon, and INDERENA[69,70] is an excellent point from which to expand to new communities.
4. Support for the inception of an aggressive public awareness campaign using tools such as T-shirts, stickers, posters, radio, television and print media, which would focus on both the illegality and impracticality of capturing and maintaining cotton-tops as pets, as well as the long-term dangers of habitat destruction to both man and biological diversity (Figure 9).
5. Encouragement of stricter enforcement of wildlife regulations by INDERENA and local authorities pertaining to the capture, sale, purchase, and maintenance of cotton-tops and other wildlife by the Colombian pet trade.
6. Support for experimentation with, and refining of, methodologies for recuperation of forest through reforestation or natural regeneration.
7. Support for experimentation with, and refining of methodologies for, reintroduction and translocation of cotton-top tamarins for the purposes of maintaining wild genetic diversity and for repopulating sites where they have become locally extinct.
8. Support for exploration of the possibilities of local income generation through ecotourism centered on wildlife viewing (e.g., at forested areas near population centers like Cartagena where tourists could pay to view wild tamarins, such as is done with mountain gorillas in Rwanda).

VI. CONCLUSIONS

The plight of the Colombian cotton-top tamarin provides a unique point of departure from which to take a deeper look at the situation of the world today. Of all the ills now facing mankind and the planet Earth, the most pressing issue of this decade is the loss of biological diversity. While humankind possesses or can develop the technology to cure illness, stem global warming, and control population growth, we are unable to recreate a species lost; extinctions are final and irreversible. The present rate of species loss is 400 times higher than that of the recent geologic past; if man's destructive tendencies remain unchanged, as we finish this century we face what may be the greatest series of extinction spasms since the disappearance of the dinosaurs some 65 million years ago. These extinctions will result largely from the anthropogenic destruction of high-diversity ecosystems, especially tropical rain forests.

Despite years of public outcry, the world's tropical forests are disappearing now at rates 40% higher than just ten years ago, according to statistics recently published by the United Nations Food and Agriculture Organization.[73] Eminent rainforest ecologist, Norman Myers[42] goes further to point out that in 1989 the world lost almost twice the amount of tropical moist forest as was lost in 1979. The basis of perhaps 60% of this destruction lies in the repeating pattern of large-scale development and logging companies building roads into the forest to extract precious hardwoods; then land-hungry farmers use these roads to reach the once inaccessible forests where they slash and burn the remaining trees for agriculture. The patterns of deforestation are uneven, with more than three quarters of the destruction occurring in just ten countries worldwide, and Colombia is among those top ten.[42]

Humans depend on biodiversity for survival, and essentially what we lose when tropical forests disappear are our options for the future. Sadly, we have barely begun to tap the potential that the biodiversity of the tropical forest holds for our own species. Currently 25% of all prescription drugs available in the U.S. contain plant-derived natural materials. Many of these drugs, such as the alkaloid D-turbocurarine (widely used as a muscle relaxant in abdominal surgery) cannot currently be synthesized in the laboratory.[74,75] Yet, Brazilian chemist Otto Gottlieb wrote that "Nothing at all is known about the chemical composition of 99.6% of our flora."[76] It is most frightening to think that the cures for human cancer might be going up in smoke before even being described by science; and medicinals are merely the tip of the iceberg — less than 20 plant species now produce most of the world's food.[77] Many of these species such as corn, rice, tomatoes, sugarcane, and cassava originated in the tropics and rely on continuous cross-breeding with semidomesticated and wild tropical varieties in order to maintain high yields, nutritional quality, durability, responsiveness to different soils and climates, and resistance to pests and disease.[78] Yet, as forests disappear, so do the relatives of important crop species and chances of discovering more wonder drugs and crops, not to mention an unimaginable number of other industrially valuable products.

In terms of what tropical forest animals can provide, let us consider just briefly the role of primates in science. Studies of primates have taught us a great deal about the intricacies of our own behavior, they have clarified questions about our evolution and our origins, and they have played a significant role in biomedical research, helping to unravel the mysteries of a plethora of human ailments such as hepatitis, malaria, colon cancer, and now, acquired immunodeficiency syndrome (AIDS).

In the case of the cotton-top tamarin, maintenance of the species in the wild and especially of its native forests in Colombia will be important in solving the puzzle of colon carcinogenesis. Some cancer researchers believe that colitis and colon cancer result from a combination of factors, including genetics, diet, and stress. Also, it is virtually impossible to replicate wild conditions in captive settings; hence, it is logical that research on colon carcinogenesis may increasingly rely upon control data gathered by minimally invasive techniques using wild cotton-top tamarins in their natural habitat, the only setting in which these animals could be free of artifically (though not naturally) induced stress.

Indeed, studies of cotton-tops in the wild in northern Colombia are currently being conducted by a team of medical researchers;[79] an initial report suggests that moderate or severe colitis does not occur frequently in wild tamarins. Wood et al.[78] indicate in their title that ''Captivity Promotes Colitis in the Cotton-Top Tamarin;'' this implies that something about the nature of the wild, be it diet, social contact, or any combination of an infinitely wide variety of other variables, may reduce the susceptibility of animals to colitis and, thus, affect death rates in wild populations. The cotton-top's ability to survive in the wild may derive from its association with another native plant or animal species possessing prophylactic or therapeutic properties. While this may seem a far-fetched hypothesis at present, it nonetheless cannot be ignored in such an important pursuit as the search for a cure to human cancer.

It behooves the medical profession to pay close attention to the conservation of the cotton-top's native forests. The same argument might apply also to the native forests of other biomedically important species like the chimpanzee, the rhesus monkey, night monkeys of the genus *Aotus,* the squirrel monkeys (genus *Saimiri*), and the common marmoset (*Callithrix jachus*). The habitats of all these biomedically important species are under substantial threat today.

So the biomedical community and those interested in conserving biological diversity in the tropics share a common goal and mandate. There are many ways in which the biomedical community can play a greater role in tropical conservation.

There is little doubt that the trade in wild captured animals for biomedical use was to some degree responsible for the current endangered status of the cotton-top tamarin. Despite the fact that Colombian, U.S., and international

Policy Statement on Use of Primates for Biomedical Purposes

The ECG and WHO recognize that nonhuman primates play an important role in biomedical research and testing, and that their use as experimental animals has made a significant contribution to advances in human health and disease control.

The ECG and WHO are committed to maintaining the current diversity of the Order Primates and to ensuring the survival of representative, self-sustaining populations of all species in their natural habitats.

A total of 76 primate taxa are currently considered *endangered, vulnerable* or *rare* by the IUCN. Since these taxa are either in serious decline or already at very low and precarious population levels, any exploitation of them threatens their continued survival. Therefore, the ECG and WHO strongly recommend that:

(1) *endangered, vulnerable* and *rare* species be considered for use in biomedical research projects only if they are obtained from existing self-sustaining captive breeding colonies (i.e. in captive breeding, all animals are required to be at least F2 generation);

(2) species categorized as *status unknown* or *indeterminate* also not be considered for use in such research projects until adequate data indicate that they are not *endangered, vulnerable* or *rare*.

Members of more than 30 species of nonhuman primates, the majority of them wild-caught, are currently being used worldwide in biomedical research and testing. However, sustained yield trapping strategies for wild primates, based on long-term ecological field studies and adequate demographic data, have not yet been developed for any primate species. Continuing habitat loss in most areas where primates occur makes demographic projections difficult and unreliable in most cases. The ECG and WHO therefore recommend that:

(1) wild-caught primates be used primarily for the establishment of self-sustaining captive breeding colonies, the eventual goal of which should be to captive-breed most or all (depending on species) of the primates used in research;

(2) populations of the apparently common primate species be trapped only in:

(a) special management areas where demographic data are available, where the populations are continually monitored to avoid overexploitation, and where sustained yield trapping strategies are being developed and tested;

(b) areas where the animals are living in agricultural or other man-modified environments and have been shown to be agricultural nuisances that would otherwise be destroyed; or

(c) areas where the habitat is already being destroyed, where the primates would otherwise be killed or would die from starvation or stress, and where translocation is not a viable alternative.

To minimize impact on free-living populations, the ECG and WHO urge that trapping, holding and shipping techniques be perfected to the point that accidental death, destruction of habitat, disruption of family groups, and other forms of wastage are kept to an absolute minimum.

The ECG and WHO urge researchers and their funding agencies to assist in the control of international commerce in primates by requiring proper export and import documentation on all animals that they purchase or otherwise obtain, and to refuse animals obtained in contravention of CITES and/or protective legislation in the source countries.

FIGURE 11. Policy statement on use of primates for biomedical purposes.

law have curtailed the export of these animals, there have nonetheless been alleged abuses since Colombia's banning of cotton-top exportation in 1969. Petersen[56] reports that 2500 cotton-tops per year were still sold in the U.S. market after 1974 and that animal importers were able to circumvent the legal ban by trading through intermediate nations such as Bolivia and Panama. It is illegal to import animals to the U.S. from countries which prohibit their export (Panama and Bolivia do not prohibit export of *Saguinus oedipus*). Hence, importation to the U.S. was legal despite the fact that cotton-tops are not native to either Panama or Bolivia and may have been exported illegally from Colombia to these transshipment points.

Notwithstanding laws to the contrary, if there is money to be made through the capture and sale of wild species, there will be someone willing to take the risk to earn that money. The best way to curtail the threat posed by live capture is to eliminate all demand for wild-captured animals. Those who deal in the exchange of live animals for biomedical research should be fully knowledgeable of the wild status of the species with which they work, as well as all the laws pertaining to the movement of those species. Animals should not be purchased, traded, or transported if there is even the remotest possibility of illegal capture or shipment in their history. This again applies not only to the cotton-top, but to all primate species.

Figure 11 reproduces in its entirety the *Policy Statement on Use of Primates for Biomedical Purposes,* drafted by the IUCN/SSC Primate Specialist Group between 1979 and 1981 and later adopted by the World Health

Organization and the Ecosystem Conservation Group (including UNESCO, UNEP, FAO, and IUCN). An additional reference of value to biomedical researchers is the International Primatological Society's International Guidelines for the Acquisition, Care and Breeding of Nonhuman Primates, available from the Institute of Primate Research, National Museums of Kenya (ISBN 9966-9847-2-0).

Biomedical research institutes and scientists should attempt to develop closer ties with foreign governments and NGOs (nongovernmental organizations) involved with conservation of the species with which they work. Partnerships such as those developed by Anne Savage (Rhode Island Zoo) and INDERENA counterparts, and Jack Wood (Ohio State University) and Colombian associates (including representatives from INDERENA and private Colombian landholders) have resulted in fruitful collaborative research, training, and conservation initiatives thus far in Colombia.

The private and government agencies responsible for the protection of species and natural habitats in Colombia and most other tropical countries are plagued by a paucity of funding with which to achieve their conservation goals. Biomedical researchers seeking support for studies utilizing cotton-tops or other living models should, whenever possible, include in their grant requests funds for conservation of those species and their habitats in the wild. Those funds can be channelled to any number of conservation NGOs or government agencies in the U.S. or Colombia and converted directly into conservation action on the ground. A 5 to 10% add-on to a biomedical research grant, if spent effectively in the field, could have an immense positive effect in conserving tropical habitats.

VII. SUMMARY

This paper discusses the taxonomy, distribution, natural history, and conservation status of the cotton-top tamarin (*Saguinus oedipus*) in the wild. The authors recommend several actions to ensure the long-term survival of the species and the integrity of its natural habitat. Rationale and general guidelines are provided regarding ways in which biomedical researchers can play a greater role in conserving the natural habitats of cotton-tops and other primate species used in biomedical research.

VIII. RESUMEN

Este documento analiza la taxonomía, distribución, historia natural y estado de conservación del mico tití blanco (*Saguinus oedipus*) en su medio natural. Los autores recomiendan varias acciones dirigidas a garantizar la sobrevivencia en el tiempo de la especie y la integridad de su habitat natural. A su vez, los autores proveen justificación y directrices generales relacionadas a la forma en que los investigadores en biomedicina pueden realizar un papel más eficáz en la conservación de los habitat naturales de la especie y de otras especies de primates utilizados en la investigación biomédica.

ACKNOWLEDGMENTS

Several people provided valuable assistance in the preparation and review of this manuscript and we would like to extend our gratitude to Zorayda Calle, John Carr, Neal Clapp, Thomas Defler, Ardith Eudey, Jorge Hernandez Camacho (especially for his valuable contributions to Table 1), Bill Konstant, Betsy Lovejoy, Ella Outlaw, Mark Plotkin, Stephen Nash, Owen Peck, Anne Savage, Suzette Tardif, and especially all the Colombian scientists who are helping to conserve that country's diverse forests and fauna. This chapter is dedicated to the memory of Juan Manuel Paez (1965–1992), one of the dedicated Colombian scientists whose tireless efforts have contributed greatly to our knowledge of the wild cotton-top tamarin, and whose untimely death marks a great loss to the Colombian conservation movement.

REFERENCES

1. **Clapp, N. K., Lushbaugh, C. C., Humason, G. L., Gangaware, B. L., Henke, M. A., and McArthur, A. H.,** The marmoset as a model of ulcerative colitis and colon cancer, in *Colorectal Cancer and its Precursors,* Ingalls, J. F. and Mastromarino, A., Eds., Alan R. Liss, New York, 1985, 247.
2. **Clapp, N. K. et al.,** Natural history, time course, and Pathogenesis of idiopathic colitis in cotton-top tamarin (*Saguinus oedipus*), This volume, chap. 4.
3. **Clapp, N. K. and Henke, M. A.,** Spontaneous colonic carcinoma observations in the Oak Ridge Associated Universities' 26-year-old cotton-top tamarin (*Saguinus oedipus)* colony, This volume, chap 11.
4. **King, N. W., Johnson, L. D., and Sehgal, P. K.,** The prevalance of idiopathic colitis in the New England Regional Primate Research Center cotton-top tamarin *(Saguinus oedipus)* colony, This volume, chap. 5.
5. **Tardif, S. D.,** Status of the cotton-top tamarin (*Saguinus oedipus)* in captivity, *Primate Conservation,* 39(6), 38, 1985.
6. **Tardif, S. D. and Colley, R.,** *International Cotton-Top Tamarin Studbook,* 3rd ed., Oak Ridge Associated Universities, Oak Ridge, TN, 1989.
7. **Aquilina, G. D.,** *N. A. Regional Cotton-Top Tamarin Studbook,* Buffalo Zoological Gardens, New York, 1992.
8. **Mast, R. B. and Patiño, A. F.,** Aid for a native Colombian, *Nature Conservancy Magazine,* January/February, 1988.
9. **Mittermeier, R. A., Schwarz, M., and Ayres, J. M.,** A new species of marmoset, genus *Callithrix* erxleben, 1777 (Callitrichidae, Primates) from Rio Maués Region, State of Amazonas, Central Brazilian Amazon, *Goeldiana,* No. 14, October 12, 1992.
10. **Lorini, M. L. and Persson, V. G.,** Nova especie de *Leontopithecus* lesson, 1840, do Sul do Brasil, *Bol. Mus. Nac. Nova Ser. Rio de Janeiro Zool.,* No. 338, June 11, 1990.
11. **Mittermeier, R. A. and Coimbra-Filho, A. F.,** Systematics: species and subspecies, in *Ecology and Behavior of Neotropical Primates,* Vol. 1, Coimbra-Filho, A. F. and Mittermeier, R. A., Eds., Academia Brasileira de Ciencias, Rio de Janeiro, 1981.
12. **Snowdon, C. T. and Soini, P.,** The tamarins, genus *Saguinus* , in *Ecology and Behavior of Neotropical Primates,* Vol. 2, Mittermeier, R. A., Rylands, A. B., Coimbra-Filho, A., and da Fonseca, G. A. B., Eds., World Wildlife Fund, Washington, D.C., 1988, 223.

13. **Hershkovitz, P.,** *Living New World Monkeys* (Platyrrhini): *With an Introduction to Primates,* Vol. 1, University of Chicago Press, Chicago, 1977.
14. **Mast, R. B.,** Marmoset, in *The World Book Encyclopedia,* Vol. M, Edition 89-A, 174, World Book Publishers, Chicago, 1989.
15. **Kavanagh, M.,** *A Complete Guide to Monkeys, Apes, and Other Primates,* Viking Press, New York, 1983.
16. **Coimbra-Filho, A. and Mittermeier, R. A.,** Tree-gouging, exudate-eating and the ''short-tusked'' condition in *Callithrix* and *Cebuella,* in *The Biology and Conservation of the Callitrichidae,* Kleiman, D. G., Ed., Smithsonian Institution Press, Washington, D.C., 1977.
17. **Mittermeier, R. A., Kinzey, W. G., and Mast, R. B.,** Neotropical primate conservation, *J. Hum. Evol.,* No. 18, 597, 1989.
18. **Barbosa, C. C., Patiño, A. F., and Giraldo, H.,** Proyecto sobre Evaluacion del Habitat y Status del Mono Titi Cebeza Blanca *(Sanguinus oedipus)* en Colombia, Unpublished paper, INDERENA, Santafé de Bogotá, Colombia, February 1988.
19. **Hernandez Camacho, J. and Defler, T. R.,** Algunos aspectos de la conservación de primates no humanos em Colombia, in *La Primatologia en Latinoamerica,* Saavedra, C. A., Mittermeier, R. A., and Santos, I. B., Eds., World Wildlife Fund, Washington, D.C., 1983, 31.
20. **Hernandez Camacho, J. and Defler, T. R.,** Some aspects of the conservation of non-human primates in Colombia, *Primate Conservation,* No. 6, July, 1985, 42.
21. The designation of *Saguinus oedipus* and *Sanguinus geoffroyi* as members of a super-species is consistent with the view that the two could be full species and is a point worthy of discussion. A superspecies consists of a monophyletic group of entirely or essentially allopatric species that are morphologically too different to be included in a single species. The principal feature of the superspecies is that it essentially presents the picture of a polytypic species for which the allopatric populations are so different morphologically or otherwise that reproductive isolation between them can be assumed.
22. **Hernandez Camacho, J. and Cooper, R. W.,** The nonhuman primates of Colombia, in *Neotropical Primates: Field Studies and Conservation,* Thorington, R. W. and Heltne, P. G., Eds., National Academy of Sciences, Washington, D.C., 1976, 35.
23. A field survey of *Saguinus leucopus* is now being carried out by a Colombian primatol-ogist, Zorayda Calle, in the Rio La Miel watershed in the departments of Caldas and Tolima on the east flank of the central cordillera of the Colombian Andes. Her work, which is being supported by a Colombian company planning a hydroelectric project in the vicinity (ISA), Conservation International, and the Cali-based Fundación Herencia Verde, will provide some of the first data on wild distribution, ecology, and conservation of the white-footed tamarin.
24. **Skinner, C.,** Justification for reclassifying Geoffroy's tamarin from *Saguinus oedipus geoffroyi* to *Saguinus geoffroyi, Primate Rep.,* No. 31, October, 1991.
25. **Epple, G.,** Maintenance, breeding and development of marmoset monkeys (Callitrichi-dae) in captivity, *Folia Primatol.,* 12, 56, 1970.
26. **Hernandez Camacho, J.,** personal communication.
27. **Neyman, P. F.,** Aspects of the ecology and social organization of free-ranging cotton-top tamarins *(Saguinus oedipus)* and the conservation status of the species, in *The Biology and Conservation of the Callitrichidae,* Kleiman, D. G., Ed., Smithsonian Institution Press, Washington D.C., 1977.
28. **Mittermeier, R. A. and Coimbra-Filho, A. F.,** Distribution and conservation of New World primate species used in biomedical research, in *Reproduction in New World Pri-mates,* Hearn, J., Ed., MTP Press, Lancaster, 1983, 1.
29. **Dawson, G. A.,** Some Aspects of the Population Ecology of the Panamanian Marmoset, *Saguinus oedipus geoffroyi,* Ph.D. dissertation, Michigan State University, East Lansing, Michigan, 1976.

30. **Dawson, G. A.,** Composition and stability of social groups of the tamarin, *Saguinus oedipus geoffroyi* in Panama: Ecological and behavioral implications, in *The Biology and Conservation of the Callitrichidae,* Kleiman, D. G., Ed., Smithsonian Institution Press, Washington, D.C., 1979, 23.
31. The maps in Figures 3A and 3B were produced by Stephen Nash, based on Hershkovitz,[13] Ramirez-Cerquera,[32] Barbosa et al.,[18] INDERENA,[33] and Hernandez Camacho.[26]
32. **Ramirez Cerquera, J.,** S.O.S. for the cotton-top tamarin, *Primate Conservation,* No. 6, July, 1985.
33. Instituto Geográfico Augustín Codazzi (IGAC), Instituto Nacional de Recursos Naturales y del Ambiente (INDERENA), and Corporación Nacional de Investigacion Fomento Forestal (CONIF) *Mapa de Bosques Memoria Explicativa,* Santafé de Bogotá, 1984.
34. Neymann[27,35] proposes an altitudinal range for *Sanguinus oedipus* up to 500 m, and also reports that, based on interviews with local Indians,[36] the range of the species may not be continuous even up to 500 m; apparently the cotton-top does not inhabit steep riverine habitat but is rather confined to broader valleys. In contrast, Barbosa et al.[18] report interviews with both local guerrillas and Indians of the Emberá-Katío linguistic group in the upper Sinú and San Jorge River valleys (Department of Córdoba) indicating that cotton-tops are found, at least in this area, at altitudes approximating 1000 m. Neither Neyman's observations nor those of Barbosa et al. were accompanied by sightings of wild animals. To provide a liberal view of the animal's range, the authors have chosen here to base the proposed distribution of *Saguinus oedipus* on Camacho and Defler's[19,20] calculated altitudinal limits of 1500 m. Further field observations of wild cotton-tops in the Andes will be necessary to fully elaborate the actual altitudinal tolerances of the species.
35. **Neyman, P. F.,** The Protection and Management of Primates in Sucre and Cordoba (Colombia), Unpublished report to the New York Zoological Society, December, 1977.
36. **Mayr, J.,** personal communication.
37. **Lippold, L. K.,** Mona monkeys of Grenada, *Primate Conservation,* No. 10, December 1989, p. 22.
38. **Scott, J., Struhsaker, T. T., Glander, K., and Chiriví, H.,** Primates and their habitats in Northern Colombia with recommendations for future management and research, in *First Inter-American Conference on Conservation and Utilization of American Nonhuman Primates in Biomedical Research,* Scientific Publication No. 317, Pan American Health Organization, 1976, 30.
39. **Baker, A.,** personal communication.
40. **Mittermeier, R. A. and Mast, R. B.,** Conservación y diversidad biológica en Colombia y el mundo, in *Ecobios Colombia 88,* Rodriguez, J. V. and Sanchez Paez, H., Eds., Biblioteca Andres Posada Arango, Bogotá, No. 1990, 143.
41. **Alderman, C. L.,** A general introduction to primate conservation in Colombia, *Primate Conservation,* no. 10, December, 1989, p. 44.
42. **Myers, N.,** Tropical deforestation: the latest situation, *Bioscience,* 41 (No. 5), 282, 1989.
43. **International Union for the Conservation of Nature,** *1990 IUCN Red List of Threatened Animals,* Gland, Switzerland, 1990.
44. CITES. Convention on International Trade in Endangered Species of Wild Flora and Fauna, Appendices I, II, and III, February 20, 1990.
45. **Mittermeier, R. A.,** Primate diversity and the tropical forest: case studies from Brazil and Madagascar and the importance of megadiversity countries, in *Biodiversity,* Wilson, E. O., Ed., National Academy Press, Washington, D.C., 1988, 145.
46. **Marsh, C. W., Johns, A. D., and Ayres, J. M.,** Effects of habitat disturbance on rain forest primates, in *Primate Conservation in the Tropical Rain Forest,* Marsh, C. W. and Mittermeier, Eds., Alan R. Liss, New York, 1987, 83.
47. **Mast, R. and Cubberly, P. S.,** SOS for the cotton-top tamarin, *Focus,* 9 (No. 2), 5, 1987.

48. **LeDec, G.,** personal communication.
49. Interconexión Eléctrica S. A. (ISA) Oficina de Divulgación. Nuevo Plan de Expansión para el Sectór, *Internoticias,* No. 109, December 1988, p. 3.
50. World Resources Institute in collaboration with the United Nations Environment Programme and the United Nations Development Programme, *World Resources 1992–93,* Oxford University Press, New York, 1992.
51. **Mittermeier, R. A.,** Hunting and its effects on wild primate populations in Suriname, in *Neotropical Wildlife Use and Conservation,* Robinson, J. G. and Redford, K. H., Eds., University of Chicago Press, Chicago, IL, 1991, 93.
52. **Mittermeier, R. A.,** Effects of hunting on rain forest primates, in *Primate Conservation in the Tropical Rain Forest,* Marsh, C. W. and Mittermeier, R. A., Eds., Alan R. Liss, New York, 1987, 109.
53. **Defler, T. R.,** The status and some ecology of primates in the Colombian Amazon, *Primate Conservation,* No. 10, December, 1989.
54. **Thorington, R. W., Jr.,** Importation, breeding and mortality of New World primates in the United States, in *International Zoo Yearbook,* Vol. 12, Duplaix, N., Ed., 1972, 18.
55. **Mack, D. and Mittermeier, R. A.,** *The International Primate Trade,* Vol. 1, *Legislation, Trade and Captive Breeding,* TRAFFIC (USA) and International Union for the Conservation of Nature, Washington, D.C., 1984.
56. **Peterson, D.,** *The Deluge and the Ark: A Journey into Primate Worlds,* Houghton Mifflin, Boston, 1989.
57. **Calle, Z.,** personal communication.
58. **Hershkovitz, P.,** Mammals of Northern Colombia, preliminary report No. 4: Monkeys (Primates), with taxonomic revisions of some forms, *Proc. U.S. Natl. Museum,* 98, 323, 1949.
59. **Neyman, P. F.,** Ecology and Social Organization of the Cotton-Top tamarin *(Saguinus oedipus),* Ph.D. thesis, University of California, Berkeley, 1979.
60. In 1985, Roderic Mast was Program Officer for Species Conservation at the World Wildlife Fund — U.S., José Vicente Rodriguez was Chief of the Fauna Division of INDERENA, and Russell Mittermeier was Vice President of World Wildlife Fund and Director of WWF's Primate Conservation Program.
61. Shortly after initial discussions concerning the inception of such an effort, Dr. Ramirez Cerquera tragically disappeared along with his family and 23,000 other Colombians when the town of Armero was obliterated by a mudslide resulting from a seismic disturbance on the slopes of the Ruiz Volcano.
62. **Savage, A., Burger, W. T., and Giraldo, H.,** Field techniques for trapping and individual identification of small primates, *Am. J. Primatol.,* submitted.
63. **Savage, A., Snowdon, C. T., Giraldo, H., and Rodriguez, J. V.,** Group composition, patterns of emigration and home range size of cotton-top tamarins *(Saguinus oedipus oedipus)* in Colombia, *Natl. Geographic Res.,* submitted.
64. **Savage, A.,** Reproductive Biology of the Cotton-top Tamarin *(Saguinus oedipus oedipus)* in Colombia, Ph.D. dissertation, University of Wisconsin, Madison, WI, 1990.
65. **Snowdon, C. T., Savage, A., and Giraldo, H.,** Survival of cotton-top tamarins: captive breeding and field conservation, American Association of Zoological Parks and Aquaria Annual Conference Proceedings, Washington, D.C., 1989.
66. **Tardif, S. D., Forman, L., Savage, A., Rush, J. R., and Snowdon, C. T.,** Status of the endangered cotton-top tamarin *(Saguinus oedipus oedipus)* in captivity, American Association of Zoological Parks and Aquaria Annual Conference Proceedings, 1989.
67. **Savage, A., Snowdon, C. T., Giraldo, H., and Clavijo, J.,** The ecology and biology of the cotton-top tamarin *(Saguinus oedipus oedipus)* in Colombia, American Association of Zoological Parks and Aquaria Annual Conference Proceedings, 1988.
68. **Savage, A.,** From teens to tamarins: conservation efforts in Colombia, *Zoolife,* 3, 50, 1992.

69. **Savage, A. and Giraldo, H.,** "Proyecto Tití": The development of a conservation education program in Colombia, in *First Pan American Conference on the Conservation of Wildlife Through Education Proceedings,* in press.
70. **Savage, A., Snowdon, C. T., and Giraldo, H.,** Proyecto Tití: A hands-on approach to conservation education in Colombia, American Association of Zoological Parks and Aquaria.
71. **Seal, U. S., Ballou, J. D., and Padua, C. V.,** *Leontopithecus Population Viability Analysis Workshop Report,* IUCN Captive Breeding Specialist Group Publication, International Union for the Conservation of Nature, Cambridge, U.K., June, 1990.
72. IUCN Captive Breeding Specialist Group, *CBSG News,* Vol. 3, No. 2, August, 1992.
73. **Booth, W.,** Tropical forests disappearing at a faster rate, *The Washington Post,* September 9, 1991.
74. **Plotkin, M. J.,** Conservation, ethnobotany, and the search for new jungle medicines: pharmacognosy comes of age . . . again, *Pharmacother. J. Hum. Pharmacol. Drug Ther.,* No. 8, 257, 1988.
75. **Plotkin, M. J.,** The outlook for new agricultural and industrial products from the tropics, in *Biodiversity,* Wilson, E. O., Ed., National Academy Press, Washington, D.C., 1988, 106.
76. **Gottlieb, O.,** New and underutilized plants in the Americas: solutions to problems of inventory through systematics, *Interciencia,* 6(1), 22, 1981.
77. **Vietmeyer, N.,** Lesser-known plants of potential use in agriculture and forestry, *Science,* No. 232, 1379, 1986.
78. International Union for the Conservation of Nature, *World Conservation Strategy,* Gland, Switzerland, 1980, 55.
79. **Wood, J. D., Peck, O. C., Sharma, H. M., Mekhjan, H. S., Stone, D. W., Stonerook, M., Weiss, H. S., Hernandez, J., Rodriguez, J. V., and Rodriguez, M. A.,** Captivity promotes colitis in the cotton-top tamarin *(Saguinus oedipus), Gastroenterology,* No. 98, 1408, 1990.

Chapter 2

BREEDING THE COTTON-TOP TAMARIN *(Saguinus oedipus)* IN CAPTIVITY

Suzette D. Tardif and Neal K. Clapp

TABLE OF CONTENTS

0-8493-5363-7/93/$0.00 + $.50

I. INTRODUCTION

Efforts to breed large numbers of marmosets and tamarins (Family Callitrichidae) for biomedical research began in the 1960s.[1-3] The species most commonly used and bred included the cotton-top tamarin (*Saguinus oedipus*), the saddle-backed tamarin (*S. fuscicollis*), the white-lipped tamarin (*S. mystax*), and the common marmoset (*Callithrix jacchus*). Breeding efforts intensified in the 1970s because the animals became less readily available from the wild and researchers desired animals that were of known age and parasite-free. Successful captive breeding of the cotton-top tamarin became particularly crucial as this species was declared endangered by its country of origin, Colombia, in 1972 and then by the U.S. in 1976.[4] Because of its endangered species status, use of the cotton-top tamarin as a general research resource in fields such as virology was reduced in the 1970s; however, this species was at this point recognized as a unique biomedical resource for the study of colon cancer, given its propensity to develop this important human cancer spontaneously.[5-7]

During the past 20 years, substantial improvements have occurred in callitrichid production and better definition of the reproductive potential of callitrichids in general and the cotton-top tamarin in particular have been recognized. This chapter summarizes the available information on husbandry and reproduction of the cotton-top tamarin. The future of the cotton-top tamarin as a research resource is also discussed.

II. REPRODUCTIVE PARAMETERS

Callitrichids are the most fecund simian primates. Cotton-top tamarin females may ovulate as early as 10 to 14 months of age,[8,9] but viable offspring are generally not produced before 26 to 30 months of age, due to frequent abortions and parental incompetence in younger animals.[10-12] Female tamarins are capable of reproduction at 14 to 15 years of age.[13,14] Cotton-top tamarins, in common with other callitrichids, usually produce fraternal twins. The percentage of twin deliveries varies from 60 to 85%, with the remaining deliveries being singletons or triplets.[1,10,11,15-21] Singletons are frequently the result of abortion and resorption of the second fetus.[3] Large litters (triplets and quadruplets) are generally more frequent in common marmosets;[22,23] however, in some colonies of cotton-top tamarins, triplets account for 10 to 30% of deliveries.[10,11,24,25] Triplet deliveries may result in delivery complications[22] or low birth-weight infants.[26] It is rare for all three infants to be successfully parent-reared, but hand-rearing techniques are well established.[27-32] Litter size in captive callitrichids has been postulated to be related to nutrition. Kirkwood and Underwood[33] have suggested that the occurrence of triplets in the Bristol, England colony was related to increased dietary protein. Other studies[34] suggest that increased litter sizes result with breeding of captive-born animals.

Abortions occur rather commonly in cotton-top tamarins; however, frequency varies greatly between colonies, ranging from 5 to 35% of deliveries[10,11,15,19-21,35] (percentages may vary with inclusion of stillbirths in these data). Pregnancy failures both early and late in pregnancy are common. Stressful housing conditions, such as small cages, frequent moving, and exposure to conspecifics, have been suggested as increasing the incidence of abortion.[1] The overall incidence of abortions and premature deliveries in the Oak Ridge colony decreased from approximately 45% to 20% when the breeding animals were moved into more spacious cages with minimum exposure to other social groups.[20,24] The results of Kirkwood et al.[10] suggest that an early age (prior to 29 months) for first conception may also increase the frequency of abortion.

Gestation in the cotton-top tamarin is approximately 184 days,[36] 28% longer than the 145 days that had previously been observed in the common marmoset.[37] Females frequently become pregnant during the postpartum estrus, occurring 10 to 30 days after delivery.[39] The reported average interbirth intervals range from approximately 230 to 290 days.[10,15,18-20,24] The interbirth intervals in the colonies at Bristol, England and Oak Ridge, Tennessee follow a bimodal distribution with peaks at around 240 and 360 days. Kirkwood et al.[19] and Evans[18] found that those females that nursed and weaned young had a longer interbirth interval (mean of 289 to 358 days) than those that lost their young in the neonatal period (mean of 207 to 220 days). However, others, including a subsequent report from Kirkwood, have reported no relation between the number of young nursed or weaned and the length of the interbirth interval.[10,20,38] Ziegler et al.[39] found that lactation did influence the interval from birth to ovulation, but this influence did not translate into significant effects on the interbirth interval.

Another factor that may affect the interbirth interval in captivity is seasonality. Most colonies report that births may occur in any month, but there is a peak occurrence reported from February to June in several colonies exposed to temperate lighting.[1,10,19,24,40,41] Brand[41] found a clear seasonality in cotton-top tamarin births in British colonies exposed to natural lighting, with a peak in March to June and a trough in July to September. However, seasonal birth peaks have also been recorded in colonies not exposed to natural lighting.[24,40]

Mortality of live offspring is frequently high. Within the first six months of life, approximately 45 to 65% of live offspring die.[10-12,17-21,24,35] The most frequently cited causes of neonatal mortality include parental abuse or neglect and loss of one triplet, probably due to inadequate lactation or poor birth condition.[10-12,17,19,21,24,42] Poor parental behavior is observed less frequently now that the social requirements for successful breeding of the species are more fully understood (see Section IV). Review of mortality figures from the *International Cotton-Top Tamarin Studbook* (N = 1581 births from 1976 to 1984) indicates a consistent improvement in infant survival each year.[43] (Table

TABLE 1
Infant Survival to 1 Year (1976–1984)

Year	No. born	No. surviving to 1 year	Percent
1976	120	32	26.7
1977	208	53	25.5
1978	139	53	38.1
1979	177	68	38.4
1980	171	69	40.3
1981	187	79	42.2
1982	178	79	44.4
1983	229	106	46.3
1984	172	89	51.7

1). Production of viable offspring in major colonies averages 0.8 to 1.2 per female per year.[44]

III. PHYSICAL REQUIREMENTS

Cotton-top tamarins have been housed in a wide variety of cage sizes that have ranged from 0.11 to 12.3 m^3.[1,3,12,15-21] Generally, fewer abortions and higher infant survival are associated with the use of larger cages.[21,45,44] The improved reproductive performance associated with housing in larger cages may be due to a combination of factors, including reduced crowding stress and larger, more complex family groups. Johnson et al.[12] found that cage size alone had minimal effect on infant survival, but survival was higher in groups with older siblings present. Cages are usually supplied with appropriate surfaces for an arboreal primate, including tree branches, dowels, ropes, and shelves. While metal or plastic surfaces may be preferred for sanitation, these arboreal, clawed animals locomote much more easily on wood surfaces.[21] If given a choice, cotton-top tamarins will preferentially utilize the higher portions of cages.[1,21] Use of cages that provide the animals with usable space at least 1.0 to 2.2 m above the ground is preferred. The housing in most colonies includes some type of nest box, which allows animals to retreat from exposure to humans and other animals. Removable nest boxes are also frequently used as a means of capturing animals, if necessary,[45] thereby reducing disturbance to other animals in the group.

Callitrichids are generally housed at a relatively high temperature (optimum, 27°C) and humidity (optimum, greater than 50%).[39] However, for animals with access to a large enclosure, acceptable temperatures may be much lower.[1,45,46]

In order to minimize both disturbance to the animals and the chances of their contracting a human infection, most colonies strictly limit human contact with the animals, with the exception of the caretaking staff.[45] There is much variation between colonies in the preventive measures required of caretakers and investigators to minimize chance of human-to-animal infection; some managers require protective clothing and masks and disinfectant foot baths, whereas others do not.

Callitrichid nutrition is more thoroughly examined in Chapter 3. However, some points concerning feeding should be mentioned here. Most colonies feed a diverse diet, that consists of a pelleted or canned prepared diet supplemented with a variety of fruits, insects, milk products, and/or eggs.[21,33,46-51] A diverse diet may play an important behavioral as well as nutritional role for animals in a relatively monotonous environment. Provisioning with a wide variety of foods increases behavioral diversity as well.[46] The protein portion of the diet should be presented in an easily consumable form. Early experience with captive callitrichids fed a hard pellet combined with fruit indicated that animals would frequently forgo feeding on the pellet and subsist largely on a fruit diet, resulting in an unbalanced diet and in weight loss.[52,53] However, tamarins will readily consume a number of protein sources, including canned marmoset diets, insects, eggs, and milk products such as cheese and yogurt. Competition for prized food items will occur in social groups, but the effects of such competition may be minimized by providing more than one feeding station.[54] Food should be presented at a relatively high location, as cotton-top tamarins are hesitant to approach the bottom of the cage even to obtain food.[21,45]

IV. SOCIAL REQUIREMENTS

Callitrichids are ideally housed as a mated pair with a number of their offspring (through 18 to 24 months of age); multifemale housing is not recommended as in some other primate species. Recent fieldwork suggests that a monogamous social organization may not be the only or most common social organization of tamarins in the wild.[55-57] However, complications associated with strong intrasexual aggression in captive situations makes monogamous housing the safest and most efficient means of breeding these animals.[58] Visual screening between cotton-top tamarin breeding groups is recommended.[21,44,45,48] In family groups, there is only one functionally reproductive pair. Adult female offspring in the groups are generally reproductively suppressed, both behaviorally and physiologically.[8,9,59-61]

All subadult and adult family members may participate in caring for infants, including carrying the infants and provisioning them with solid food. Studies indicate that experience in caring for infants is essential to development of desirable parental behavior.[12,21,62-65] This experience with infant siblings needs to occur after the older offspring is old enough, at least 12 to 14 months of age, to actively participate in infant care.[66] Experience is important for both sexes.[12,13,65]

Incompatibility of mates is rare, and both males and females are easily remated if an original mate must be removed. Mating of individuals who have no previous reproductive history with individuals who have reared their own offspring provides the best reproductive performance.[11]

V. THE FUTURE OF THE COTTON-TOP TAMARIN IN CAPTIVITY

The cotton-top tamarin can be maintained indefinitely in a self-sustaining captive population if proper care is taken at this point to manage the population effectively. The third edition of the *International Cotton-Top Tamarin Studbook*[43] indicates that, as of December 31, 1988, the captive population of cotton-top tamarins exceeded 1700 animals. Of these, 63.5% were in research institutions. As indicated previously, the reproductive performance of this population has continuously improved over the years 1976 to 1984. A demographic analysis of the second edition of the studbook[63] indicated that the population had 188 known founders as of December 31, 1986; of these, 164 were proven. An additional 400 animals had unknown parents, suggesting that the number of identified founders may increase with improved data collection. Sixty-five percent of the population was wild-caught or first-generation, suggesting that substantial change in the demographic and genetic character of the population is possible and future management may be extremely important.

For future successful propagation, care should be exerted to maintain this broad genetic base so that problems arising through generations of restrictive breeding may be avoided. Maintenance of this genetic base should be possible now that research and experience have provided an understanding of the physical, nutritional, and social environment in which this species will thrive. Social housing, which allows for experience through assisting in infant care, is particularly important.

The cotton-top tamarin presents a unique opportunity for biomedical and conservation interests to coalesce. The research interests in the cotton-top tamarin as a model for Epstein-Barr virus and colonic disease studies may now aid in the conservation of the species on two fronts, by enhancing interest in field studies, particularly of feeding ecology, and by maintaining a large, diverse captive population. Research programs have and may continue to provide economic incentive for preservation of the cotton-top tamarin.

ACKNOWLEDGMENTS

The authors thank Charles T. Snowdon for his thoughtful review of this chapter. This work was supported by National Institutes of Health grant R01-RR-02022 (SDT), ORAU Corporation, and National Cancer Institute contract N01 CP21004. The Marmoset Research Center at Oak Ridge Associated Universities is an AAALAC-accredited facility.

REFERENCES

1. **Hampton, J. K., Hampton, S. H., and Landwehr, B. T.,** Observations on a successful breeding colony of the marmoset, *Oedipomidas oedipus, Folia Primatol.*, 4, 265, 1966.
2. **Deinhardt, J. B., Devine, J., Passovoy, J., Pohlman, R., and Deinhardt, F.,** Marmosets as laboratory animals. I. Care of marmosets in the laboratory, pathology and outline of statistical evaluation of data, *Lab. Anim. Care,* 17, 11, 1967.
3. **Gengozian, N.,** Marmosets. Their potential in experimental medicine, *Ann. N.Y. Acad. Sci.*, 162, 336, 1969.
4. **Mittermeier, R. A. and Coimbra-Filho, A. F.,** Distribution and conservation of New World primate species used in biomedical research, in *Reproduction in New Worl Primates,* Hearn, J. P., Ed., MTP Press, Lancaster, 1983, 1.
5. **Lushbaugh, C. C., Humason, G. L., Swartzendruber, D. C., and Richter, C. B.,** Spontaneous colonic adenocarcinoma in marmosets, *Primates Med.*, 10, 119, 1978.
6. **Chalifoux, L. V. and Bronson, R. T.,** Colonic adenocarcinoma associated with chronic colitis in cotton-top marmosets, *Saguinus oedipus, Gastroenterology,* 80, 942, 1981.
7. **Clapp, N. K., Lushbaugh, C. C., Humason, G. L., Gangaware, B. L., and Henke, M. A.,** Natural history and pathology of colon cancer in *Saguinus oedipus oedipus, Dig. Dis. Sci.*, 30, 107S, 1985.
8. **Tardif, S. D.,** Social influences on sexual maturation of female *Saguinus oedipus oedipus, Am. J. Primatol.*, 6, 99, 1984.
9. **Ziegler, T. E., Savage, A., Scheffler, G., and Snowdon, C. T.,** The endocrinology of puberty and reproductive functioning in female cotton-top tamarins *(Saguinus oedipus)* under varying social conditions, *Biol. Reprod.*, 37, 618, 1987.
10. **Kirkwood, J. K., Epstein, M. A., Terlecki, A. J., and Underwood, S. J.,** Rearing a second generation of cotton-top tamarins (*Saguinus oedipus oedipus)* in captivity, *Lab. Anim.*, 19, 69, 1985.
11. **Tardif, S. D., Carson, R. L., and Clapp, N. K.,** Breeding performance of captive-born cotton-top tamarin *(Saguinus oedipus)* females: proposed explanations for colony differences, *Am. J. Primatol.*, 11, 71, 1986.
12. **Johnson, L. D., Petto, A. J., and Sehgal, P. K.,** Factors in the rejection and survival of captive cotton-top tamarins *(Saguinus oedipus), Am. J. Primatol.*, 25, 91, 1991.
13. **Epple, G. and Katz, Y.,** The saddle-back tamarin and other tamarins, in *Reproduction in New World Primates,* Hearn, J. P., Ed., MTP Press, Hingham, MA, 1983, 115.
14. **Tardif, S. D. and Ziegler, T. E.,** Features of female reproductive senescence in the tamarin, a New World primate, *J. Reprod. Fertil.*, in press.
15. **Wolfe, L. G., Deinhardt, F., Ogden, J. D., Adams, M. R., and Fisher, L. E.,** Reproduction of wild-caught and laboratory-born marmoset species used in biomedical research *(Saguinus* sp., *Callithrix jacchus), Lab. Anim. Sci.*, 25, 802, 1975.
16. **Brand, H. M.,** Husbandry and breeding of a newly-established colony of cotton-top tamarins *(Saguinus oedipus oedipus), Lab. Anim.*, 15, 7, 1981.
17. **Kilborn, J. A., Sehgal, P., Johnson, L. D., Beland, M., and Bronson, R. T.,** A retrospective study of infant mortality of cotton-top tamarins *(Saguinus oedipus)* in captive breeding, *Lab. Anim. Sci.*, 33, 168, 1983.
18. **Evans, S.,** Breeding of the cotton-top tamarin, *Saguinus oedipus oedipus:* a comparison with the common marmoset, *Zoo Biol.*, 2, 47, 1983.
19. **Kirkwood, J. K., Epstein, M. A., and Terlecki, A. J.,** Factors influencing population growth of a colony of cotton-top tamarins, *Lab. Anim.*, 17, 35, 1983.
20. **Tardif, S. D., Richter, C. B., and Carson, R. L.,** Reproductive performance of three species of Callitrichidae, *Lab. Anim. Sci.*, 34, 272, 1984.
21. **Snowdon, C. T., Savage, A., and McConnel, P. B.,** A breeding colony of cotton-top tamarins *(Saguinus oedipus), Lab. Anim. Sci.*, 35, 477, 1985.

22. **Stevenson, M. F.,** Maintenance and breeding of the common marmoset with notes on hand-rearing, *Intl. Zoo Yearb.,* 16, 110, 1976.
23. **Hearn, J. P.,** The common marmoset (*Callithrix jacchus*), in *Reproduction in New World Primates,* Hearn, J. P., Ed., MTP Press, Hingham, MA, 1983, 181.
24. **Gengozian, N., Batson, J. S., and Smith, T. A.,** Breeding of marmosets in a colony environment, *Primates Med.,* 10, 71, 1978.
25. **Jaquish, C. E., Gage, T. B., and Tardif, S. D.,** Reproductive factors affecting survivorship in captive Callitrichidae, *Am. J. Phys. Anthropol.,* 84, 291, 1991.
26. **Hershkovitz, P.,** *Living New World Monkeys (Platyrrhini),* Vol. 1, University of Chicago Press, Chicago, 1977.
27. **Hampton, S. H. and Hampton, J. K.,** Rearing marmosets from birth by artificial laboratory techniques, *Lab. Anim. Care,* 17, 1, 1967.
28. **Hearn, J. P. and Burden, F. J.,** Collaborative rearing of marmoset triplets, *Lab. Anim.,* 13, 131, 1979.
29. **Ogden, J. D.,** Hand-rearing *Saguinus* and *Callithrix* genera of marmosets, in *Nursery Care of Nonhuman Primates,* Ruppenthal, G. C., Ed., Plenum Press, New York, 1979, 313.
30. **Ziegler, T. E., Stein, F. J., Sis, R. F., Coleman, M. S., and Green, J. H.,** Supplemental feeding of marmoset *(Callithrix jacchus)* triplets, *Lab. Anim. Sci.,* 31, 194, 1981.
31. **Collier, C., Kaida, S., and Brody, J.,** Fostering techniques with cotton-top tamarins, *Saguinus oedipus oedipus* at the Los Angeles Zoo, *Intl. Zoo Yearb.,* 21, 224, 1981.
32. **Dronzek, L. A., Savage, A., Snowdon, C. T., Whaling, C. S., and Ziegler, T. E.,** Techniques of hand-rearing and reintroducing rejected cotton-top tamarin infants, *Lab. Anim. Sci.,* 36, 243, 1986.
33. **Kirkwood, J. K. and Underwood, S. J.,** Energy requirements of captive cotton-top tamarins, *Saguinus oedipus oedipus, Folia Primatol.,* 42, 180, 1984.
34. **Rothe, H., Konig, A., Darms, K., and Siess, M.,** Analysis of litter size in a colony of the common marmoset, *Z. Saeugetierk.,* 52, 227, 1987.
35. **Hampton, S. H., Gross, M. J., and Hampton, J. K.,** A comparison of captive breedig performance and offspring survival in the family Callitrichidae, *Primates Med.,* 10, 88, 1978.
36. **Ziegler, T. E., Bridson, W. E., Snowdon, C. T., and Eman, S.,** Urinary gonadotropin and estrogen excretion during the post-partum estrus, conception, and pregnancy in the cotton-top tamarin *(Saguinus oedipus oedipus), Am. J. Primatol.,* 12, 127, 1987.
37. **Chambers, P. L. and Hearn, J. P.,** Peripheral plasma levels of progesterone, oestradiol-17B, oestrone, testosterone, androstenedione, and chorionic gonadotropin during pregnancy in the marmoset monkey, *Callithrix jacchus, J. Reprod. Fertil.,* 56, 23, 1979.
38. **French, J. A.,** Lactation and fertility: an examination of nursing and inter-birth intervals in cotton-top tamarins *(Saguinus oedipus oedipus), Folia Primatol.,* 40, 276, 1983.
39. **Ziegler, T. E., Widowski, T. M., Larson, M. L., and Snowdon, C. T.,** Nursing does effect the duration of the post partum interval in cotton-top tamarins *(Saguinus oedipus), J. Reprod. Fertil.,* 90, 563, 1990.
40. **Ogden, J. D., Wolfe, L. G., and Deinhardt, F. W.,** Breeding *Saguinus* and *Callithrix* species of marmosets under laboratory conditions, *Primates Med.,* 10, 71, 1978.
41. **Brand, H. M.,** Influence of season on birth distribution in marmosets and tamarins, *Lab. Anim.,* 14, 301, 1980.
42. **Epple, G.,** Reproductive and social behavior of marmosets with special reference to captive breeding, *Primates Med.,* 10, 50, 1978.
43. **Tardif, S. D. and Colley, R.,** *International Cotton-Top Tamarin Studboodk* 3rd ed., Oak Ridge Associated Universities, Oak Ridge, TN, 1990.
44. **Price, E. C. and McGrew, W. C.,** Cotton-top tamarins *(Saguinus o. oedipus)* in a semi-naturalistic captive colony, *Am. J. Primatol.,* 20, 1, 1990.
45. **Richter, C. B.,** Biology and diseases of Callitrichidae, in *Laboratory Animal Medicine,* Fox, J. F., Cohen, B. J., and Loew, F. M., Eds., Academic Press, Orlando, FL, 1984, 353.

46. **Epple, G.,** Maintenance, breeding and development of marmoset monkeys (Callitrichidae) in captivity, *Folia Primatol.,* 12, 56, 1970.
47. **King, G. J.,** Comparative feeding and nutrition in captive non-human primates, *Br. J. Nutr.,* 40, 55, 1978.
48. **Escajadillo, A., Bronson, R. T., Sehgal, P., and Hayes, K. C.,** Nutritional evaluation in cotton-top tamarins, *Lab. Anim. Sci.,* 31, 161, 1981.
49. **Flurer, C., Scheid, R., and Zucker, H.,** Evaluation of a pelleted diet in a colony of marmosets and tamarins, *Lab. Anim. Sci.,* 33, 264, 1983.
50. **Clapp, N. K. and Tardif, S. D.,** Marmoset husbandry and nutrition, *Dig. Dis. Sci.,* 30, 17S, 1985.
51. **Tardif, S. D., Clapp, N. K., Henke, M. A., Carson, R. L., and Knapka, J. J.,** Maintenance of cotton-top tamarins fed an experimental pelleted diet versus a highly diverse sweetened diet, *Lab. Anim. Sci.,* 38(5), 588, 1988.
52. **Stellar, E.,** The marmoset as a laboratory animal: maintenance, general observations of behavior and simple learning, *J. Comp. Physiol. Psychol.,* 53, 1, 1960.
53. **Shimwell, M., Warrington, B. F., and Fowler, J. S. L.,** Dietary habits relating to "wasting marmoset syndrome", *Lab. Anim.,* 13, 139, 1979.
54. **Tardif, S. D. and Richter, C. B.,** Competition for a desired food in family groups of the common marmoset *(Callithrix jacchus)* and the cotton-top tamarin *(Saguinus oedipus), Lab. Anim. Sci.,* 31, 52, 1981.
55. **Neyman, P. F.,** Aspects of the ecology and social organization of free-ranging cotton-top tamarins *(Saguinus oedipus)* and the conservation status of the species, in *Biology and Conservation of the Callitrichidae,* Kleiman, D. G., Ed., Smithsonian Institution Press, Washington, D.C., 1978, 39.
56. **Garber, P. A., Moya, L., and Malaga, C.,** A preliminary field study of the moustached tamarin monkey *(Saguinus mystax)* in northeastern Peru: questions concerned with the evolution of a communal breeding system, *Folia Primatol.,* 42, 17, 1984.
57. **Terborah, J. and Goldizen, A. W.,** On the mating system of the cooperatively breeding saddle-backed tamarin *(Saguinus fuscicollis), Behav. Ecol. Sociobiol.,* 16, 293, 1985.
58. **Price, E. and McGrew, W. C.,** Departures from monogamy in colonies of captive cotton-top tamarins, *Folia Primatol.,* 57, 16, 1991.
59. **Savage, A., Ziegler, T. E., and Snowdon, C. T.,** Sociosexual development, pairbond formation and mechanisms of fertility suppression in female cotton-top tamarins *(Saguinus oedipus oedipus), Am. J. Primatol.,* 14, 345, 1988.
60. **Abbott, D. H.,** Behavioral and physiological suppression of fertility in subordinate marmoset monkeys, *Am. J. Primatol.,* 6, 169, 1984.
61. **French, J. A., Abbott, D. H., and Snowdon, C. T.,** The effect of social environment on estrogen excretion, scent marking, and sociosexual behavior in tamarins *(Saguinus oedipus), Am. J. Primatol.,* 6, 155, 1984.
62. **Epple, G.,** Parental behavior in *Saguinus fuscicollis* ssp. (Callitrichidae), *Folia Primatol.,* 24, 221, 1975.
63. **Tardif, S., Forman, L., Savage, A., Rush, J., and Snowdon, C.,** Status of the endangered cotton-top tamarin *(Saguinus oedipus)* in captivity, *AAZPA Annual Conference Proceedings,* (1989), 602, 1989.
64. **Hoage, R. J.,** Parental care in *Leontopithecus rosalia rosalia:* sex and age differences in carrying behavior and the role of prior experience, in *Biology and Conservation of the Callitrichidae,* Kleiman, D. G., Ed., Smithsonian Institution Press, Washington, D.C., 1978, 293.
65. **Tardif, S. D., Richter, C. B., and Carson, R. L.,** Effects of sibling rearing experience on future reproduction success in two species of Callitrichidae, *Am. J. Primatol.,* 6, 377, 1984.
66. **Cleveland, J. and Snowdon, C. T.,** Social development during the first twenty weeks in the cotton-top tamarins *(Saguinus oedipus oedipus), Anim. Behav.,* 32, 432, 1984.

Chapter 3

CALLITRICHID NUTRITION

Dennis Barnard and Joseph J. Knapka

TABLE OF CONTENTS

0-8493-5363-7/93/$0.00 + $.50

I. INTRODUCTION

The marmosets and tamarins, members of the family Callitrichidae, have great potential as laboratory animal models for human diseases. Given their small size and their ability to regularly produce twins that mature sexually in two years, healthy callitrichids can be housed and bred in large numbers at lower costs than larger species of nonhuman primates. Another important biological characteristic is that in the callitrichids, fraternal twinning involves the development of placental vascular anastomoses between twins.[1] This anatomical characteristic leads to hemopoietic chimerism and immunological tolerance between twins, which make these nonhuman primate species unique models for immunological research. Certain species of callitrichids also appear to be good models for diseases of the colon.[2] Colitis has been frequently reported in callitrichid colonies.[3-7] Spontaneous colon cancer has been reported in the *Saguinus oedipus*.[3,5,6,8,10-12] However, progress in the use of various tamarin species in research has been inhibited by poor reproduction and the occurrence of what has been termed ''wasting marmoset syndrome'' (WMS).

The occurrence of WMS in callitrichid colonies has appeared to decrease recently.[12] However, the etiology of the syndrome has not yet been determined. It is believed to be due to behavior, infection, and/or nutrition. Results of a recent study indicate that nutritional intervention reversed WMS-like symptoms in a colony of *S. mystax*.[13]

The inability to determine the etiology of WMS is an example of what can occur when the requirements of a species are not clearly defined. Adequate animal husbandry requires at least a basic knowledge of the behavioral and nutritional requirements of the species. Ignorance of these factors can lead to unacceptable marginally healthy animals.

Determination of the nutritional requirements for a wild animal species involves assimilation of information from four areas of study: (1) observation of the diet consumed by related species; (2) field observations of food consumption by the species being studied; (3) anatomical features of the species that influence nutritional requirements; (4) controlled research of the nutritional requirements of the species. The current knowledge of the nutritional requirements of the Callitrichidae has been established using these methods.

II. NUTRITION OF FERAL CALLITRICHIDAE

Observations from field studies indicate that the kinds of foods consumed vary greatly between and within primate species. Clutton-Brock states that there is no evidence that any primate species shows a high criterion for food-species specificity.[14] Evidence suggests that there are sex, age, temporal, and geographic variations in food consumption by primates.[14,15] It is also believed that caloric value is only one of many factors affecting food selection.[15]

Field studies of callitrichid feeding behavior indicate that these variations in food consumption are found in the callitrichids. Nelson[16] observed juvenile

S. geoffroyi eating prior to adults and Kaumann[17] observed female *S. mystax* eating only after the males had eaten. Exudate feeding by *Saguinus* has been determined to be seasonal and linked to periods of gestation and lactation.[18,19] These observations provide examples of variations in food consumption by callitrichids due to age, sex, and temporal variation.

Diurnal variation in feeding patterns has also been observed. *Saguinus* has been observed to concentrate on fruit feeding early in the morning and spend more time foraging for insects during the remainder of the day.[20] This variation complicates the interpretation of data obtained by stomach content analysis. For example, Fooden[21] and Enders[22] both reported finding only fruits in the stomachs of two species of *Saguinus,* incorrectly suggesting that these animals are frugivorous.

Consumption of fruits and exudates from various plant and tree species due to different geographical locations of the monkeys has been observed in the Callitrichidae.[17-19,23,24] Variation in the type of food consumed due to established ecological niches between species has also been observed. An example of this has been reported in the sympatric relationship between *S. fuscicollis* and *S. labiatus.*[17,25,26] This relationship has resulted in the two species foraging for insects at different levels of the forest; *S. fuscicollis* foraged in the lower layer (from ground level to 5 m above the ground) and *S. labiatus* foraged in the foliage from 5 to 20 m above the ground.[17,25] The differences in foraging behavior and prey size between these species were influenced by the areas utilized. Recognition of these intrageneric variations in feeding behavior is important when conclusions are drawn about the nutritional requirements from the literature on food consumption by wild populations or designing a field study in which dietary habits are to be examined.

The four genera of the Callitrichidae can be divided into two major groups based on the relationship between the lower canines and the lower incisors.[27] The terms "short-tusked" and "long-tusked" have been used to describe such differences.[28] *Saguinus* and *Leontopithecus* comprise the "long-tusked" genera in which canines are much longer than incisors. The "short-tusked" genera, which consist of *Callithrix* and *Cebuella,* have long incisors that are almost equal in length to the canines. It has been shown that *Callithrix* uses its lower anterior dentition for gouging holes in trees to induce the flow of exudates.[29,30] Exudates may include sap and/or gums. Fonseca reported that between August and November of 1980, *Callithrix jacchus penicillata* located in Cerradao, Brazil, engaged in exudate feeding over 70% of the total time spent feeding.[31] However, if exudate feeding is seasonal, this level of exudate feeding may not represent a true picture of the monkeys' dietary habits since it only represents four months of the year.

Tree gouging which resulted in the flow of exudates has never been observed during captive or field studies of *Saguinus* and *Leontopithecus.*[19] However, the consumption of exudates by these species has been documented.[32-34] Ramirez suggested that tamarins make opportunistic use of exudate holes gouged by *Cebuella,* rodents, and insects.[19] According to

Coimbra-Filho and Mittermeier,[27] *Callithrix, Cebuella,* and *Phaner furcifer* (forked-marked mouse lemur) are the only primates that use teeth to gouge holes in trees to elicit exudate flow.

Another anatomical feature of the Callitrichidae which enables them to be exudativorous are their claw-like nails, called tegulae. The tegulae enable Callitrichidae to ascend and then cling to large vertical tree trunks to consume tree exudates.[35] Garber[35] and Coimbra-Filho and Mittermeir[27] suggest that the significance of exudate feeding for the Callitrichidae is that it provides an energy source that is not utilized by other animals; thus, they avoid competition for fruit, which is a major energy source for other arboreal mammals and birds. Also, exudates are probably a more dependable food source than seasonal fruit.[35]

There are other morphological characteristics involving dentition and body size that relate to the insectivorous nature of the callitrichids. These include tritubercular molars, which are very effective in crushing the chitinous covering of arthropods.[36] Unlike other New World primates, they lack third molars in their upper and lower jaws.[29] This abbreviated dentition is found in other insectivorous animals and is thought to be sufficient for trituration of arthropods, but inappropriate for the mastication of plant fibers.[29]

There is a causal relationship between the small body size of callitrichids and their insectivorous habits.[29,36,37] For example, callitrichids forage for insects in the low shrub layer of the forest understory, which consists of a network of thin, flexible nonwoody supports and dense vine tangles.[29,37] Therefore, small body size is required for the cryptic movement used to stalk insects. Metabolic costs of maintenance and locomotor activity are relatively high in small primates. Therefore, the Callitrichidae feed on insects, a food source in which the caloric density is high.[24]

Gut transit rates are also decreased in small-bodied as compared to large-bodied primates.[39] The physiological reason for this, as explained by Milton,[39] is that "as body size increases, metabolic costs per unit body weight decrease exponentially while gut volume remains proportionate to body mass." In other words, in small animals, the size of the gut cannot process the amount of food required for their disproportionately high energetic requirements per unit body weight without decreased food transit time. Therefore, the apparently short gut transit times seen in tamarins explain observations that they seek out nutritionally concentrated food and rarely eat fibrous plants which require long transit times to digest.

Observations in the field and captivity suggest that the Callitrichidae are primarily insectivorous.[15,21,25,26,29,32,35,36,40] However, they have been observed, depending on the genus, to feed on other animals, including small birds, mammals, lizards, and eggs, as well as large quantitites of fruit and exudates.[26,27,31,40] There have been many field studies in which the amounts of insects, fruits, and tree exudates eaten have been estimated using either stomach content analysis or time spent feeding on these foods. Hladik and

Hladik,[41] Dawson,[42] and Garber[35] estimated that insects constituted 30 to 64% of the tamarin diet.

A field study by Ramirez suggests that the diet of most Callitrichidae includes predominantly insects (up to 70% of feeding time was spent foraging for them) and fruits (approximately 40% of feeding time).[19] Exudates, nectar, seeds, flowers, and leaf buds constitute a small percentage of their diet. In the upper Amazon (northeast Peru), *Saguinus* appeared to feed on exudates during the dry season. However, exudate feeding by the *S. fuscicollis illigeri* did not appear to be seasonal.[19] Exudate feeding averaged 17% of plant feeding from mid-dry to early-wet season for *S. mystax*. However, the average exudate feeding increased to 37% of plant feeding at the onset of the wet season but decreased rapidly as preferred fruit became available. Exudate feeding occurred almost exclusively on trees currently being used by *Cebuella*. The excudates consumed by the *S. mystax* appeared to be mostly gums.[19]

S. mystax located at the Tahuayo River in Peru were studied for 70 days between October 1981 and November 1982.[40] They fed on a variety of fruits (approximately 90 species), exudates (approximately 10 species) and invertebrates (insects and spiders). Foraging for invertebrates accounted for about 50% of the feeding time, Orthoptera and Lepidoptera being the most common insects eaten. During fruit consumption, the mesocarp or aril from drupes and berries were eaten most often.[40] The most frequented fruit sources (involving 33% of time spent feeding on plants) included tree and liana species (*Maripa* sp., *Parkia* sp., *Pourona* sp.) with long and/or synchronous fruiting periods. Thirteen percent of plant feeding time was spent on tree species producing large fruit crops (*Byrsonema* sp., *Ficus* sp.).[40]

Yoneda observed *S. fuscicollis* in the Pando, in northern Bolivia, from July to December, the dry season.[20] Observations indicate that these monkeys spend almost all day foraging insects. However, Yoneda suggested that the tamarins depended on fruit (from the Moraceae family) for most of its caloric intake. Fruit feeding occurred most often during the early morning. Exudate feeding was observed very infrequently. Infants appeared to begin feeding on fruit by themselves and sharing insects obtained by the mother at about 5 weeks of age and continued until about 10 weeks of age.[20]

A field study of *S. mystax* and *S. fuscicollis* in the Amazon Basin of northeastern Peru indicated that their diets were composed principally of ripe fruits, insects, and plant exudates.[43] The fruits were characterized by large seeds surrounded by either a thin aril or a gelatinous and adhesive pulpy coat. These fruits were legumes of the genera *Inga* or *Parkia* and drupes of various liana species. Redford et al.[44] suggest that ingestion of fruits by primates involves significant and deliberate ingestion of insects infesting the fruit. They speculate that when insects and fruit are consumed together, the protein derived from the insect can be utilized for vital functions other than energy.

Garber studied *S. oedipus geoffroyi* from January through August in a dry tropical forest on the Pacific coast of Panama.[32] He concluded that tamarins spent 39.4, 38.4, and 14.4% of their feeding time on insects, fruits, and exudates, respectively. Garber considers insect protein as the primary component of the tamarin diet.[35] Irrespective of the time of year, Orthoptera contributed between 65.7 and 77.3% of the total volume of insects on a dry weight basis in the stomach ingesta. According to Dawson[42] and Garber,[35] grasshoppers (Tettigoniidae) are the most common prey item even though many varieties of Orthoptera are available. Thus, it appears that the Panamanian *S. oedipus geoffroyi* is very selective in its choice of insect prey.

Garber's study of the Panamanian *S. oedipus* indicates that exudate feeding constituted 23% of the noninsect portion of their diet, a significant part of its total diet.[35] All observations of exudate feeding occurred during the wet season (May to July) at this location (Pacific coast of Panama 8.57°N, 79.37°W), when there is an abundance of fruits and insects. Therefore, the increased consumption of exudates is not due to a reduction in the availability of a more preferred food.[32] Garber postulates that the importance of exudates as a food source lies in its calcium content, which can offset the high phosphorus content of a diet composed predominantly of insects.[32]

The seasonal pattern of exudate feeding observed in *S. oedipus geoffroyi* coincides with increased demands for calcium during the terminal phase of gestation and during lactation.[32] Reproduction in the Callitrichidae is characterized by twinning.[45] It has also been determined that the neonates average between 14.1 and 23.6% of the maternal body weight.[46] This neonate-to-maternal body weight ratio is greater than in any other primate species.[46] The combination of these two factors, along with a suggestion that callitrichids require high daily amounts of calcium, indicates a high potential requirement for calcium.[32,47]

The nutrient composition of the tamarin's dietary components has not been completely determined. However, the nutrient composition of closely related insect, fruit, and tree exudate species are available for comparison. Evidence indicates that insects may be the most important component of the diet because they provide a food source that has a high caloric density.[19,25,29,32,35,41,42] A review of the nutritional composition of Orthoptera insects by Uvarov showed that all species were characterized by high concentrations of protein and fat.[48] The adults of this species had protein levels of 50 to 75% and lipid levels of 7 to 18%. Fat and proteins provide more energy than carbohydrates,[49] the major nutrient component in the tamarin's other significant food sources, which are fruit and tree exudates.

The mineral composition of the Orthoptera is characterized by a low calcium and high phosphorous content. The calcium is located in the indigestible chitin-containing tissues. Thus, the insects provide a high phosphorous/low calcium diet that could lead to problems of mineral metabolism if an additional source of calcium were not available.[50] Since fruits are relatively low in calcium, tree exudates most likely serve as the source of this element.[18,32]

The nutrient composition of *Acacia* gum excudates consists of carbohydrates, protein, and minerals.[27,51-53] Mineral analyses of *Anacardium excelsum* exudate, a primary food source for tamarins, indicated that calcium, phosphorous, sodium magnesium, and potassium were present; an important observation is the high calcium (average 54.3 mg/100 g dry weight) and low phosphorous concentration (8 mg/100 g weight). Analysis of the protein concentration of *Anacardium excelsum* shows a seasonal variation.[32] The greatest concentration (approximately 9.64%) occurs during the wet season (May) and coincides with seasonal patterns of exudate feeding.[32] Nutrient analysis of *Anacardium occidentale* has shown that there are 76.0% water-soluble substances, 7.8% water-insoluble substances, 1.05% minerals, and 16.2% moisture with a pH of 1.9.[27] Ash content consisted of iron, aluminum, calcium, magnesium, silica, potassium, and traces of manganese and sodium. The exudate contained the water-soluble carbohydrate arabin, which is composed of arabinose and galactose. Also, two water-insoluble carbohydrates were found: cerasin and bassorin. Cerasin is composed of arabinose and arabin, and bassorin is composed of galactose, xylose, and methylpentose.

III. NUTRITION OF CAPTIVE CALLITRICHIDAE

Captive Callitrichidae have consistently been described as fastidious eaters.[26,54] The result is that most callitrichid colony managers use complicated schedules to feed commercial primate diets supplemented with various foodstuffs, vitamins, and minerals.[1,26,55-65] Many observations in the literature regarding callitrichid nutrition are subjective and unconfirmed by controlled experimentation, since nutrition per se was not the primary objective for most investigators. The necessity for controlled nutritional research to determine the nutrient requirements for many species of nonhuman primates was documented by Harris 18 years ago.[66] However, this need still remains mostly unfulfilled for the Callitrichidae.

It is generally believed that feeding the monkeys a commercial primate diet supplemented with various foods and nutritional supplements is a sure way to prevent deficiencies when nutritional requirements are not known. It is also believed that this type of dietary regimen helps satisfy the behavioral needs of the monkeys.[55,67-69]

Documentation of the monkeys' response to diets supplemented with various foods has provided valuable information regarding the animals' taste preferences as well as insights into their nutritional requirements. Fitzgerald[70] and Lucas et al.[71] appear to be the first investigators to document the response of captive callitrichids to various foods. Recently, Epple reported that *S. geoffroyi* ate between 15 and 20 crickets (*Gryllus bipunctata*) a day while also feeding on fruit and cereal. She also observed that the soft consistency of feces produced by these monkeys was reversed by consumption of indigestible material such as feathers or hair.[67] When small animals were fed to

S. geoffroyi that had not been fed an animal food source for two weeks, the monkeys ate the pelage before the meat, but complete consumption of the hair was not observed in monkeys fed an animal food source regularly. Epple reported that *Leontipithecus rosalia* with dull, unthrifty pelage regained their red color after eating grasshoppers; she suggested that the fat composition of the grasshopper was responsible.

Kaumann observed the feeding behavior of a pair of *S. mystax* in an open-air enclosure at the Estacion de Conservacion y Reproducion de los Primates (ECRP) in Iquitos, Perus.[17] Each morning at 6 o'clock they were offered fruits and a gruel. They ate immediately for a few minutes, but spent most of the day foraging for insects and small animals. It was estimated that their food intake consisted of two thirds fruit and gruel and one third insects and small animals.

King pooled dry matter, energy, protein, and fat intake data collected from *C. jacchus, S. midas,* and *S. oedipus,* which had been given a commercial primate diet, plant products (vegetables and fruits), and animal products (eggs, milk, insects, etc.).[72] Daily voluntary dry matter intake was 52 g/kg body weight. This consisted of approximately 16% primate diet, 77% plant products, and 7% animal products. The protein intake consisted of approximately 38% primate diet, 42% plant products, and 27% animal products. Fat intake was 13.6% of the total calories. The sources of dietary fat consisted of approximately 15% primate diet, 55% plant products, and 30% animal products.

Benirschke and Richart fed a colony of callitrichids a variety of fruits, nuts, and animal protein food sources.[68] They reported that sweetened milk and fresh eggs were consumed eagerly. The monkeys rarely ate vegetables, fish, or meat, and never ate cooked food. Insects, including grasshoppers, cicadas, Japanese beetles, praying mantises, flies, and spiders were devoured avidly. It was noted that male callitrichids would frequently allow females to take food from them, except for insects. The authors reported that the monkeys maintained constant body weight and had normal hair coats while consuming this diet. A general conclusion derived from observations of callitrichids fed diets based on plant products, insects, and animal products was that they had a nutritional requirement for an animal protein source and had a preference for fruits and insects.

Potential problems when the dietary regimen of large callitrichid colonies involves a variety of natural food sources include: (1) possible bacterial contamination of the food; (2) transmission of intestinal parasites via insects; (3) increased cost due to wastage; (4) unknown and uncontrolled nutrient intake; and (5) labor-intensive procedures for diet preparation and cage cleaning. Therefore, investigators began to develop complete diets.[54,58,75] Stellar formulated a diet which had the consistency of dough.[54] Proximate analysis of the dry mixture indicated that the protein, carbohydrate, fat, fiber, and moisture concentrations were 24.5, 51, 14.5, 1.5, and 3.8%, respectively. It was reported that 30 to 50 g of diet were consumed daily with 30 to 40 ml of water. The monkeys gained 70 g after being transferred from a dietary regimen consisting only of natural food sources to the complete diet. Stellar suggested that adaptation to the complete diet was an important factor in the reduction of fatal respiratory disorders.

Levy and Artecona provided the recipe for a high-protein bread which was successfully fed to *S. oedipus* and *C. jacchus*.[58] It provided food of consistent and known nutrient concentrations, but its preparation and feeding as well as the cleaning of the cages were labor intensive. Therefore, investigators began to study the possibility of using commercial primate diets as a replacement or complement to diets consisting of insects, mice, fruit, and vegetables.[57-62]

Deinhardt et al. conducted a comparative study of various diets fed to three species of *Saguinus*.[57] The diets included one composed of fresh fruits, vegetables, insects, and animal products; the Stellar diet;[54] a high-protein bread modified from Levy and Antecoma;[58] and a commercial primate diet. These were fed individually or in combinations. It was concluded that body weights increased and were maintained better for those monkeys fed fresh foods and either the protein bread, Stellar diet, or commercial primate diet. It was suggested that the monkeys showed a preference for fruit, and thus it was necessary to carefully balance the quantities of fruit with the other food offered. For convenience, a combination of commercial primate diet and fresh foods was adopted as the colony diet.

Gengozian[56] modified the primate diet developed by Deinhardt et al.[57] He fed various species of *Saguinus* a commercial primate diet softened with milk and supplemented with a multivitamin preparation and supplemental ascorbic acid. Fruit, vegetables, and hard-boiled eggs were also fed sparingly at regularly determined intervals. The monkeys gained weight and appeared healthy while being fed this diet. Hampton et al. reported feeding a similar diet to *S. mystax* and *C. jacchus*.[61]

Flurer et al. evaluated a pelleted diet fed to five callitrichid species. The results indicated that sweet and fruity tastes were preferred, but saccharin and artificial banana flavor were not.[74] The monkeys disliked diets with bitter tastes that were caused by feed-grade rolled oats, undebittered brewers yeast, or alfalfa meal. The pelleted diet contained 23.4% protein, 6.6% fat, 3.6% crude fiber, and 9.4% water. It was determined that the mean daily pellet intake ranged from 3.0 to 5.5% of body weight for *C. jacchus* and *S. fuscicollis* and 2.7 to 4.0% for other species. However, some colony-born *S. fuscicollis* consumed up to 6.5% of their body weight daily. The monkeys were fed 20 g of banana daily; this may have influenced the pellet intake data. It was reported by Barnard et al. that *S. mystax* consumed 7.5% of their weight daily when fed a pelleted diet exclusively.[13] Morin surveyed 36 Callitrichidae colonies in 1978, and the results indicated that all the colonies were fed commercial primate diets supplemented with numerous kinds of feedstuffs.[75]

Problems have occurred using the supplemented diets, regardless of whether a commercial primate diet was used or not. Many investigators have reported

TABLE 1
Components of the Oak Ridge Associated Universities (ORAU) Callitrichid Diet

1. Chow slurry[a]
   - 4,500 g ground monkey chow[b]
   - 2,700 ml cold water
   - 3,200 g bananas
   - 4,200 g applesauce
   - 650 ml Karo syrup
2. Canned diet[c]
   - Presented in slices of 16.5 g
3. Supplements
   - Hard boiled egg (3 × weekly)
   - Small marshmallows (2 × weekly)
   - Roasted peanuts in shell (once weekly)
   - Meal worms (once weekly)
   - Raisins (once biweekly)
   - Lettuce (once biweekly)
   - Sweet potatoes, raw (once biweekly)

[a] Slurry is fortified with the following vitamins and minerals on a weekly basis: folic acid (2×); vitamin D_3 (2×); multiple vitamins, $CuSO_4$, and ascorbic acid once weekly.
[b] High-protein Monkey Chow 5045, 25% protein: Ralston Purina Co., St. Louis, MO.
[c] Zu/Preem Marmoset Diet, Hills Division, Riviana Foods, Topeka, KS.

From Tardiff, S., *Lab. Animal Sci.*, 38, 588, 1988. With permission.

that callitrichids develop preferences to fruit, which resulted in decreased consumption of more nutritious food.[13,17,54,57,72,76-78] This appeared to be a problem more often in the tamarins than the marmosets.[13,17,57,76,77] Both Kaumanns[17] and Deinhardt et al.[57] reported a marked preference for bananas by tamarins. Kirkwood and co-workers[76,77] reported that a colony of *S. oedipus* fed a diet consisting of one fourth apple, one fourth banana, one eighth orange, and ad lib monkey pellets for 5 years had a high incidence of diarrhea. The monkeys always consumed the fruit prior to, and in preference to, the pellets. Upon introduction of hard-boiled eggs (one fifth egg per monkey daily) and reduction of the fruit by one half, there was increased consumption of the commercial diet, resulting in a 50% increase in protein intake. A decrease occurred in the incidence of chronic diarrhea, followed by an increase in body weight, new hair growth on alopecic monkeys, and an increased incidence of triplet births.[76,77] Fruits, including bananas and applesauce, have also been successfully combined with commercial pelleted diets and delivered in a porridge consistency; this presentation method requires the animals to consume needed nutrients while eating preferred fruits (Table 1).[79]

Barnard et al. used nutritional intervention to reverse an apparent wasting syndrome in *S. mystax*.[13] The results of the study indicated that the protein concentration and caloric density of a commercial marmoset diet may have been deficient for *S. mystax*. This deficiency was compounded when a fruit

TABLE 2
Formulation for the NIH 48 Open Formula Pelleted Diet

Ingredient	Amount per kg (in grams)
Fish meal (60% protein)	100
Soybean meal (48.5% protein)	120
High fat milk solids[a]	90
Rice gel[b]	200
Casein	70
Glucose	140
Apple pomace, dried	100
Beet pulp	70
Soy oil	20
Soy lecithin	20
Mineral premix[c]	50
Vitamin premix[d]	20
	1000

[a] Manufacturer, Merrick Food Inc., Milwaukee, Wisconsin.

[b] Manufacturer, Rivianna Incorporated, Houston, Texas.

[c] Mineral premix composition (g/kg): calcium carbonate, 299. 74; cupric sulfates · $5H_2O$, 3.00; potassium phosphate dibasic, 206.23; ferric ammonium citrate, 27.47; magnesium sulfate, 101.91; manganous sulfate, 4.99; calcium phosphate dibasic, 74.93; potassium iodide, 0.06; zinc sulfate, 0.34; sodium chloride, 167.35; and carrier-limecrest, 113.98.

[d] Vitamin premix composition (g/kg): vitamin A/D_3 (650/325k IU/g), 0.33; vitamin A (650k IU/g), 1.47; vitamin E (500 IU/g), 11.01; Hetrazeen (45.5% menadione), 1.21; vitamin B_{12} (2200 mg/kg), 3.63; thiamin mononitrate USP (92%), 1.10; riboflavin (50%), 2.20; *d*-calcium pantothenate USP (92%), 5.50; pyridoxide HCl USP (82%), 1.10; folic acid USP, 0.83; biotin (1%), 2.75; ascorbic acid coated (97.5), 110.10; choline chloride (60%), 45.91; niacinamide USP, 8.26; ethoxyquin (66.6%), 11.01; carrier sucrose, 793.59.

From Addcox, N., *Lab. Animal Sci.*, 38, 282, 1988. With permission.

mash was fed with the commercial diet, resulting in a 31-g reduction in the daily consumption of the commercial diet. In contrast, a colony of *C. jacchus* was maintained on the same commercial marmoset diet for 2 years with low morbidity and a good reproductive performance.

Barnard et al. fed a highly palatable pelleted open formula diet.[13] Proximate analysis of the diet indicated that the crude protein, ether extract, crude fiber, and nitrogen free extract (NFE) concentrations based on dry weight were 26.2, 12.3, 5.9, and 43.4%, respectively. The moisture content of the diet was 10.3%. The formulation of the diet is presented in Table 2. Consumption of the open formula diet for 2 months resulted in a mean weight gain of 56 g. This diet was fed successfully to healthy adult *S. mystax* with and without supplementation for 5 months with a maintenance of weight and no adverse effects;[79] previously, animals had been fed a diverse mash diet.[64]

A long-term feeding study in which *C. jacchus* were fed a pelleted diet was conducted by Wirth and Buselmaier.[80] Proximate analysis of the diet showed that the crude protein, ether extract, crude fiber, and NFE values based on dry weight were 25.9, 6.9, 2.8, and 64.4%, respectively. The marmosets preferred pellets that were 10 mm in diameter. The results indicated that the monkeys could live and reproduce adequately while being fed this diet without supplements.

Nutritional quality and palatability are two important factors to be considered when formulating diets. The palatability of various nutrient sources and the effect of their concentration on other nutrients have been examined. Krombach et al. studied the effects of fiber in a pelleted diet on food intake, transit time, consistency of feces, digestibility of dry matter, energy, and crude fiber.[81] It was determined that when dehydrated alfalfa meal, beet pulp, and malt sprouts were used as fiber sources the palatability of the diet was reduced and resulted in diarrhea. Coarse cellulose, microcellulose, wheat bran, and shrimp meal (chitin as fiber) were used as fiber sources in diets at levels of 2, 4, and 6%. The results showed that digestibility of commercial cellulose was low but there was no significant depression of energy digestibility. Wheat bran at 4% and 6% concentrations was more digestible than the other two fiber sources but resulted in the depression of dry matter and energy digestibility. This may have been due to the decreased transit time. Wheat bran at the 6% concentration also increased fecal volume. Shrimp meal was highly digestible and there was no significant depression of energy digestibility. It was suggested that microbiological degradation partially explained the digestibility of chitin. However, these results may indicate that callitrichids have the ability to synthesize chitinolytic enzymes. The possibility that callitrichids have the ability to synthesize chitinolytic enzymes would alter Garber's theory concerning their utilization of insect phosphorous and calcium and their increased requirement for calcium from tree sap.[32]

The ability of an animal to utilize fibrous food is related to the morphology of the cecum. Coimbra-Filho et al. studied the morphology and physiology of the ceca from *C. jacchus, S. midas,* and *Leontopithecus rosalia* in an effort to determine the ability of these monkeys to digest fibrous foods.[82] The results indicated that the *C. jacchus* have a cecum that is better adapted to the degradation of poorly digestible products than *Saguinus* or *Leontopithecus*.

Flurer et al. studied the effects that four protein sources had on palatability, digestibility, body weight, and consistency of feces when fed in pelleted diets to *C. jacchus* and *S. fuscicollis*.[83] The protein sources included lactalbumin, casein, soy protein concentrate, and soybean meal. They were incorporated in the diet at crude protein concentrations of 12, 17, and 22% (dry weight). However, the animals were also given a banana supplement which reduced the total protein content to 10.7, 14.7, and 18.3%. The results of this study indicated that a diet containing 10.7% total crude protein (based on dry weight) had no unfavorable effects on adult Callitrichidae when fed for three weeks.[83] The monkeys consumed more of the 12% protein diets than the 22% protein diets. The digestibility of protein was highest in diets containing lactalbumin and casein. Protein digestibility decreased with increasing concentration of dietary protein. This may relate to the decrease in efficiency of protein utilization as intake of high-quality protein increases.[84] Digestibility of dry matter was not significantly affected by varying the protein concentration in the diet.

Flurer et al. also showed that increasing levels of crude fiber (2.4 to 7.2% cellulose) decreased apparent digestibility of protein and dry matter.[83] Protein digestibility was not significantly affected until the crude fiber concentration of the diet was above 4%. However, there was a more constant decline in the digestibility of dry matter. The authors concluded that the Callitrichidae's ability to digest crude fiber is comparable to that in other monogastric animals.

These studies show that when callitrichids are fed primate diets supplemented with other foods, the proportions of each foodstuff must be controlled so the monkeys consume a balanced diet.

IV. NUTRITION OF CALLITRICHIDAE IN THEIR COUNTRIES OF ORIGIN

The survival rate of newly imported Callitrichidae depends on their health upon arrival; the health of the monkey and its resistance to opportunistic pathogens correlate with its nutritional status. The trapping methods and husbandry of callitrichids in their countries of origin have improved over the past 10 years. However, since these countries do not have primate feed manufacturers, diets must be formulated at the primate centers,[55] where trained nutritionists are usually unavailable for supervision. This is a major concern.

Reports from two South American primate centers indicate they have had satisfactory success with diets produced on-site.[17,55] Centro Primatologia de Rio de Janeiro (CPRJ) feeds a bread foritified with various supplements during the morning. The afternoon feeding consists of fruit and various sources of animal protein.[55] It was suggested the 54% neonatal survival rate was evidence of a satisfactory diet. The staff of Estacion de Conservacion y Reproducion de los Primates (ECRP) baked their own primate diet.[17] The ingredients of the baked primate diet were 195 g soya flour, 125 g fish flour, 120 g wheat flour, 80 g sugar, 50 g vegetable oil, and 20 g vitamin and mineral premix per 1000 g of diet.[17] Kaumanns[17] reported that *S. labiatus* appeared to be healthier than the *S. mystax* when this diet was fed.

V. DIETARY RECOMMENDATIONS FOR NEWLY IMPORTED PRIMATES

In 1969, New World monkeys were normally held in their country of origin from 2 to 6 weeks before shipment. During this time the diet was usually protein deficient and consisted solely of fruit. Since that time, the dietary management of captive primates in the countries of origin has improved dramatically. However, newly imported primates may still be malnourished upon arrival or become so during quarantine. Causes may include loss of appetite due to parasitism, stress of captivity and shipment, and a deficient diet. Early diagnosis of malnutrition in newly imported monkeys is important because the immune system of malnourished monkeys can be compromised, and infectious disease usually develops before deficiency disease appears. Thus, careful monitoring of the monkeys' health must be performed during the quarantine period. Although callitrichids are generally viewed as very fragile animals that survive best when disturbance is minimal, passive husbandry may not allow for timely diagnosis and treatment of potential health problems, resulting in significant morbidity and mortality.

Several measures can be taken that require minimal handling of monkeys but still provide information on their health status. These include (1) maintaining a record of monkey weights beginning at the time of arrival, (2) maintaining a record of the condition of the pelage, (3) measuring dehydration by skin fold response, and (4) recording daily observations of stool consistency and food consumption.

More extensive screening of the monkeys' health would include analyses of serum albumin, total protein, hematocrit, complete blood count, and an immune response assay. Although the results of these blood analyses can be influenced by many factors, active screening of the monkeys can be justified since it is the only means of nutritional or health evaluation that may indicate a problem before a severe outbreak of disease.

Transition from one diet to another is a factor that can lead to nutritional problems in fastidious eaters like the Callitrichidae. Moreland suggested that to reduce stress before introducing a new diet, the dietary regimen used by the monkey supplier should be evaluated for adequacy and should be continued for a few days at the new monkey facility if this is practical.[107]

The most common method used to transfer Callitrichidae to a new diet is to mix fruit with the new diet so that the monkey must eat the diet with the fruit. The fruit is gradually withdrawn over a short period of time. However, the feeding of fruit must be minimized and monitored during the quarantine period. The most important consideration concerning the management of newly imported primates is their hydration. Monkeys may arrive dehydrated, or they may become dehydrated from diarrhea or the inability to use the watering device. Investigators have suggested providing a 5 to 10% glucose solution or water with a vitamin solution added to increase water consumption.[57,61] Fruit may also be used to rehydrate monkeys; however, it may lead to problems as discussed previously.

Epple and Katz[1] reported the most common health problems of newly imported callitrichids involve protein, vitamin, and calcium deprivation. They administered these nutrients by soaking living insects in a mixture of calcium and a vitamin supplement before feeding them to the monkeys. When some very active insects (such as the grasshopper) are fed, they may escape a caged monkey. Immobilizing the insects by cooling them in a refrigerator increases the monkey's chance of capturing them.

VI. FEEDING BEHAVIOR

Several investigators reported social interactions within callitrichid families which could affect their nutritional status. Tardif and Richter[85] studied competition for a desired food in family groups of *C. jacchus* and *S. oedipus*. The results showed that, in both species, competition caused disparities in consumption of a desired food, adult females consuming more than other group members and adult males less. The use of two food cups reduced the inequalities in consumption of the *S. oedipus* families. Snowdon et al.[86] reported that *S. oedipus* preferred to eat from feeders placed 1 m above the cage floor. Epple observed competition for food between weaned callitrichid infants and their parents.[67] Petry et al. determined that food intake for *C. jacchus* was continuous throughout the day, with variable intensity.[87] These observations indicate that nutritional studies must be designed so that results are not affected by behavioral factors.

VII. NEONATAL NUTRITION

A high correlation has been reported between increased fecundity and nutrition in callitrichids.[1,55,74,76,88] Callitrichids frequently produce triplets, but rarely raise all of them successfully. Usually one infant will die within the first 4 days. In an effort to save such neonates, infant dietary regimes have been developed. Turton et al. analyzed *C. jacchus* milk to determine values for crude protein, lactose, total lipids, and minerals.[89] The milk provided 114 kcal/100 ml, with 12.6% of the calories from protein. The authors suggested that when a human milk formulation is used, it should be modified by increasing the level of protein, carbohydrate, and total lipids. Fatty acid analysis of marmoset milk indicated higher concentrations of palmitoleic acid and polyunsaturated fatty acids with 20 and 22 carbon atoms than in human milk formulations. Thus, it was suggested to add a small amount of fish oil to the human milk formulation.

Dronzek et al. fed *S. oedipus* neonates a nonhuman primate infant formula (Primalac) which supplied 17.4% of the total calories as protein and 0.9 IU vitamin D_3/ml.[90] Hampton and Hampton reported successfully hand-rearing *S. oedipus* using a human infant formula (SMA, Wyeth Labs).[91] The caloric intake of the neonates plateaued at 220 to 300 cal/kg/day by 6 days of age. This level of intake was measured for 20 days, and it was reportedly continued after introduction of other foodstuffs.[91] A comparison of the body weight increase between neonates fed the human infant formula and those reared by the parents showed no significant difference. A comparison of the body weight curves between neonates fed the nonhuman primate formula and those fed human infant formula also showed no difference.[89,91]

Both Dronzek et al.[90] and Hampton and Hampton[91] introduced foodstuffs other than infant formula when the monkeys were about 30 days of age. Stellar[54] and Epple[67] reported that parent-reared neonates began to be weaned at 30 days of age. Observations indicate that after weaning, parents and juveniles compete for food so that the juveniles' food consumption depends on the amount they can take from their parents.[67] Two examples were cited in which twins developed normally until they were weaned. Within 8 weeks of age, an infant from each set of twins apparently starved to death.[67] Administration of vitamins and calcium to other sets of twins prevented this problem.

VIII. VITAMIN AND MINERAL REQUIREMENTS

There is little published information regarding the vitamin and mineral requirements of the Callitrichidae. Most of the vitamin and mineral concentrations used in callitrichid diets, with the exception of that for vitamin D, are extrapolated requirements of other primate species.[92] Bone diseases have been common among the callitrichids since their introduction as laboratory animals. In 1927, Lucas et al.[71] documented the vitamin D requirement in the marmoset diet to prevent "cage paralysis", a synonym for rickets and osteomalacia. Gengozian described the gross signs as slow jerky movements, slight curvature of the spine and femurs, and a thin and unkempt appearance.[56] These signs are not evident until between 7 and 12 months after arrival at the colony.[56] The Jersey Zoological Park reported that osteomalacia occurred in adults at 12-month intervals and in infants during the first 3 to 5 months of life.[63]

Hampton et al. determined that daily dietary supplementation with 500 IU of vitamin D_3 (cholecalciferol) would prevent osteomalacia.[61] This result was also observed at the Jersey Zoological Park.[63] Takahashi et al. suggested that the high requirement of vitamin D_3 is necessary due to an end-organ resistance to cholecalciferol.[93] Flurer and Zucker[94] studied the vitamin D_3 requirement of *S. fuscicollis* by examining serum levels of 25(OH)D, alkaline phosphatase, and parathormone. The results of this study indicate that a dietary vitamin D_3 content of 2000 IU/kg diet, or a daily intake of 33 IU per 400 g body weight meets the requirement for *S. fuscicollis.*

Another study in which vitamin and mineral data were reported involved pooled food and nutrient intake data collected from *C. jacchus, S. midas,* and *S. oedipus.*[72] It was reported that retinol, cholecalciferol, calcium, and phosphorous intakes were 171 g/kg body weight, 2.8 g/kg body weight, 206 mg/kg body weight, and 194 mg/kg body weight, respectively.

The zinc status of tamarins has been studied. Chadwick et al. used zinc to control alopecia and skin lesions in *S. mystax.*[95] These apparent zinc deficiency signs reversed when the tamarins were fed a diet containing 150 mg zinc/kg plus 40 ppm zinc in the water. However, addition of 80 ppm zinc to the water resulted in no significant reversal of the zinc deficiency signs. Barnard et al. fed *S. mystax* suffering from wasting syndrome a diet containing

200 mg zinc/kg diet without any deleterious effects.[13] However, Chandra has recently determined that high levels of zinc may affect the immune system.[96]

Flurer et al. demonstrated that the optimal ascorbic acid intake for *C. jacchus* was 27 mg of ascorbic acid per day and the minimum requirement was 20 mg of ascorbic acid/kg body weight.[97] This ascorbic acid requirement for *C. jacchus* is severalfold higher than that for humans. However, these monkeys appear to tolerate extreme ascorbic acid deficiency for several weeks without clinical signs. Flurer and Zucker also determined that *C. jacchus* and *S. fuscicollis* fed the same diet had significantly different ascorbic acid serum levels, .54 ± .29 mg/dl and 2.56 ± 1.07 mg/dl, respectively.[97] This may reflect differences in ascorbic acid requirements between these genera.

King suggests that the potential harmful effects of fat-soluble vitamins must be considered when vitamin supplementation is part of the maintenance diet.[72] This problem is compounded by the observations that species of low body weight may consume higher levels of nutrient per unit of body weight.[72]

IX. PROTEIN AND ENERGY REQUIREMENTS

Energy and protein requirements of smaller species are greater on a per unit body weight basis than those of larger species. Pregnancy, lactation, and growth increase energy requirements. Energy requirements for primates appear to be directly related to body weight.[99] However, Portman reported that some carnivorous New World monkeys consume fewer calories if a high nondigestible-residue diet is fed rather than one with a caloric density.[66] King suggested that Callitrichidae have higher energy intake than other primate species.[72]

Many investigators have studied Callitrichidae energy and protein consumption. Kirkwood et al. determined that, for *S. oedipus,* the daily intake of metabolizable energy (ME) and protein was 130 kcal/kg body weight and .6 g protein/kg body weight, respectively.[76,77] They concluded that these levels were sufficient to maintain the monkeys, providing the protein was of a high quality. Escajadillo et al. determined that *S. oedipus* consumed 160 kcal/kg body weight daily.[100] Flurer et al. hypothesized from data collected from many species of callitrichids that a 400-g tamarin would consume 225 kcal/kg body weight per day and 9.75 g protein/kg body weight per day.[74] Barnard et al. reported that *S. mystax* consumed 82 g of diet/kg of body weight daily, which was equivalent to 335 kcal GE/kg body weight and 21.5 g protein/kg body weight.[13] Nicolosi and Hunt suggested that, based on ad lib intake, infants of New World primates required 300 to 500 cal/kg body weight daily, and the adult energy requirements are only 30 to 50% of requirements for infants.[101] Tardif et al.[79] reported energy levels for maintenance of healthy adult *S. oedipus* ranging from 189 to 219 kcal/kg body weight in three different dietary regimens. King pooled food and nutrient intake data collected from several species and genera of Callitrichidae and determined that, on an ad lib basis, the average caloric intake was 677 kJ/kg body weight$^{0.75}$ per day.[72]

Kirkwood and Underwood measured food intake of *S. oedipus* at various stages of the life cycle.[102] They determined that energy intake required for maintenance of adults was approximately 152 kcal/kg body weight/day with a range of 112 to 253 kcal/kg/d. The mean intake for pregnant females in the last 7 weeks of pregnancy was approximately 139 kcal/kg body weight/day, which was not significantly different from that of nonpregnant monkeys. During lactation the daily caloric intake increased significantly to 260 kcal/kg/d. It was postulated that the ME provided by the breast milk was 17.8 kcal/d. Daily energy intake at 100 days of age was 106 kcal/kg body weight.

Flurer and Zucker studied the effects of different concentrations of dietary protein (12, 18, and 24%) on *C. jacchus* and *S. fuscicollis.*[103] There was no apparent protein deficiency at any of the dietary protein concentrations fed to the monkeys based on serum albumin concentrations, body weight, and reproductivity. However, growing *S. fuscicollis* did not thrive as well as *C. jacchus* offspring when these monkeys were fed the diet containing 12% protein. The results indicated that adult callitrichids can be maintained on a semipurified diet with a high-quality protein equal to 15% of gross energy. This corresponds to 5 g protein/kg body weight daily. The study also showed that *S. fuscicollis* may be able to tolerate 2.8 g protein/kg body weight/day. It is important to note that the protein values provided by this study are based on consumption of high-quality protein in a semipurified diet. Thus, other dietary components are less likely to interfere with the availability of protein for digestion and absorption. Another factor that influences protein requirement is the caloric density of the diet.[84] It has been shown that increased caloric density of the diet decreases apparent protein requirements as determined by nitrogen balance studies.[104] These diets fed to the monkeys have a high caloric density and thus may have influenced the protein requirement.

Flurer et al. used the nitrogen-balance procedure to compare nutritional adequacy of high-quality protein at different concentrations and to determine the appropriate essential amino acid requirements of *C. jacchus.*[105] It was determined that the minimal protein requirement was 1.65 g protein/kg body weight$^{0.75}$/day, which was equivalent to a dietary protein content of 5.9% when the feed intake was 3.5% of body weight.

Flurer et al. also used the ''factorial method'' to determine the minimum protein requirement of *C. jacchus.*[105] The results indicated that the daily minimum requirement was 1.96 g protein/kg body weight$^{0.75}$, thus confirming their results from the previous study (Reference 103). However, these are minimum requirements based on the consumption of high-quality proteins incorporated into a semipurified diet of high caloric density. They represent the dietary protein requirements needed to replace obligatory losses of nitrogen. Correction factors for possible changes in efficiency of protein utilization due to decreased protein concentration in the study and for the biologic quality of the protein consumed may be applied to these values.[84] The calculated maintenance level for protein intake would be 3.47 g protein/kg body weight$^{0.75}$/day.

Flurer et al. determined that the average daily essential amino acid requirement is between 1.5 and 3.6% of the diet, based on dry matter.[106] Essential amino acids fed at 2.5% of the dry matter resulted in a positive nitrogen balance. The results showed that either arginine or histidine or both are not synthesized in required quantities by the adult marmoset, thus indicating their essentiality.

X. SUMMARY

This review of Callitrichidae nutrition indicates that these monkeys are primarily insectivorous, but they complement their diet with fruits and tree exudates in the wild. However, different morphological characteristics between *Callithrix* and *Saguinus* suggest potential differences in dietary requirements or preferences. The most evident morphological difference involves their dentition. The ''short-tusked'' dentition of the *Callithrix* allows them to gouge into trees for exudates, while the *Saguinus,* with their ''long-tusked'' dentition, are not capable of tree gouging. The dentition of the *Saguinus* appears to be best suited for an insectivorous type of diet, while that of the *Callithrix* is much better adapted to excudate feeding. Results of a study examining the correlation between dental and cecal morphology of several species of callitrichids support this theory.[82] It was concluded from this study that the cecum of the *Callithrix* was better adapted to the degradation of poorly digestible products than that of the *Saguinus.* These anatomical differences may indicate differences in nutritional requirements such as protein. A colony of *Callithrix* thrived on a diet that appeared to be protein and calorie deficient for *Saguinus.*[13] Flurer and Zucker[103] determined that growing *S. fuscicollis* did not thrive as well as *C. jacchus* on a diet containing 12% protein. Flurer et al. also determined that the minimum protein requirement for *C. jacchus* is 1.96 g protein/kg body weight[.75], which is a low protein requirement.[106] Thus, there is evidence that there may be a difference in protein requirement between the *Callithrix* and *Saguinus* genera.

A large variation in caloric and protein intake by the callitrichids has been reported by different investigators. This variation may be due to factors involving diet and experimental design. One possible confounding variable was that several studies were conducted using monkeys caged together as families or breeding pairs; feeding behavior of the cagemates may have affected the results. Some studies pooled the results from different genera and species; this may also result in inaccurate interpretation of the data because of differences in interspecies dietary requirements or preferences. Also, the differences in dietary regimens among the studies may be responsible for the apparent variations. For example, some studies used diets that included large amounts of fruit and other supplements, but others fed only commercial primate diet. There is evidence that excessive dietary supplementation results in the callitrichids eating preferred foods which may be less nutritious, such as banana, and neglecting the more nutritious foods. These observations

TABLE 3
Proximate Analysis of Callitrichid Diets

	Diet source (percent of dry weight)				
Nutrient	**ORAU**[a]	**Flurer**[b]	**Barnard**[c]	**Commercial**[c]	**Escajadillo**[d]
Crude protein	19.8	25.8	26.2	23.4	20.0
Ether extract	7.0	7.3	12.3	5.2	15.0
Crude fiber	6.4	4.0	5.9	2.3	10.0
Ash	5.3	4.2	12.2	7.3	5.0
Nitrogen free extract[e]	61.4	58.7	43.4	61.8	49.5

[a] Data from Reference 79.
[b] Data from Reference 74
[c] Date from Reference 13.
[d] Data from Reference 100.
[e] Nitrogen free extract determined by difference.

suggest that the feeding of dietary supplements may influence the results not only of nutritional studies but of all studies. Therefore, feeding dietary supplements should be monitored carefully to ensure that a nutritionally balanced diet is consumed. This is most important for newly imported monkeys since they are most susceptible to disease and malnutrition during quarantine.

As knowledge of the callitrichid feeding behavior and nutritional requirements has increased there has been a corresponding decrease in mortality and increase in productivity. However, the present understanding of Callitrichidae nutrition is still limited. A 1978 international dietary survey of callitrichid colonies determined that most monkeys were fed commercial primate diets supplemented with a variety of foods.[75] More recent literature indicates that this dietary regimen is still typical. This type of dietary regimen presents several potential problems, such as: (1) the nutrient concentration may be inconsistent and/or unknown; (2) the feed stuff may have potential for bacterial contamination; (3) the monkeys may select and eat only the less nutritious but preferred food; (4) group competition for desired food may occur; (5) procedures for diet preparation and cage cleaning may be labor intensive; and (6) dietary control during experimentation may be impossible.

Although several callitrichid colonies have been maintained by using varied diets with supplements (Table 3), the ideal callitrichid diet may be a palatable, nutritionally balanced diet that can be fed without supplementation. However, dietary supplementation can be used as a means for environmental enrichment.

Primate diets specifically formulated for callitrichids have been described by investigators. Thus, the practice of supplementing the primate diet with various foods, vitamins, and mineral mixes indicates that a single palatable nutritionally balanced callitrichid diet has yet to be developed or has yet to be accepted by the scientific community. More nutritional research using better experimental design is needed to confirm and to expand upon the available information on callitrichid nutrition.

REFERENCES

1. **Epple, G. and Katz, Y.,** The saddle back tamarin and other tamarins: reproduction in New World primates, in *New Models in Medical Science,* Hearn, J. P., Ed., MTP Press, Hingham, MA, 1983, chap. 4.
2. **Clapp, N. K., Lushbaugh, C. C., Humason, C. L., Gangaware, B. L., Henke, M. A., and McArthur, A. H.,** The marmoset as a model of ulcerative colitis and colon cancer, in *Carcinoma of the Large Bowel and Its Precursors,* Ingall, J. R. F. and Mastromarino, A. J., Eds., Alan R. Liss, New York, 1985, 247.
3. **Lushbaugh, C. C., Humason, G. L., and Clapp, N. K.,** Histology of colitis in *Saguinus oedipus oedipus, Dig. Dis. Sci.,* 30 (Suppl. 12), 45S, 1985.
4. **Chalifoux, L. V. and Bronson, R. T.,** Colonic adenocarcinoma associated with chronic colitis in cotton-top marmosets, *Saguinus oedipus, Gastroenterology,* 80, 942, 1981.
5. **Clapp, N. K., Littlefield, L. G., and Lushbaugh, C. C.,** Colon carcinoma in subhuman primates, *Gastroenterology,* 83, 519, 1982.
6. **Madara, J. L., Podolsky, D. K., King, N. W., Sehgal, P. K., Moore, R., and Winter, H. S.,** Characterization of spontaneous colitis in cotton-top tamarins *(Saguinus oedipus)* and its reponse to sulfasalazine, *Gastroenterology,* 88, 13, 1985.
7. **Lushbaugh, C. C., Humason, C. L., Swartzendruber, D. C., Richter, C. B., and Gengozian, N.,** Spontaneous colonic adenocarcinoma in marmosets, Proceedings of the Conference on Marmosets in Experimental Medicine, in *Primates in Medicine,* Gengozian, N. and Dienhardt, F., Eds., S. Karger, Basel, 1978, 119.
8. **Lushbaugh, C. C., Humason, G. L., and Clapp, N. K.,** Histology of colon cancer in *Saguinus oedipus oedipus, Dig. Dis. Sci.,* 30 (Suppl. 12), 119S, 1985.
9. **Clapp, N. K., Lushbaugh, C. C., Humason, G. L., Gangaware, B. L., and Henke, M. A.,** Natural history and pathology of colon cancer in *Saguinus oedipus oedipus, Dig. Dis Sci.,* 30 (Suppl. 12), 107S, 1985.
10. **Clapp, N. K., Lushbaugh, C. C., Humason, C. L., Gangaware, B. L., and Henke, M. A.,** The cotton-top tamarin was an animal model of colorectal cancer metastasis, in *The Biology and Treatment of Colorectal Cancer Metastasis,* Mastromarino, A., Ed., Martinus Nijhoff, Hingham, MA, 1985, chap. 3.
11. **Richter, C. B., Lushbaugh, C. C., and Swartzendruber, D. C.,** Cancer of the colon in cotton-top tamarins, in *the Comparative Pathology of Zoo Animals,* Montali, R. J. and Migaki, G., Eds., Smithsonian Institution Press, Washington, D.C., 1980, 567.
12. **Morin, M.,** A different approach in examining a wasting syndrome, *Lab. Anim.,* 12(3), 36, 1983.
13. **Barnard, D., Knapka, J., and Renquist, D.,** The apparent reversal of a wasting syndrome by nutritional intervention in *Saguinus mystax, Lab. Anim. Sci.,* 38(3), 282, 1988.
14. **Clutton-Brock, T. H.,** Some aspects of intraspecific variation in feeding and ranging behavior in primates, in *Primate Ecology: Studies of Feeding and Ranging Behavior in Lemurs, Monkeys and Apes,* Clutton-Brock, T. H., Ed., Academic Press, London, 1977, chap. 18.
15. **Thorington, R. W.,** Feeding behavior of nonhuman primates in the world, in *Feeding and Nutrition of Nonhuman Primates,* Harris, R. S., Ed., Academic Press, London, 1970, chap. 2.
16. **Nelson, T. W.,** Quantitative observations on feeding behavior in *S. geoffroyi, Primates,* 16(2), 223, 1975.
17. **Kaumann, W.,** Behavioral observations of moustached tamarins *(S. mystax). Z. Koln. Zoo,* 25(4), 107, 1982.
18. **Garber, P. A.,** Proposed nutritional importance of plant exudates in the diet of the Panamanian tamarin *Saguinus oedipus geoffroyi, Int. J. Primatol.,* 5(1), 1, 1984.
19. **Ramirez, M.,** Exudate feeding in Upper Amazonian *Saguinus* and *Cebuella, Am. J. Phys. Anthropol.,* 66(2), 216, 1985.

20. **Yoneda, M.,** Ecological study of the saddle backed tamarin *(S. fuscicollis)* in Northern Bolivia, *Primates,* 25(1), 1, 1984.
21. **Fooden, J.,** Stomach contents and gastro-intestinal proportions in wild-shot Guianan monkeys, *Am. J. Phys. Anthropol.,* 22, 227, 1964.
22. **Enders, R. K.,** Notes on some mammals from Barro Colorado Island, Canal Zone, *J. Mammal.,* 11, 280, 1930.
23. **Garber, P. A.,** Nectar feeding in two species of callitrichid primates: *S.mystax* and *S. fuscicollis, Am. J. Phys. Anthropol.,* 66(2), 172, 1985.
24. **Garber, P. A.,** Use of habitat and positional behavior in a neotropical primate, *S. oedipus,* in *Adaptations for Foraging in Nonhuman Primates,* Rodman, P. S. and Cant, J. C. H., Eds., Columbia University Press, New York, 1984, chap. 4.
25. **Yoneda, M.,** Comparative studies on vertical separation, foraging, behavior and traveling mode of saddle-backed tamarins *(S. fuscicollis)* and red-chested moustached tamarins *(S. labiatus)* in northern Bolivia, *Primates,* 25(4), 414, 1984.
26. **Hershkovitz, P.,** *Living New World Monkeys (Platyrrhini),* Vol. 1, University of Chicago Press, London, 1977, 764.
27. **Coimbra-Filho, A. F. and Mittermeier, R. A.,** Tree-gouging, exudate-eating and the "short-tusked" condition in callithrix and cebuella, in *The Biology and Conservation of the Callitrichidae,* Kleiman, D. C., Ed., Smithsonian Institution Press, Washington, D.C., 1977, 106.
28. **Napier, J. R. and Napier, P. H.,** *A Handbook of Living Primates,* Napier, J. R. and Napier, P. H., Eds., Academic Press, London, 1967.
29. **Moynihan, M.,** Natural history, in *The New World Primates,* Moynihan, M., Ed., Princeton University Press, Princeton, 1976, chap. 3.
30. **Coimbra-Filho, A. F.,** Aspectos ineditos do comportamento de saguis do genero Callithrix, *Rev. Brasil. Biol.,* 32(4), 505, 1972.
31. **Fonseca, G. A. B.,** Exudate-feeding by *Callithrix jacchus penicillata* in semideciduous woodland (Cerradao) in Central Brazil, *Primates,* 25(4), 441, 1984.
32. **Garber, P. A.,** Proposed nutritional importance of plant exudates in the diet of the Panamanian tamarin, *Saguinus oedipus geoffroyi, Int. J. Primatol.,* 5(1), 1, 1984.
33. **Hladik, A. and Hladik, C. M.,** Rapports trophiques entre vegetation et primates dans la foret de Barro Colorada (Panama), *Terre Vie,* 1, 25, 1969.
34. **Izawa, K.,** Foods and feeding behavior of monkeys in the Upper Amazon Basin, *Primates,* 16(3), 295, 1975.
35. **Garber, P. A.,** Locomotor behavior and feeding ecology of the Panamanian tamarin, *Int. J. Primartola,* 1, 185, 1980.
36. **Hershkovitz, P.,** The recent mammals of the neotropical region: a zoogeographic and ecological review, *Q. Rev. Biol.,* 44(1), 1, 1969.
37. **Temerin, L. A., Wheatley, B. P., and Rodman, P. S.,** Body size and foraging in primates, in *Adaptations for Foraging in Nonhuman Primates,* Rodman, P. S. and Cant, J. G. H., Eds., Columbia University Press, New York, 1984, chap. 9.
38. **Lindstedt, S. L. and Calder, W. A.,** Body size, physiological time, and longevity of homeothermic animals, *Q. Rev. Biol.,* 56, 1, 1981.
39. **Milton, K.,** The role of food-processing factors in primate food choice, in *Adaptations for Foraging in Nonhuman Primates,* Rodman, P. S. and Cant, J. G. H., Eds., Columbia University Press, New York, 1984, chap. 9.
40. **Ramirez, M.,** Feeding ecology of the moustached tamarin, *S. mystax, Am. J. Phys. Anthropol.,* 66(2), 216, 1985.
41. **Hladik, A. and Hladik, C. M.,** Rapports trophiques entre vegetation et primates dans la foret de barro Colordao (Panama), *Terre Vie,* 23, 25, 1969.
42. **Dawson, G. A.,** Behavioral Ecology of the Panamanian Tamarin, *Saguinus oedipus geoffroyi* (Callitrichidae, Primates), Ph.D. thesis, Michigan State University, East Lansing, 1976.

43. **Garber, P. A.,** Seed dispersal in two species of callitrichid primates: *S. mystax* and *S. fuscicollis, Am. J. Phys. Anthropol.,* 69(2), 202, 1986.
44. **Redford, K. H., Fonseca, G. A. B., and Lacher, T. E.,** The relationship between frugivory and insectivory in primates, *Primates,* 25(4), 433, 1984.
45. **Eisenberg, J. F.,** Comparative ecology and reproduction of New World Monkeys, in *The Biology and Conservation of the Callitrichidae,* Kleiman, D. G., Ed., Smithsonian Institution Press, Washington, D.C., 1977, 13.
46. **Leutenegger, W.,** Evolution of litter size in primates, *Am. Nat.,* 144, 525, 1979.
47. **King, G. J.,** Comparative feeding and nutrition in captive nonhuman primates, *Br. J. Nutr.,* 40, 55, 1978.
48. **Uvarov, B.,** *Grasshoppers and Locusts: A Handbook of General Acridology,* Vol. I, Cambridge University Press, Cambridge, England, 1966.
49. **Maynard, L. A., Loosli, J. K., Hintz, H. F., and Warner, R. G.,** *Animal Nutrition,* McGraw-Hill, New York, 1979.
50. **Snyder, S. B., Omdahl, J. L., Law, D. H., and Froelich, J. W.,** Osteomalacia and nutritional secondary hyperparathyroidism in a semi-free-ranging troop of Japanese monkeys, in *The Comparative Pathology of Zoo Animals,* Montali, R. J. and Migaki, C., Eds., Smithsonian Institution Press, Washington, D.C., 1980, 51.
51. **Anderson, D. M. W. and Gill, M. C. C.,** The composition of Acacia gum exudates from species of the subseries, *Phytochemistry,* 14, 739, 1975.
52. **Anderson, D. M. W., Hendries, A., and Munro, A. C.,** The amino acid and amino sugar composition of some plant gums, *Phytochemistry,* 11, 723, 1972.
53. **Beader, S. K. and Martin, R. D.,** Acacia gum and its use by Lesser Bushbabies, *Galago senegalenesis, Int. J. Primatol.,* 1, 103, 1980.
54. **Stellar, E.,** The marmoset as a laboratory animal: maintenance, general observations of behavior and simple learning, *J. Comp. Physiol. Psychol.,* 53(1), 1, 1960.
55. **Coimbra-Filho, A. F., Silva, R. R., and Pissinatti, A.,** The diet of Callitrichidae in captivity, *Rev. Bioterioes,* 1, 83, 1981.
56. **Gengozian, N.,** Marmosets: their potential in experimental medicine, *Ann. N.Y. Acad. Sci.,* 162, 336, 1969.
57. **Deinhardt, J. B., Devine, J., Passovoy, M., Pohlman, R., and Deinhardt, F.,** Marmosets as laboratory animals. I. Care of marmosets in the laboratory, pathology and outline of statistical evaluation of data, *Lab. Anim. Care,* 17, 11, 1967.
58. **Levy, B. M. and Artecona, J.,** The marmoset as an experimental animal in biological research: care and maintenance, *Lab Anim. Care,* 14, 20, 1964.
59. **Cooper, R. W.,** A description of a unique outdoor primate colony, *Lab Anim. Care,* 18, 474, 1964.
60. **Hampton, J. K.,** Laboratory requirements and observations of *Oedipomidas oedipus, Am. J. Phys. Anthropol.,* 22, 239, 1964.
61. **Hampton, J. K., Hampton, S. H., and Landwehr, B. T.,** Observations on a successful breeding colony of the marmoset, *Oedipomidas oedipus, Folia Primatol.,* 4, 265, 1966.
62. **Shadle, A. R., Mirand, E. A., and Grace, J. T.,** Breeding responses in tamarins, *Lab Anim. Care,* 15, 1, 1965.
63. **Mallinson, J. C.,** Maintenance of marmosets and tamarins at Jersey Zoological Park with special reference to the design of the new marmoset complex, in *The Biology and Conservation of the Callitrichidae,* Kleiman, D. G., Ed., Smithsonian Institution Press, Washington, D.C., 1977, 323.
64. **Clapp, N. K. and Tardif, S. D.,** Marmoset husbandry and nutrition, *Dig. Dis. Sci.,* 30(12), 175, 1985.
65. **Morin, M. L.,** Colony management problems encountered in using marmosets and tamarins in biomedical research, *Dig. Dis. Sci.,* 30(12), 145, 1985.
66. **Harris, R. S.,** *Feeding and Nutrition of Nonhuman Primates,* Academic Press, New York, 1970.

67. **Epple, G.,** Maintenance, breeding, and development of marmoset monkeys (Callitrichidae) in captivity, *Folia Primatol.,* 12, 56, 1970.
68. **Benirschke, K. and Richart, R.,** The establishment of a marmoset breeding colony and its four pregnancies, *Lab. Anim. Care,* 13(2), 70, 1963.
69. **Deinhart, F.,** Nutritional requirements of marmosets, in *Feeding and Nutrition of Nonhuman Primates,* Harris, R. S., Academic Press, New York, 1970, 175.
70. **Fitzgerald, A.,** Rearing marmosets in captivity, *J. Mammal.,* 16, 181, 1935.
71. **Lucas, N. S., Hume, E. M., and Smith, H. H.,** On the breeding of the common marmoset *(Hapale jacchus Linn.)* in captivity when irradiated with ultraviolet rays, *Proc. Zool. Soc.,* 30, 447, 1927.
72. **King, G. J.,** Comparative feeding and nutrition in captive nonhuman primates, *Br. J. Nutr.,* 40, 55, 1978.
73. **Ratcliffe, H. L.,** Diets for zoological gardens: aids to conservation and disease control, *Int. Zoo Yearb.,* 6, 4, 1963.
74. **Flurer, C., Scheid, R., and Zucker, H.,** Evaluation of a pelleted diet in a colony of marmosets and tamarins, *Lab. Anim. Sci.,* 33(3), 264, 1983.
75. **Morin, M.,** unpublished data, 1978.
76. **Kirkwood, J. K.,** Effects of diet on health, weight and litter-size in captive cotton-top tamarins, *Saguinus oedipus oedipus, Primates,* 24(4), 515, 1983.
77. **Kirkwood, J. K., Epstein, M. A., and Terlecki, A. J.,** Factors influencing population growth of a colony of cotton-top tamarins, *Lab. Anim.,* 17, 35, 1983.
78. **Shimwell, M., Warrington, B. F., and Fowler, J. S. L.,** Dietary habits relating to wasting marmoset syndrome (WMS), *Lab Anim.,* 13, 139, 1979.
79. **Tardif, S. D., Clapp, N. K., Carson, R. L., and Knapka, J.,** Maintenance of cotton-top tamarins *(Saguinus oedipus)* fed an open formula pelleted diet versus a highly diverse sweetened diet, *Lab. Anim. Sci.,* 38(5), 588, 1988.
80. **Wirth, H. and Buselmaier, W.,** Long term experiments with a newly-developed standardized diet for the new world primates, *Callithrix jacchus jacchus* and *Callithrix jacchus pencillata* (marmosets), *Lab. Anim.,* 16, 175, 1982.
81. **Krombach, F., Flurer, C., and Zucker, H.,** Effects of fibre on digestibility and passage time in Callitrichidae, *Lab. Anim.,* 18, 275, 1984.
82. **Coimbra-Filho, A. F., Rocha, N. C., and Pissinatti, A.,** Morphophysiology of the cecum and its correlation with odontological type in Callitrichidae (*Platyrrhini,* Primates), *Rev. Bras. Biol.,* 40(1), 177, 1980.
83. **Flurer, C., Krombach, F., and Zucker, H.,** Palatability and digestibility of soya-milk protein in Callitrichidae, *Lab Anim.,* 19, 245, 1985.
84. **Muro, H. N. and Crim, M. C.,** The proteins and amino acids, in *Modern Nutrition in Health and Disease,* Goodhart, R. S. and Shils, M. E., Lea & Febiger, Philadelphia, 1980, chap. 3.
85. **Tardif, S. D. and Richter, C. B.,** Competition for a desired food in family groups of the common marmoset *(C. jacchus)* and the cotton-top tamarin *(S. oedipus), Lab Anim. Sci.,* 31, 52, 1981.
86. **Snowdon, C. T., Savage, A., and McConnell, P. B.,** A breeding colony of cotton-top tamarins *(S. oedipus), Lab Anim. Sci.,* 35, 477, 1985.
87. **Petry, V. H., Riehl, I., and Zucker, H.,** Spontaneous activity and eating behavior in common marmoset *(Callithrix jacchus), Z. Versuchstierkd.,* 29, 15, 1987.
88. **Hiddleston, W. A.,** The production of the common marmoset (*Callithrix jacchus*), as a laboratory animal, in *Recent Advances in Primatology,* Vol. 1, Chivers, D. J. and Herbert, J., Eds., Academic Press, London, 1978, 173.
89. **Turton, J. A., Ford, D. J., Bteby, J., Hall, B. M., and Whiting, R.,** Composition of the milk of the common marmoset (*C. jacchus*) and milk substitutes used in hand-rearing programs with special reference to fatty acids, *Folia Primatol.,* 29, 64, 1978.

90. **Dronzek, L. A., Savage, A., Snowdon, C. T., Whaling, C. S., and Ziegler, T. E.,** Technique for hand-rearing and reintroducing rejected cotton-top tamarin infants, *Lab Anim. Sci.,* 36(3), 243, 1986.
91. **Hampton, S. H. and Hampton, J. R.,** Rearing marmosets from birth by artificial laboratory techniques, *Lab Anim. Care,* 17, 1, 1967.
92. National Research Council, Committee on Animal Nutrition, Agricultural Board, Nutrient Requirements of Nonhuman Primates, National Academy of Sciences, Washington, D.C., 1978.
93. **Takahashi, N., Suda, S., Shinki, T., Horinchi, N., Shiina, Y., Tanioka, Y., Koizumi, H., and Suda, T.,** The mechanism of end-organ resistance to 1,25-dihydroxy cholecalciferol in the common marmoset, *Biochem. J.,* 227, 555, 1985.
94. **Flurer, C. I. and Zucker, H.,** Evaluation of serum parameters relevant to vitamin D status in tamarins, *J. Med. Primatol.,* 16, 175, 1987.
95. **Chadwick, D. P., May, J. C., and Lorenz, D.,** Spontaneous zinc deficiency in marmosets, *S. mystax, Lab Anim. Sci.,* 29, 482, 1979.
96. **Chandra, R. K.,** Excessive intake of zinc impairs immune responses, *JAMA,* 252(11), 1443, 1984.
97. **Flurer, C. I., Kern, M., Rambeck, W. A., and Zucker, H.,** Ascorbic acid requirement and assessment of ascorbate status in the common marmoset *(Callithrix jacchus), Ann. Nutr. Metabol.,* 31, 245, 1987.
98. **Flurer, C. I. and Zucker, H.,** Difference in serum ascorbate in two species of Callitrichidae, *Int. J. Vit. Nutr. Res.,* 57, 297, 1987.
99. **Clarke, H. E., Coates, M. E., Eva, J. K., Ford, D. J., Milner, C. K., O'Donoghue, P. N., Scott, P. P., and Ward, R. J.,** Dietary standards for laboratory animals: report of the Laboratory Animals Centre Diets Advisory Committee, *Lab. Anim.,* 11, 1, 1977.
100. **Escajadillo, A., Bronson, R. T., Sehgal, P. K., and Hayes, K. C.,** Nutritional evaluation in cotton-top tamarins *(S. oedipus), Lab Anim. Sci.,* 31, 161, 1981.
101. **Nicolosi, R. J. and Hunt, R. D.,** Dietary allowances for nutrients in nonhuman primates, in *Primates in Nutritional Research,* Hayes, K. C., Ed., Academic Press, New York, 1979, 11.
102. **Kirkwood, J. K. and Underwood, S. J.,** Energy requirements of captive cotton-top tamarins *(S. oedipus oedipus), Folia Primatol.,* 42, 180, 1984.
103. **Flurer, C. and Zucker, H.,** Long-term experiments with low dietary protein levels in Callitrichidae, *Primates,* 26(4), 479, 1985.
104. **Inoue, G., Fujita, Y., and Niiyama, Y.,** Studies on protein requirements of young men fed egg protein and rice protein with excess and maintenance energy intakes, *J. Nutr.,* 103, 1673, 1973.
105. **Flurer, C. I., Sappl, A., Adler, H., and Zucker, H.,** Determination of the protein requirement of marmosets *(Callithrix jacchus)* by nitrogen balance with regard to the concentration of essential amino acids in the diet, *J. Anim. Physiol. Anim. Nutr.,* 57(1), 23, 1987.
106. **Flurer, C. I., Krommer, G., and Zucker, H.,** Endogenous N-excretion and minimal protein requirements for maintenance of the common marmoset *(C. jacchus), Lab Anim. Sci.,* 38, 183, 1988.

B. Inflammatory Bowel Disease in Callitrichids

Chapter 4

NATURAL HISTORY, TIME COURSE, AND PATHOGENESIS OF IDIOPATHIC COLITIS IN COTTON-TOP TAMARINS *(Saguinus oedipus)*

Neal K. Clapp, Marsha A. Henke, Robert M. Hansard, Robert L. Carson, Linas J. Adams, and Ronald V. Nardi

TABLE OF CONTENTS

0-8493-5363-7/93/$0.00 + $.50

I. INTRODUCTION

Idiopathic ulcerative colitis is a devastating disease that occurs frequently (1/1000) in the human population of the western world and increases the risk of afflicted individuals to develop colonic carcinoma.[1] While the disease has been identified and studied for centuries, the lack of an animal model has made understanding of the natural history and pathogenesis of the disease difficult. Reluctance on the part of patients to submit to colonoscopic examination on a regular basis and the concern that repeated colonoscopic examinations might be considered excessive have added to the dilemma. This report examines the time course of cotton-top tamarin (CTT) spontaneous colitis pathogenesis and progression to determine (1) how closely these events mimic the human disease and (2) the potential value of the CTT disease as an animal model.

Recognition of a spontaneously occurring idiopathic ulcerative colitis in cotton-top tamarins (*Saguinus oedipus*) (CTT)[2-10] has made possible study of this animal disease in light of the human counterpart, including mucin production,[10,11] response to chemotherapy,[9] presence of colonic antigen,[12] alteration of T cell subsets,[13] and presence of inflammatory mediators.[14] Further, repeated observations by visualization (colonoscopy) and histologic examinations (colonic mucosal biopsy) have been accomplished over several years. Adapting the use of a commercially available pediatric bronchoscope to visualize and biopsy colons of these animals has enabled us to describe and follow changes in the tamarin's mucosa from an asymptomatic inactive stage of colitis through exacerbations of varying intensities and duration and into remission. The state of the colon can be histologically graded qualitatively (acute or chronic), and scored semiquantitatively. The stage of the colitis is evaluated by determining the types and number of inflammatory cells present, as well as their location within the colonic mucosa. Correlations can be made between the onset of symptoms and variables such as age, sex, microbial flora, etc. Further, in a closed tamarin research colony, most environmental factors can be readily controlled or stabilized beyond levels possible in human studies.

This chapter reports observations made on 40 CTTs that have been examined endoscopically at 2- to 3-month intervals for a 6-year period (1985 to 1991). The animals were first identified for the study based upon the presence of colon cancer in their first-degree relatives and independent of colitic state. The experimental protocol was designed to look diligently for the presence and/or development of dysplastic changes that should be histologically identifiable as colonic cancer develops; this aspect of the study continues under investigation. The resulting study of the pathogenesis of tamarin colitis offers, to the best of our knowledge, the first exhaustive information about the time course and patterns of exacerbations and remissions of this spontaneously occurring disease in any species. Correlations and possible cause/effect relationships are still being studied and evaluated, and comparisons are being made with the emerging knowledge regarding biochemical changes (e.g., inflammatory mediators, mucin production, antigens, etc.) associated with the development of this disease. Mechanisms associated with disease development as well as protective aspects may be identified, and targeted therapeutics can then be developed that would ease the devastation of ulcerative colitis in man and animal.

II. METHODS

A. ANIMAL SELECTION

Forty CTTs 4 to 7 years of age of both sexes (20 M and 20 F) were selected for the study; 30 had first-degree relatives with histologically confirmed colon cancer and 10, at the beginning of the study, had no history of colon cancer in their families. The histological condition of the colon was unknown in these animals at the start of the experiment and was determined only after the first colonoscopic and biopsy examination. The following histological considerations were to be evaluated in the study: (1) recognize and describe what changes occur within the colon histologically during exacerbations and remissions of colitic episodes; (2) identify the etiologic mechanisms of CTT colitis and relate them to the known situations in the human form of the disease; (3) identify the development, presence, and characteristics of associated dysplastic changes that precede the presence of frank carcinoma. Observations regarding item one are being reported in this chapter.

B. COLONOSCOPY

Instrument — A 5.0-mm fiberoptic pediatric bronchoscope (Fujinon BRO-YP_2) was used for this procedure. This endoscope was adapted for video display using the EPX-301A electronic video endoscopy processor (Fujinon). Digital image capture and image analysis was accomplished with a bias system using Pharmapath® software (Loats Associates). This unit includes a color video monitor and VCR. Biopsy forceps were passed through the 2-mm channel to obtain tissue samples of the colonic mucosa. A hypodermic syringe and plastic tube with a three-way valve was adapted to the instrument so the colon could be inflated with air during insertion of the tube and as needed during visualization.

Procedure — This procedure has been reported in detail elsewhere,[15] but will be described briefly. Fasted animals that had been given a tap water enema were anesthetized with ketamine hydrochloride (~20 to 25 mg IM/kg body weight) plus butorphanol (1.0 to 1.25 mg/kg body weight) and then taped to a mylar board for restraint in a ventral-dorsal position. Lubricating jelly was applied to the sides of the fiberoptic tube which was then inserted through the anal sphincter into the colon. As the tube was gently passed proximally in the colon, air was introduced to distend the colon for better visualization of the colonic mucosa. Grossly visible changes in the appearance of the colonic mucosa were described and recorded as the scope was advanced proximally. After the blind end of the cecum was reached, a second visualization of the colon was made as the tube was extracted and biopsy samples were obtained. Biopsies were routinely taken at 15-cm (transverse colon) and 5-cm (descending colon) distances from the anus during the exiting process. Biopsy specimens were oriented on filter paper and fixed in 10% formalin. Histological sections (5 μm) from paraffin blocks were mounted and stained for grading colitis. Any focal abnormalities, e.g., ulcers, nodules, hemorrhages, etc., were described and biopsy samples taken. (Note: Initially, biopsies were taken at 5-, 10-, 15-, and 20-cm distances from the anus. However, the inflammatory state of the colon was relatively consistent from cecum through the descending colon and it was decided not to subject the animals to excessive mucosal biopsies to describe the colon.)

C. HISTOLOGICAL EVALUATION OF COLITIS

This protocol has been described elsewhere in detail.[3] The number and types of cells infiltrating into the lamina propria and epithelium were counted and epithelial and crypt morphological changes were noted. Two to three crypts and associated lamina propria were evaluated per specimen; cells were identified (400× magnification) and counted (250×). Grading of each colon was expressed by a letter which indicated the type and number of cells present: normal (N), acute (A) (or active), or chronic (C) (or inactive). Acute colitis was categorized as mild (A1) or severe (A2). Normal colons had no increased cellular infiltrate in the lamina propria but were relatively rare in these CTT age groups. When the infiltrate was composed predominantly of chronic inflammatory cells (plasma cells, lymphocytes, monocytes, histiocytes, etc.), the grade was designated chronic (inactive). If some polymorphonuclear leukocytes (PMNs) were also present in the lamina propria and/or the epithelium or an occasional crypt abscess was present, mild acute (A1) was assigned. When the infiltrate included large numbers of PMNs (including microabscesses) in the lamina propria and/or crypt epithelium and crypt abscesses were common, the condition was considered severe acute (A2). Architectural abnormalities of the crypt epithelium and any other unusual observations were also recorded.

The presence of active colitis was almost always superimposed upon the chronic condition. Thus, the presence of increased PMNs in the lamina propria occurred in the presence of increased numbers of mononuclear cells that remained from prior active episodes and repair processes. In addition, architectural changes in the mucosa were seen that included branching crypts, tortuosity of crypts, and atrophy in length and numbers. All CTTs had histological evidence of prior colitic episodes.

For this study, the most severe state seen in the biopsies was used to describe the condition of the colon. For example, if an animal's colon was graded as mild acute at 15 cm and chronic at 5 cm (regular sampling points), a biopsy at 10 cm of a focal lesion with severe acute colitis and ulceration would cause the colon to be graded as A2 (severe acute colitis).

D. FREQUENCY OF EXAMINATION

Animals were examined by endoscopy and by colonic mucosal biopsy at 2- to 3-month intervals beginning in 1985; this report covers observations through October 1991.

E. OTHER DATA COLLECTED

Body weights were obtained during each colonic examination and stool consistency was recorded.

Stool consistency was graded in four levels: firm, loose, puddly, and diarrhea. The following descriptions were used:

Firm:	formed stool
Loose:	semiformed, stool did not hold its shape after being passed but was not watery
Puddly:	semiliquid, stool lost its shape quickly after being passed but could not be described as a solution or suspension
Diarrhea:	liquid, stool was watery with no form at all and resembled a dilute suspension

Relationships were attempted in order to define and explain the sequence of events that led from asymptomatic, but histologically detectable, changes through debilitating and life-threatening weight loss with persistent nonformed stools and associated fluid imbalances.

III. RESULTS

A. GENERAL OBSERVATIONS

The cotton-top tamarins tolerated both the procedure and the associated anesthesia very well. A related study in this volume[16] reported that mortality was not greater (actually less) in age-matched groups subjected to large numbers of biopsies (X = 14.6 biopsies) as compared with groups with ~1 biopsy over 5 years (mortality was ~45% vs. 63%, respectively). Recovery from anesthesia occurred within 1 to 2 hours, animals begain eating when food was given, and no signs of postbiopsy stress or pain was evident.

B. NUMBERS OF OBSERVATIONS

Body weights — Animals were weighed at the time of each colonoscopy/colon biopsy. Consequently, each animal's weight was recorded at least four times per year.

Stool evaluations — During the 6-year period, recorded stool samples (504) from the 40 CTTs were graded as: firm — 351, loose — 107, puddly — 45, and diarrhea — 1.

Colonoscopies and mucosal biopsies — During the 6-year observation period, a total of 673 colonoscopies were performed and colonic mucosal biopsies taken. Only rarely was a colonoscopy procedure not performed as scheduled; exceptions were made for certain clinical conditions: unusual illness such as anorexia, weight loss of 50 to 100 g, moribund state prior to euthanasia, etc. Consequently, animals that survived through October 1991 have had ~24 biopsy procedures. Of the 673 procedures, 420 (62.4%) were chronic (C) (inactive but with increased infiltration of mononuclear inflammatory cells), 152 (22.6%) were mild acute (A1) (active with infiltration of PMNs), and 101 (15%) were severe acute (A2) (active with large infiltration of PMNs in the lamina propria and/or colonic epithelium with or without crypt abscesses). The mean age of occurrence for each disease diagnosis was chronic, 7.75 years, mild acute, 7.9 years, and severe acute, 9.0 years.

C. COLITIC EPISODES

While the majority of histological observations were chronic in nature, all 40 animals had at least one acute colitic episode during the 6-year observation period. Whithin the 40 animals, the average age for the first A1 event was 6.5 years and the first A2 event was 8.2 years.

Interanimal patterns of colitis development were quite variable. Some (37.5% = 15/40) never developed severe acute colitis (A2). Acute colitis occurred in spikes (a single observation at that particular grade) or in plateaus (defined as two or more consecutive observations at the same grade of colitis). Some animals had spikes, either single or repeated at varied intervals, while others had large numbers of biopsies that were repeatedly graded at A2. Some had more or less alternating acute spikes followed by a period(s) of remission, a return to chronic (inactive) status. Generally, the older the animal, the more severe was the colitic episode and the more frequent were the acute episodes. Examples of some of the various developmental patterns are shown in Figures 1 to 10, along with observations of weight and stool condition at the time of biopsy.

Tamarin acute colitis occurred in two different clinical situations; some CTTs were symptomatic (e.g., loose stools, weight loss, lethargy, etc.) and others were asymptomatic as far as could be determined. Of the 15 "A1-only" animals that never reached A2, 5 (33%) were asymptomatic, whereas only 2/25 (8%) of A2s were asymptomatic. Of the 15 "A1-only" CTTs, 14 had one or more plateaus even though an A2 condition was not diagnosed in these animals; 5 animals had two to four plateaus, and they ranged from two to six consecutive biopsies. Of the 25 animals that were graded as A2 one or more times, 10 had one A2 event (spike), 1 had three separate spikes, and 1 each had either two or four consecutive biopsies (plateaus); however, 12 had more than five A2 grades and each animal had at least one plateau. Twelve of the plateaus were >3 biopsies and one plateau had 8 consecutive A2 biopsies.

D. TIME COURSE EXAMPLES: COLITIC STATE, STOOL CONDITION, AND BODY WEIGHT WITH TIME AND AGE

Figures 1 and 2 are examples of animals that never developed severe acute colitis (A2) over 5½-year periods that included ages 5.5 to 11 and 7.5

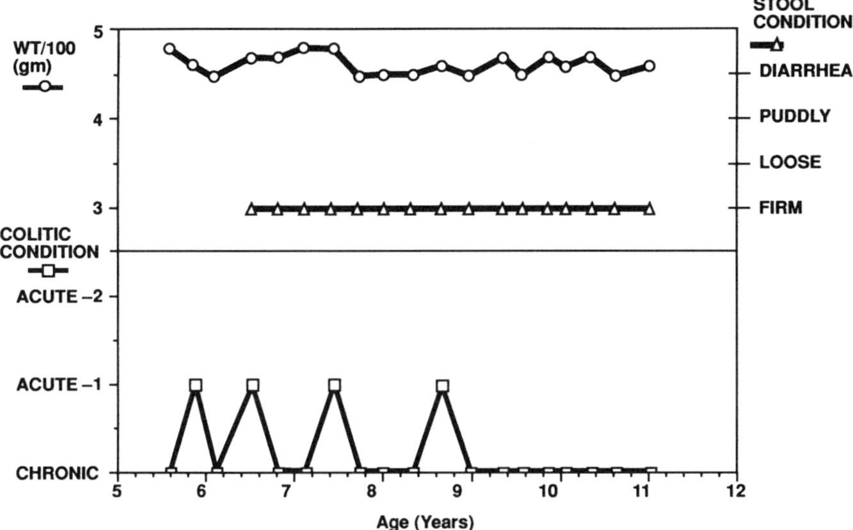

FIGURE 1. Cotton-top tamarin (FO-4267). Changes in colitic condition, body weight, and stool condition.

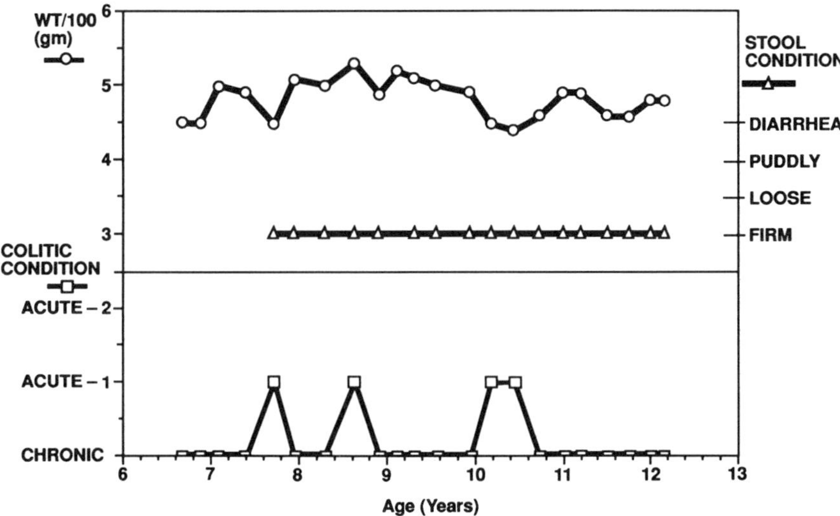

FIGURE 2. Cotton-top tamarin (MO-4060). Changes in colitic condition, body weight, and stool condition.

to 12.5 years, respectively. CTT 4267 (Figure 1) had only A1 spikes of mild acute colitis (no plateaus) with firm stools and no body weight changes during the observation period. Figures 3 and 4 show data on two animals that had spikes of severe acute colitis (A2) followed by a plateau that persisted until

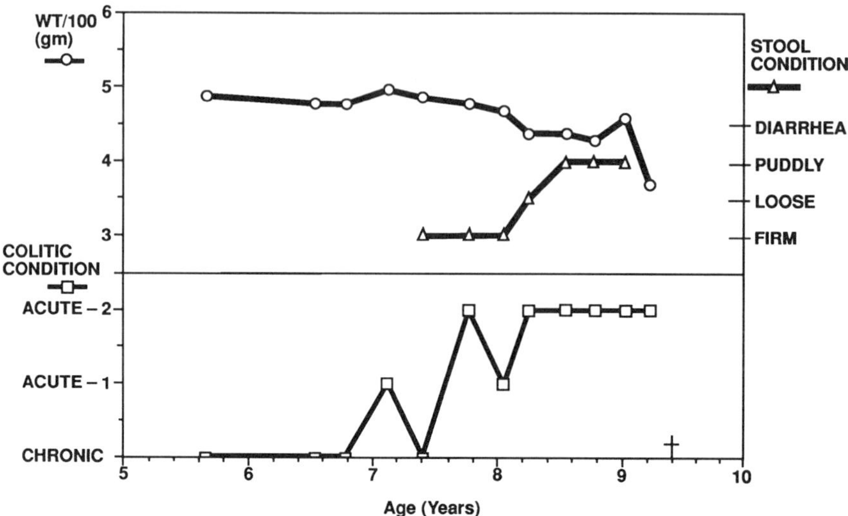

FIGURE 3. Cotton-top tamarin (MO-4137). Changes in colitic condition, body weight, and stool condition.

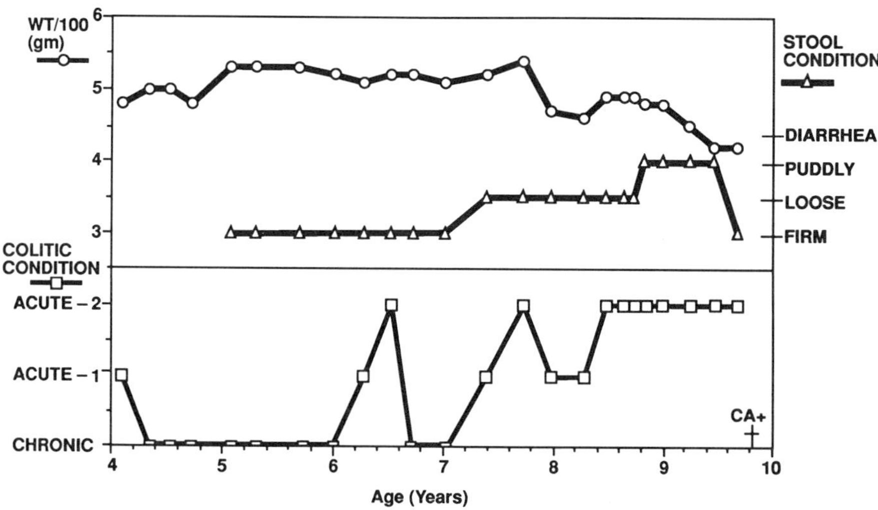

FIGURE 4. Cotton-top tamarin (MO-4462). Changes in colitic condition, body weight, and stool condition.

death (>1 year). Weight loss and nonfirm stools were associated with prolonged severe acute colitis. Figure 5 shows a CTT (4282) that had 16 A1 observations, 8 A2s, and only 4 Cs. With only minor fluctuations, body weight declined steadily during the 6-year period, and stool condition varied in close correlation with the severity of colitis.

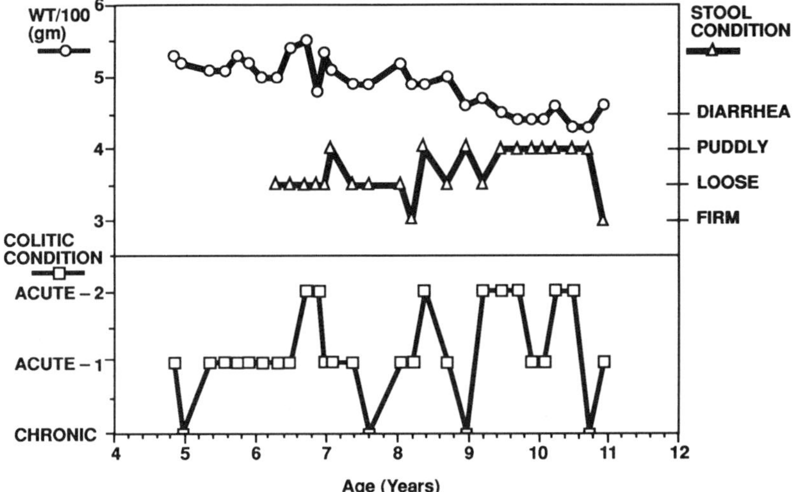

FIGURE 5. Cotton-top tamarin (MO-4282). Changes in colitic condition, body weight, and stool condition.

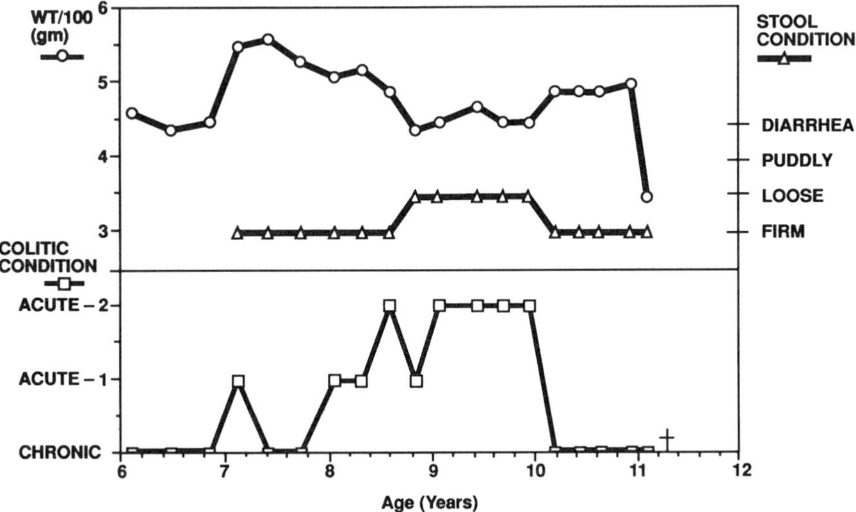

FIGURE 6. Cotton-top tamarin (MO-4149). Changes in colitic condition, body weight, and stool condition.

Figures 6 to 10 show other patterns that were observed. In Figure 6, 4149 had a 1-year plateau of A2 colitis with loose stool and ~50 g weight loss. Following that period the colitis was in remission for ~1 year, the stool became firm, and body weight increased ~50 g. An undetermined event unrelated to changes in colitic status (probably pneumonia) caused a dramatic

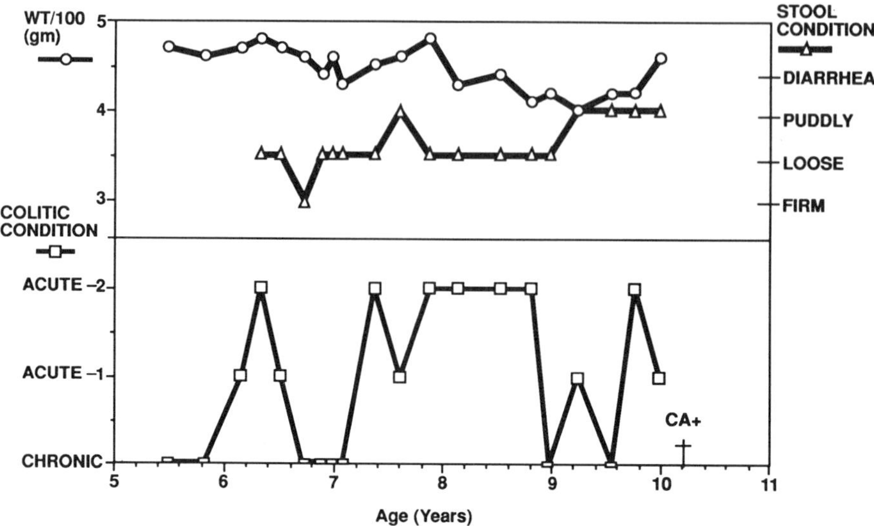

FIGURE 7. Cotton-top tamarin (FO-4283). Changes in colitic condition, body weight, and stool condition.

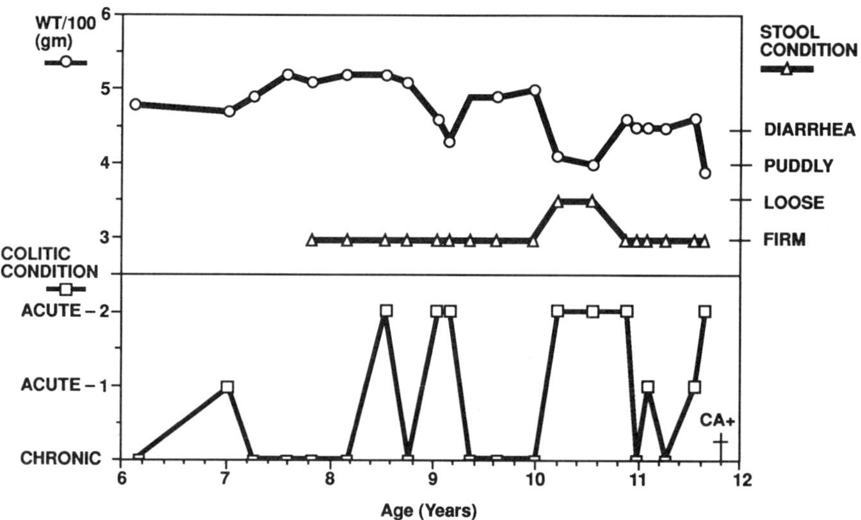

FIGURE 8. Cotton-top tamarin (MO-4053). Changes in colitic condition, body weight, and stool condition.

150-g weight loss and death. The CTT (FO-4283) pattern in Figure 7 showed A2 spikes, remissions, an A2 plateau for 1 year and a varied status until death due to colon cancer. Weight loss and loose-to-puddly stools generally correlated with severe acute colitis. Figure 8 shows data on 4053, which had a varied colitic status that correlated well with changes in stool condition and

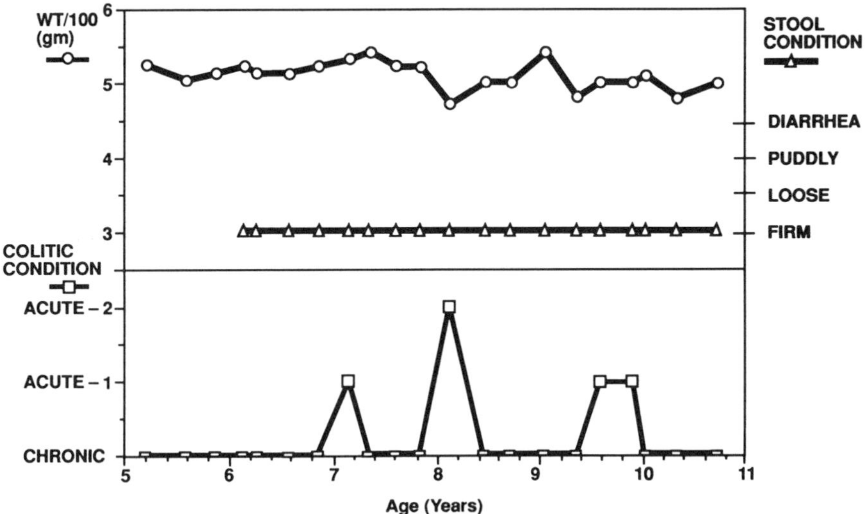

FIGURE 9. Cotton-top tamarin (FO-4302). Changes in colitic condition, body weight, and stool condition.

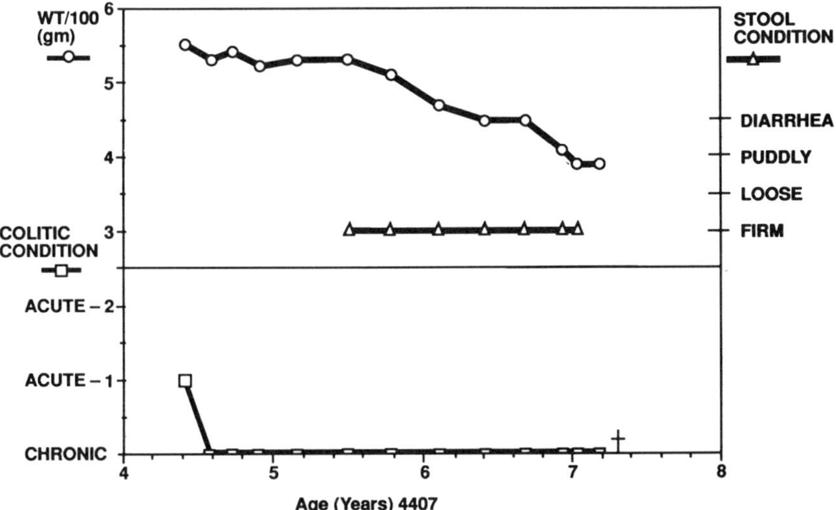

FIGURE 10. Cotton-top tamarin (MO-4407). Changes in colitic condition, body weight, and stool condition.

body weight. This animal eventually developed three right-sided colonic polyps, one of which became malignant and was the cause of death.[17] Figure 9 shows a tamarin with colitic flares interspersed with periods of remission and associated weight changes but all colonic changes occurred while the stool condition remained firm. CTT 4407 (Figure 10) had only a single A1 acute colitis followed by 3 years of chronic colitis and no change in stool condition; however, a gradual but continuing 175-g weight loss of undetermined cause occurred prior to death.

IV. DISCUSSION

The sampling of CTT colons at 2- to 3-month intervals provided insight into the development of colitis over time (5 to 6 years) that is generally not available in any animal population, including humans. It appears that the characteristics of CTT spontaneous colitis — pathogenesis, time course, and progression — resemble very closely the intermittent exacerbations and remissions that are well known in the human disease, idiopathic ulcerative colitis.

Since the CTTs were examined routinely (at 2- to 3-month intervals), acute (active) colitis was often diagnosed histologically in animals that were asymptomatic (e.g., absence of weight loss, diarrhea, etc.). Thus, acute colitis occurred before the animals would have reason to be examined by a clinician. This situation would parallel the human condition in that a subclinical onset of inflammation may occur, but patients usually develop some symptoms before visiting a physician.

The evaluation of the A1 episodes has been of some concern since at least three alternatives could yield mild acute colitis. First, the inflammation could have peaked with A1 as the most severe stage. Second, A1 could be observed early in an A2 event which developed after the biopsy was taken, or, third, A1 could also be observed on a declining curve after A2 had been reached in the days before biopsy and the healing process had started. Histologically, the location of PMNs in the colonic tissue could suggest whether the A2 exacerbation was early in the disease process or later during the healing process. Early onset of active colitis had PMNs primarily in the lamina propria with few crypt abscesses, whereas the healing stage had most PMNs in the epithelium and crypt abscesses and few in the lamina propria.

A. INTERPRETATIONS OF RELATIONSHIPS

Body weight vs. age — In the 15 asymptomatic CTTs, there was no apparent change in weight with age within the age ranges (4 to 12 years) in this study. Unless a life-threatening condition developed, the adult body weight was maintained throughout. This is consistent with our unreported observations that aging with associated decline in body weight and general health occurs after ~15 years of age.

Stool condition vs. age — Similarly, the 15 asymptomatic CTTs showed no change in stool condition during the time course studied (ages of 4 to 12 years); occasionally, a condition unrelated to colon status developed and clinical symptoms occurred. The symptoms mentioned in this chapter were typical but not exclusive and included weight loss, change in stool condition, and histological diagnosis of severe acute colitis.

The following relationships are based largely upon, and demonstrated by, the data from the 10 CTTs shown in Figures 1 to 10.

Body weight vs. colitis grade — Some body weight variations occurred irrespective of the colitic state of A1 (see Figures 1 and 2); however, A1 in single or multiple events had little effect upon body weights. A plateau of two consecutive A1s (see Figure 2) correlated with some weight loss during the 10-year age period, suggesting that persistence of even mild acute colitis over a 2- to 3-month period could produce some weight loss. A gradual and finally precipitous weight loss associated with a 2-year persistent active colitis, primarily A2, was seen in Figure 3. Spikes of severe active colitis had little effect on weight loss; however, this minimal effect contrasts with the severe weight loss associated with persistent A2 over eight observations (~2 years), as seen in Figure 4. In Figure 5, 1½ years of A1 (early age) caused little change in body weight but 17 biopsies of A1 or A2 (late) with only three remissions resulted in a gradual, but steady, weight decline. Figure 6 shows a CTT that had some early variations in body weight (unexplained by colitic state) but a later persisting weight loss during 1 year of A2; this loss was followed by a 1-year period of remission with some weight gain and then an unrelated sudden weight loss and death. As a result body weights during chronic colitis can vary widely.

Colitic grade vs. stool condition — Figures 1 and 2 demonstrate the general observation that A1 occurring in spikes alone did not alter the stool condition, but A2 colitis changed the stool condition toward diarrhea, especially when it persisted over several months (Figures 3 to 8). Figure 7 shows a CTT that had persistent loose stool with long-standing acute colitis that finally ended in death; only during an early period of 6 to 8 months of remission (C) was the stool firm.

Colitis vs. age — A relationship was observed between colitic state and CTT age. As reflected by the mean time of occurrence of the various colitic states (C = 7.75, A1 = 7.9, and A2 = 9.0 years), A2s occurred first primarily in the 8- to 9-year age range and tended to persist through 10 to 12 years of age. A histogram of the frequency of the three colitic grades with age is shown in Figure 11. While an occasional animal survived a long-term active colitis, most were eventually overwhelmed by the disease progression and died or were euthanized.

Generally, the following correlations were recognized.

Relationships	Correlation
Age vs. body weight or stool condition	None
Acute colitis vs. body weight	
A1	None or little
A2 (spike)	Little to slight inverse
A2 (plateau)	Consistent inverse relationship
Acute colitis vs. stool	
A1	None
A2 (spike)	Little to slight
A2 (plateau)	Loose → puddly → diarrhea

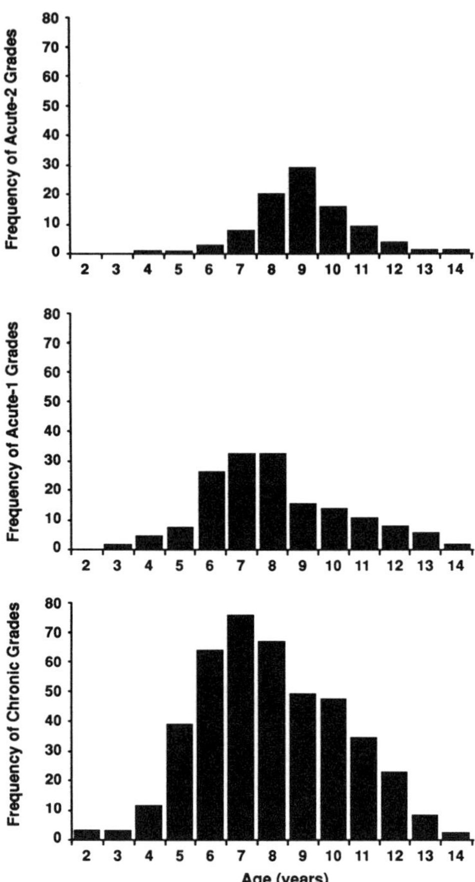

FIGURE 11. A histogram of frequency of occurrence for the three colitic grades with age.

Relationships	**Correlation**
Age vs. colitis	
<7 years	Little
8–12 years	High risk for acute colitis

Persistent severe active colitis was often accompanied by cellular changes in the crypt epithelium, including hyperplasia of epithelial cells (loss of basal orientation), mucin depletion, increased nuclear/cytoplasmic ratio, and prominent nucleoli. Because these changes were always found in the presence of active CTT colitis, a diagnosis of unequivocal dysplasia was excluded following the human criteria of Riddell et al.[18]

A hypothetical model that is consistent with the observations during the course of colitis and colon cancer development is presented in Figure 12. The first line represents the occurrence of asymptomatic active colitis; this was a

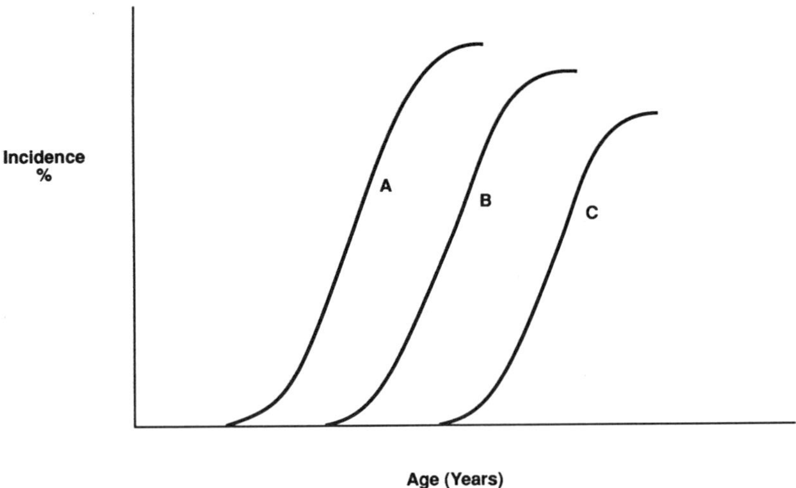

FIGURE 12. Theoretical curves of relationship between onset of colitis and the subsequent development of colon cancer in cotton-top tamarins.

common finding in CTTs and represents in humans a time when the disease has not reached sufficient severity to produce symptoms and a visit to a physician. The middle line is that time when symptoms are seen, e.g., loose stool and weight loss, and when a patient would visit a doctor. The last line represents the onset of colonic carcinoma following ulcerative colitis; this observation is consistent in both CTTs and humans. The space between the lines is variable from animal to animal. Development of targeted therapeutics would be predicated upon the fact that, in theory at least, appropriate active anticolitic agents could displace the colitis curve to the right, and possibly the cancer curve (delay of onset), and/or depress the curve(s) and ultimately reduce the numbers of colon cancers that develop following ulcerative colitis.

V. SUMMARY

In summary, a 6-year examination of 40 4- to 7-year-old CTTs at 2- to 3-month intervals has shown that CTT spontaneous colitis resembles the human disease in its time course, age dependence, varying periods of exacerbation and remission, and eventual susceptibility of the animal to colon cancer. Considerable animal-to-animal variation exists, as is seen in humans. While age had little effect on body weight and stool condition, the severity of the colitis (A2 vs. A1) and the length of the disease dramatically affected both CTT body weight and stool condition. The data collected from this study supports the fact that the CTT disease closely mimics the human disease and further demonstrates its validity as an animal model from which information can be gained to understand the human disease; the model also offers promise of helping afflicted human patients through targeted therapeutics.

ACKNOWLEDGMENTS

This research was conducted in ORAU's AALAC-accredited Marmoset Research Center at Oak Ridge (MARCOR) and was approved and monitored by ORAU's Animal Care Standards Committee.

Research was supported, in part, by the ORAU Corporation and National Cancer Institute Contract N01 CP21004.

The authors acknowledge the excellent manuscript review by S. Tardif, R. Damian, and M. Tobi, and manuscript preparation by S. Womble.

REFERENCES

1. **Goulston, S. J. M. and McGovern, V. J.,** *Fundamentals of Colitis,* Pergamon Press, New York, 1981.
2. **Chalifoux, L. V. and Bronson, R. T.,** Colonic adenocarcinoma associated with chronic colitis in cotton-top marmosets, *Saguinus oedipus, Gastroenterology,* 80, 942, 1981.
3. **Clapp, N. K., Lushbaugh, C., Humason, G. L., Gangaware, B. L., and Henke, M. A.,** The marmoset as a model of ulcerative colitis and colon cancer, in *Colorectal Cancer and Its Precurosrs,* Ingalls, J. F. and Mastromarino, A., Eds., Allen R. Liss, New York, 1985, 247.
4. **Lushbaugh, C. C., Humason, G. L., and Clapp, N. K.,** Histology of colitis: *Saguinus oedipus oedipus* and other marmoets, *Dig. Dis. Sci.,* 30, 45S, 1985.
5. **Chalifoux, L. V., Hunt, R. D., and King, N. W.,** Adenocarcinoma of the colon and chronic colitis in *Saguinus oedipus:* a possible model for analogous human disease, in *Animal Models of Intestinal Disease,* Pfeiffer, C. J., Ed., CRC Press, Boca Raton, FL, 1985, 69.
6. **Chalifoux, L. V., Brieland, J. K., and King, N. W.,** Evolution and natural history of colonic disease in cotton-top tamarins *(Saguinus oedipus), Dig. Dis. Sci.,* 30, 54S, 1985.
7. **Clapp, N. K., McArthur, A. H., Henke, M. A., Carson, R. L., Peck, O. C., and Wood, J. D.,** Is acute colitis a precursor to development of colonic cancer in cotton-top tamarins?, *Gastroenterology,* 90, 1374, 1986.
8. **Clapp, N. K., Henke, M. A., Lushbaugh, C. C., Humason, G. L., and Gangaware, B. L.,** Effect of various biological factors on spontaneous marmoset and tamarin colitis: a retrospective histopathologic study, *Dig. Dis. Sci.,* 33, 1013, 1988.
9. **Madara, J. L., Podolsky, D. K., King, N. W., Sehgal, P. K., Moore, R., and Winter, H. S.,** Characterization of spontaneous colitis in cotton-top tamarins *(Saguinus oedipus)* and its responses to sulfasalazine, *Gastroenterology,* 88, 13, 1985.
10. **Podolsky, D. K., Madara, J. L., King, N. et al.,** Colonic mucin composition in primates: selective alterations associated with spontaneous colitis in the cotton-top tamarin, *Gastroenterology,* 88, 20, 1984.

11. **Boland, C. R. and Clapp, N. K.,** Glycoconjugates in the colons of new world monkeys with spontaneous colitis: association between inflammation and neoplasia, *Gastroenterology,* 92, 625, 1987.
12. **Das, K. M., Vecchi, M., Squillante, L., Dasgupta, A., Henke, M., and Clapp, N.,** Mr 40 000 human colonic epithelial protein expression in colonic mucosa and presence of circulating anti-Mr 40 000 antibodies in cotton top tamarins with spontaneous colitis, *Gut,* 33, 48, 1992.
13. **Lee, Y.-C. C., Lawless, D., Crook, J. E., and Clapp, N.,** Analysis of T lymphocyte subsets in tamarins with colitis and colon cancer, *Am. J. Med. Sci.,* 296(7), 118, 1989.
14. **Clapp, N. K., Henke, M. A., Hansard, R. M., Walsh, R. E., Widomski, D. L., Anglin, C. P., Fretland, D. J., and Gaginella, T. S.,** Inflammatory mediators in cotton-top tamarins (CTT) with acute and chronic colitis, *Agents Actions,* 34, 1, 1991.
15. **Clapp, N. K., Henke, M. A., Holloway, E. C., and Tankersley, W. G.,** Carcinoma of the colon in the cotton-top tamarin: a radiographic study, *J. Am. Vet. Med. Assoc.,* 183, 1328, 1983.
16. **Clapp, N. K., Henke, M. A., Hansard, R. M., Carson, R. L., and Nardi, R. V.,** Do repeated colonic mucosal biopsies impact mortality in cotton-top tamarins?, This volume, Chapter 10.
17. **Clapp, N. K., Henke, M. A., Hansard, R. M., Adams, L. J., Carson, R. L., Hawkins, J. V., and Nardi, R.,** Colonic polyps associated with colitis in cotton-top tamarins *(Saguinus oedipus):* progression to colonic carcinoma?, *Dig. Dis. Sci.,* submitted.
18. **Riddell, R. H., Goldman, H., Ransohoff, D. F., Appelman, H. D., Fenoglio, C. M., Haggitt, R. C., Ahren, C., Correa, P., Hamilton, S. R., Morson, B. C., Sommers, S. C., and Yardley, J. H.,** Dysplasia in inflammatory bowel disease: standardized classification with provisional clinical applications, *Hum. Pathol.,* 14, 931, 1983.

Chapter 5

THE PREVALENCE OF IDIOPATHIC COLITIS IN THE NEW ENGLAND REGIONAL PRIMATE RESEARCH CENTER COTTON-TOP TAMARIN *(Saguinus oedipus)* COLONY

Norval W. King, Lorna D. Johnson, and Prabhat K. Sehgal

TABLE OF CONTENTS

0-8493-5363-7/93/$0.00 + $.50

I. INTRODUCTION

Captive colonies of cotton-top tamarins, *Saguinus oedipus,* develop a spontaneously occurring, idiopathic colitis characterized by intermittent episodes of acute inflammatory activity with intervening periods of inflammatory quiescence. With time, these repeated bouts of acute colitis may lead to structural changes in the mucosa that are generally associated with chronicity. The disorder may be associated with chronic diarrhea, severe wasting, and eventual death. This condition, which in the past has been considered as one possible cause of ''marmoset wasting syndrome'', continues to represent a major health problem in laboratory colonies of this endangered New World primate species.[1-7] Interestingly, animals in colonies where this condition is endemic also develop a relatively high incidence of colonic adenocarcinoma.[8-13] The apparent association of these two conditions in this nonhuman primate species has prompted considerable interest in the cotton-top tamarin as a potential model of human idiopathic ulcerative colitis and its associated colonic carcinoma.

There are a number of publications describing the clinical and pathological features of the chronic colitis and colonic adenocarcinoma of cotton-top tamarins.[1-13] Most of these, however, have been based upon either retrospective studies of autopsy specimens or studies of a relatively small number of clinical cases followed prospectively for varying periods of time with and without different forms of therapy. There have been virtually no long-term, longitudinal studies of the natural history of these conditions in which the sequential clinical and pathologic changes that occur from onset through progression to severe chronic colitis and cancer have been documented in detail.

In July, 1986 the New England Regional Primate Research Center in collaboration with the Gastrointestinal Unit of the Massachusetts General Hospital initiated a 5-year study funded by the National Institutes of Health to define the natural history of the chronic colitis and colonic carcinoma of cotton-top tamarins from infancy to adulthood. One of the components of this study was to document the prevalence of active colitis and chronic mucosal alterations in the existing colony of 269 cotton-top tamarins, based upon a one-time examination of colon biopsies from each animal. The results of the histologic examinations, including differences in the degree of severity of any acute and chronic microscopic changes, were tabulated according to age (4 groups), gender (2 groups), method of rearing (5 groups), diet (4 groups), and selected clinical findings, including endoscopy and body weight. The data presented herein represent the results of this survey.

II. MATERIAL AND METHODS

A. ANIMALS

During the first year of this prospective study of colon cancer and colitis, 269 tamarins (*Saguinus oedipus*), 144 (53.5%) males and 125 (46.5%) females

TABLE 1
Age Distribution and Method of Rearing of Cotton-Top Tamarins NERPRC Colony

	Rearing						Total	
Age group	**W**	**C**	**P**	**F**	**N**	**I**	**No.**	**%**
Infant ≤6 mos			13	8	12	23	56	(20.8)
Juvenile >6 mos to ≤2 yrs			14	30	32		76	(28.3)
Adult >2 yrs to ≤5 yrs			18	25	27		70	(26.0)
>5 years	9	27	14	16	1		67	(24.9)
Total								
No.	9	27	59	79	72	23	269	
%	3.4	10.0	21.9	29.4	26.8	8.6		(100.0)

Note: W = wild caught; C = colony inured in another colony; P = parent reared; F = family reared; N = nursery reared; I = reared in isolation nursery.

were screened with colon biopsies for colitis and colonic carcinoma. Of the 269, 56 (20.8%) were infants under 6 months of age, 76 (28.3%) were juveniles from 6 months to 2 years of age, 70 (26.0%) were adults from 2 to 5 years of age, and 67 (24.9%) were adults over 5 years of age (Table 1).

Nine (3.4%) were old, wild-caught animals who entered the colony as adults in 1975 and 1976; 27 (10.0%) adult animals were transferred from other colonies (colony-inured) and ranged in age from 8 to 12 years. The remaining animals were born in the colony: 59 (21.9%) were raised as a single litter with their parents, 79 (29.4%) were raised in families where they grew up with parents and older siblings, 72 (26.8%) were taken from parents because they were neglected or abused after birth and hand-raised in a nursery, and 23 (8.6%) were removed at birth and raised in an isolation unit. The last group of 23 tamarins were one of twins or triplets whose siblings were left with the parents as part of an ongoing prospective study of the effect of environment, diet, and genealogy on the incidence of colitis.

The tamarins are housed indoors under conditions of constant temperature and humidity with 12-hour light cycles. Mating pairs live in single cages 33 in. H × 25.5 in. W × 27 in. D containing wooden nesting boxes and perches. When the first litter is born, this space is expanded to two cages joined by a plastic tunnel. Families of six to eight individuals are housed in large cages measuring 6 ft H × 4.5 ft W × 3.5 ft D. Infants remain with the parents except those who are neglected or abused in the first week after birth. These are hand-reared in a nursery and socialized with their peers from 1 month of age until puberty at 18 to 20 months, at which time they are paired in single cages.

Animals in the colony are fed a standard diet (Diet D) consisting of canned food (Zupreem), supplemented with eggs, fruit, yogurt, and ground meat, crickets, and wax worms. Water with B complex vitamins (Visorbin and Vidaylin) is offered *ad libitum.* Vitamin D_3 is given weekly in marshmallows.

Animals in the regular and isolation nurseries are weaned at 3 months of age to the standard diet (Diet D) or to one of three semipurified diets (Diets A, B, C). Diet A, formulated to provide adequate nutrients, vitamins, and minerals for the growth of young animals and maintenance of adults, contains 30% of calories as fat, with a polyunsaturated to saturated fat ratio of 4 (P/S = 4), and 10% fiber (by weight w/w).

Diets B and C contain substantially different amounts of fat and fiber, but are otherwise adequate for growth and maintenance. Diet B contains high fat (40%, P/S = 2.0) and low fiber (5% w/w), Diet C contains low fat (20%, P/S = 0.5) and high fiber (20% w/w). The rationale for including these latter two diets in this longitudinal study is the fact that in man diets high in fat, particularly unsaturated fat, are thought to constitute a risk factor for the development of colon cancer, whereas those high in fiber have a controversial protective role in the development of colon cancer.[14,15]

B. COLONOSCOPY AND BIOPSIES

Adult animals were administered a laxative (5 mg tablet of bisacodyl orally) and had food withheld 12 hours before the biopsies were taken. To evacuate their colons, juveniles were administered 20 cc Golytely® orally and had food withheld for 12 hours. Under ketamine anesthesia, a 4.9-mm colonoscope was passed into the descending colon and the colonic mucosa was examined for abnormalities. Biopsies were taken under direct visualization including suspicious areas when present, or from two areas, one high and one low when no abnormality was noted. In all instances, only the descending colon was examined and biopsied.

The biopsies, which measured from 1 to 2 mm^3 were oriented on filter paper, and fixed in 10% neutral formalin. Paraffin sections were cut perpendicular to the epithelial surface and stained with hematoxylin and eosin. Microscopic changes denoting acute inflammatory activity, i.e., active colitis and mucosal structural alterations associated with chronicity were graded on a scale of 0 to 3 based, with slight modification, on the criteria originally devised by Madara et al.[5] Criteria used are presented in Table 2.

III. RESULTS

A. THE PREVALENCE OF ACUTE AND CHRONIC COLITIS AND COLONIC CARCINOMA

Microscopic evidence of acute inflammatory activity was found in the colons of 130 (48.3%) of the animals (Table 3). Mild colitis or grade 1 was present in 27.5%, moderate (grade 2) in 16.7%, and severe (grade 3) in 4.1%.

TABLE 2
Grading Criteria for Colonic Biopsies

Activity	Grade	Definition
Normal	(0)	Absence of single intraepithelial polymorphonuclear leukocytes (PMNs) and absence of cluster of PMNs in the lamina propria
Mild	(1)	Focal aggregates of lamina propria PMNs or the presence of isolated intraepithelial PMNs in three or fewer crypts per biopsy specimen
Moderate	(2)	Focal aggregates of lamina propria PMNs and isolated intraepithelial PMNs in more than three crypts per biopsy specimen
Severe	(3)	More than one crypt abscess per biopsy specimen
Chronicity		
Normal	(0)	No structural features of chronicity
Mild	(1)	Equivocal of crypts or surface irregularity
Moderate	(2)	Definite irregularity of crypts or surface irregularity or branching and focal loss of crypts
Severe	(3)	Definite irregularity of crypts or surface irregularity accompanied by branching and focal loss of crypts

TABLE 3
Age Distribution of Acute and Chronic Colitis

		Acute Colitis Grades			
	Total	1	2	3	Total
Age group	no.	No. (%)	No. (%)	No. (%)	No. (%)
Infants	56	12 (21.4)	4 (7.1)	1 (1.8)	17 (30.3)
Juvenile	76	22 (29.0)	6 (7.9)	2 (2.6)	30 (39.5)
Adults	70	25 (35.7)	10 (14.3)	3 (4.3)	38 (54.3)
Adults >5 yrs	67	15 (22.4)	25 (37.3)	5 (7.4)	45 (67.2)
	269	74 (27.5)	45 (16.7)	11 (4.1)	130 (48.3)
		Chronic Colitis Grades			
Infants	56	3 (5.4)	1 (1.8)		4 (7.2)
Juveniles	76	13 (17.1)	3 (4.0)		16 (21.1)
Adults	70	28 (40.0)	10 (14.3)		38 (54.3)
Older Adults	67	12 (17.9)	25 (37.3)	1 (1.5)	38 (56.7)
	269	56 (20.8)	39 (14.5)	1 (0.4)	96 (35.7)

Chronic colitis was present in 96 (35.7%) of the animals. Grade 1 was present in 20.8%, grade 2 in 14.5%, and grade 3 was extremely rare (0.4%) (Table 3).

Only 1 animal with colonic adenocarcinoma was detected in the 269 surveyed (0.37% prevalence rate). It was a 3-year-old female, parent-reared

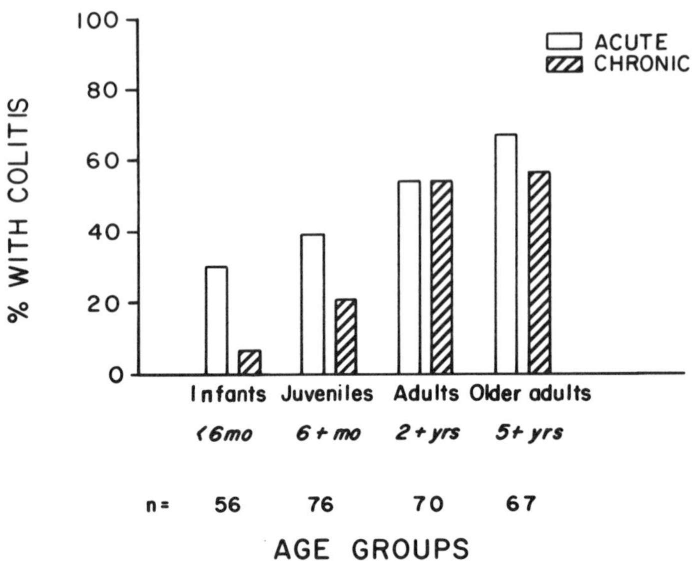

FIGURE 1. Acute and chronic colitis in relation to age groups.

animal that had been fed standard diet (diet D) since the time of weaning. It weighed 300 g and had microscopic evidence of acute and chronic colitis. It died with metastatic disease 2 weeks after biopsy.

1. Age

The prevalence of acute colitis progressively increased with age from 30.3% in infants to 67.2% in older adults (Figure 1, Table 3) (Regression: R^2 = .99). The prevalence of grade 1 activity increased progressively from 21.4% through 5 years of age and then declined in older adults to 22.4%. Grades 2 and 3 increased progressively with age and in the older adults the combined prevalence of the more severe grades of colitis (2 and 3) was higher than grade 1 acute colitis. Thus, the prevalence and the severity of the acute colitis increased with age.

Chronic colitis increased progressively with age from 7.2% among infants to 56.7% among older adults (Figure 1, R^2 = .86). The pattern of increased prevalence and severity with advancing age was similar to that of acute colitis. The prevalence of grade 1 chronic colitis progressed from 5.4% in infants to 40% in adults through 5 years of age and then declined to 17.9% over 5 years of age. Grade 2 chronic colitis increased progressively from 1.8% in infants to 37.3% in adults over 5 years of age. In the older adult group, the prevalence of grade 2 (37.3%) was more than twice the prevalence of grade 1 (17.9%).

2. Gender

The prevalence of acute and chronic colitis was similar in male and female tamarins within each of the four age groups (data not shown). Among the

TABLE 4
The Correlation of Acute and Chronic Colitis and Methods of Rearing Within Age Groups

				Acute colitis		Chronic colitis	
Age group	No.	Rearing	No.	No.	(%)	No.	(%)
Infant	56	P	13	6	(46.2)	2	(15.4)
		F	8	2	(25.0)	0	(0)
		N	12	3	(25.0)	2	(16.7)
		I	23	6	(26.1)	0	(0)
Juvenile	76	P	14	6	(42.9)	3	(21.4)
		F	30	14	(46.7)	7	(23.3)
		N	32	10	(31.3)	6	(18.8)
Adult	70	P	18	9	(50.0)	10	(55.6)
		F	25	14	(56.0)	13	(52.0)
		N	27	15	(55.6)	15	(55.6)
Adult >5 yrs	67	W	9	7	(77.8)	7	(77.8)
		C	27	20	(74.1)	15	(55.6)
		P	14	10	(71.4)	9	(64.3)
		F	16	8	(50.0)	6	(37.5)
		N	1	0	(0)	1	(100.0)
Total	269			130	(48.3)	96	(35.7)

Note: P = parent reared; F = family reared; N = nursery reared; I = reared in isolation nursery; W = wild caught; C = colony inured in another colony.

125 females, 48.0% had acute colitis and 34.4% had chronic colitis. Among the 144 males, 48.6% had acute colitis and 36.8% had chronic colitis.

3. Method of Rearing

The method of rearing was highly correlated with age (Table 1). All of the wild-caught and colony-inured animals were over 5 years of age and all of those raised in the isolation nursery were under 6 months of age. Thus, the effect of rearing was examined within age groups (Table 4).

The prevalence of acute colitis among infants, juveniles, and adults through 5 years of age was similar in the different rearing groups. Among older adults, those raised in families had a lower prevalence (50.0%) than wild-caught (77.8%), colony-inured (74.1%), or parent-raised animals (71.4%).

Among infants, juveniles, and adults, the prevalence of chronic colitis was similar in each rearing group. Among the older adults, the prevalence of chronic colitis was lower in the family-reared (37.5%) than among the older wild-caught (77.8%), colony-inured (55.6%), or parent-reared (64.3%) groups.

4. Diet

The prevalence of acute colitis among infants fed synthetic diets (B or C) or regular diet (D) was similar (Table 5). There was little difference between

TABLE 5
The Effect of Diet on Prevalence of Acute and Chronic Colitis Within Age Groups

Age group	No.	Diet	No.	Acute colitis No.	Acute colitis (%)	Chronic colitis No.	Chronic colitis (%)
Infant	56	A	0				
		B	13	3	(23.1)	1	(7.7)
		C	17	6	(35.3)	1	(5.9)
		D	26	8	(30.8)	2	(7.7)
Juvenile	76	A	11	5	(45.5)	1	(9.1)
		B	4	2	(50.0)	0	(0.0)
		C	4	0	(0.0)	1	(25.0)
		D	57	23	(40.4)	14	(24.6)
Adult	70	A	7	6	(85.7)	4	(57.1)
		B	0				
		C	0				
		D	63	32	(50.8)	34	(54.0)
Adult >5 yrs	67	D	67	45	(67.2)	38	(56.7)
Total	269			130	(48.3)	96	(35.7)

Note: Semipurified diets: (A) 30% fat, 10% fiber, P/S = 4; (B) 40% fat, 5% fiber, P/S = 2; (C) 20% fat, 20% fiber, P/S = 0.5. Standard diet: (D) See text.

diet A (45.5%) and diet D (40.4%) among juveniles. Among adults fed diet A, 85.7% had colitis compared to those fed the standard diet (50.8%).

The numbers of animals started on synthetic diets B and C is presently too small to make judgments. However, it is of interest to note that in animals fed the synthetic diet A, the prevalence of acute colitis is similar to, or higher than, those on diet D. Also, the prevalence of acute colitis increases with age in those fed diet A and those fed diet D.

B. CLINICAL OBSERVATIONS

Various grades of acute and chronic colitis were absent or present together in individual tamarins. These combinations could affect clinical observations. After examining the data in tamarins with all combinations of acute and chronic colitis, data were grouped into grades 0 or 1 and 2 or 3 (Table 6).

1. Endoscopy

Endoscopic abnormalities of the colon were described as focal or generalized hyperemia, focal hemorrhage, ulcers, plaques, focal irregularity of the surface, polyps, and strictures, as compared to the normal smooth pearly pink surface. Seventy-nine percent of all tamarins showed no endoscopic abnormalities of the descending colon (Table 7). Abnormal mucosal changes, were observed in 18.5% of 195 tamarins with mild or no colitis and in 33.3%

TABLE 6
Grades of Acute and Chronic Colitis Occurring Together in Tamarins

Acute colitis grades	Chronic colitis grades 0 or 1	2 or 3	Total
0 or 1	197	16	213
2 or 3	32	24	56
Total	229	40	269

Note: O = normal, 1 = mild, 2 = moderate, 3 = marked.

TABLE 7
Correlation of Endoscopic and Histologic Findings in the Descending Colon

Histologic colitis Grades		Endoscopic abnormalities				
		Absent		Present		
Acute	Chronic	No.	%	No.	%	Total no.
0–1	0–1	159	81.5	36	18.5	195[a]
0–1	2–3	12	75.0	4	25.0	16
2–3	0–1	24	75.0	8	25.0	32
2–3	2–3	16	66.7	9	33.3	24
		211	79.0	56	21.0	267

[a] No observation in 2.

of 24 with moderate to severe acute and chronic colitis. Between these extremes, abnormalities were observed in 25% of those which had either moderate to severe acute or chronic colitis. Thus, endoscopy findings in the descending colon correlated poorly with the presence or degree of colitis observed in biopsies.

2. Weight

The weight distribution of tamarins in all age groups and with various combinations of acute and chronic colitis was examined. In adult animals over 2 years of age, weight distributions of groups with no colitis (grade 0), moderate or severe acute *or* chronic colitis (grades 2 or 3), moderate or severe acute *and* chronic colitis are illustrated by box-and-whisker plots (Figure 2 and Table 8). Eighty tamarins with no or mild colitis had a median weight of 474.5 g, and three quartiles of the population weighed between 426 and 519 g. In the 14 with moderate or severe chronic colitis and mild or no acute colitis, the median weight was higher (513.5 g) and in three quartiles of this population the weights were between 432 and 573 g. In both groups of tamarins with moderate or severe acute colitis, however, the median weights (448 and 423 g) and first and third quartiles were lower than those with no or mild colitis.

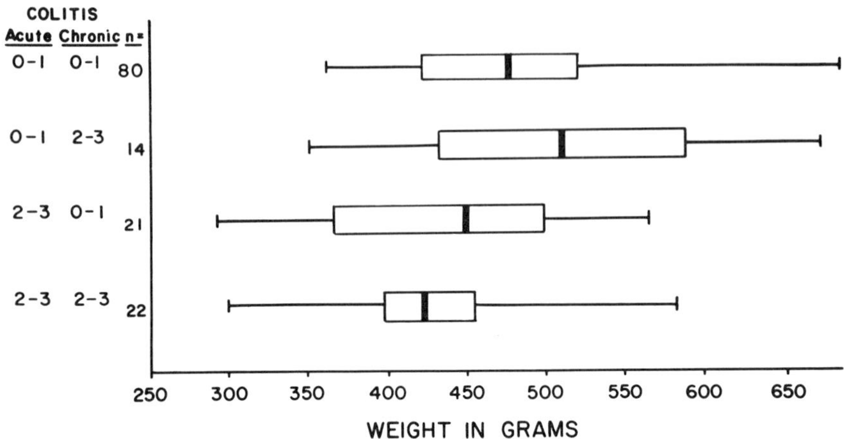

FIGURE 2. Distribution of weight among adult tamarins in relation to acute and chronic colitis.

TABLE 8
Weight Distribution Among Adult Tamarins in Relation to Acute and Chronic Colitis

Colitis grades							
Acute	**Chronic**	**No.**	**Min**	**Qtile1**	**Median**	**Qtile3**	**Max**
0–1	0–1	80	360	426	474.5	519	681
0–1	2–3	14	359	432	513.5	573	660
2–3	0–1	21	289	364	448	490	567
2–3	2–3	22	304	397	423	454	574

IV. DISCUSSION

Both acute and chronic colitis are first observed among infants under 6 months of age. More than half the adults have either acute or chronic colitis and in the older adult age group, more than one third have moderate or severe colitis. Thus, the disease occurs early in life and increases in prevalence and severity as age increases in both males and females.

The method of rearing within age groups did not appear to affect the prevalence of colitis. Among adults over 5 years of age, the lower prevalence of acute and chronic colitis in family-reared tamarins could be explained by differences in age. In family-reared adults, the median age was 6.4 years and three quartiles of the population were between 5.5 and 7.1 years. This age distribution was lower and did not overlap with the distributions of wild-caught, colony-inured, or parent-raised animals.

There was no apparent difference in the prevalence of colitis among infants on semipurified or standard diets. A difference would not be expected because animals had been on these diets for only 1 month prior to biopsy. Among juveniles and adults, the numbers of tamarins fed the three semipurified diets was too small to test for significance. It is interesting to observe, however, that the prevalence of colitis among adults fed the semipurified diet A is approximately the same or greater than the prevalence among those fed the standard diet (diet D).

There was poor correlation between endoscopic findings and histologic findings with respect to the presence or absence of colitis and its grade. Two thirds to three quarters of animals who had moderate to severe acute or chronic colitis had no endoscopic abnormality. Thus, it must be concluded that this disease is not manifested on the surface of the colon endoscopically. The weight distribution of tamarins with moderate to severe chronic colitis was higher than those with mild or no colitis, whereas the weight distribution of tamarins with moderate to severe acute colitis was lower than that of animals with mild or no colitis. In each age group, animals with the more severe grades of acute colitis weighed less than animals with no colitis, whereas the weight distribution of those with the more severe grades of chronic colitis encompassed the distribution of animals with no colitis in comparable age groups (data not shown).

V. SUMMARY

Based upon the results of this one-time whole-colony survey of 269 animals, it can be concluded that (1) acute and chronic idiopathic colitis in cotton-top tamarins begins in infancy and becomes progressively more prevalent and severe with age; (2) different types of rearing had no effect on their prevalence; (3) it is too early to determine the effect of two of the semipurified diets, i.e., high fat, low fiber and low fat, high fiber on the prevalence of acute and chronic colitis, but the third semipurified diet (diet A) was associated with a prevalence of colitis equal to or greater than that found in juvenile and adult animals fed the standard diet; (4) the prevalence of acute and chronic colitis was the same in males and females; (5) the presence of moderate to severe acute colitis is associated with lower body weight in adults, but severity of chronic colitis alone appeared not to affect body weight; and (6) there was no correlation between endoscopic findings and the histopathologic findings in biopsies.

ACKNOWLEDGMENTS

This work was supported by a National Institutes of Health Program Project Grant P01AM36350-02 and the New England Regional Primate Research Center base grant RR-00168. The authors express their appreciation for the expert technical assistance provided by Michael J. O'Connell, Monica Mattmuller, Martha Elliott, Paula Brooks, and Mary Beland, and the excellent secretarial assistance provided by Debbie Brosseau.

REFERENCES

1. **King, C. J.,** An investigation into ''Wasting Marmoset Syndrome'' at Jersey Zoo. Extract from the Jersey Wildlife Preservation Trust Thirteenth Annual Report, Isle of Jersey, United Kingdom, 1976.
2. **Richter, C. B., Tankersley, W., and Webb, A.,** Chronic recurrent colitis: a wasting syndrome in marmosets and tamarins (abstr). Twenty-ninth Annual Session of the American Association for Laboratory Animal Science, New York, 1978.
3. **Shwindell, M., Warrington, B. F., and Fowler, J. S. L.,** Dietary habits relating to wasting marmoset syndrome (WMS), *Lab Anim. (London),* 13, 139, 1979.
4. **Chalifoux, L. V., Bronson, R. T., Escajadillo, A., and McKenna, S.,** An analysis of the association of gastroenteric lesions with chronic wasting syndrome of marmosets, *Vet. Pathol.,* 19, 141, 1982.
5. **Madara, J. L., Podolsky, D. K., King, N. W., Sehgal, P. K., Moore, R., and Winter, H. S.,** Characterization of spontaneous colitis in cotton-top tamarins (*Saguinus oedipus*) and its response to sulfasalazine, *Gastroenterology,* 88, 13, 1985.
6. **Madara, J. L.,** Structural characterization of spontaneous colitis in cotton-top tamarins *(Saguinus oedipus), Dig. Dis. Sci.,* 30, 525, 1985.
7. **Chalifoux, L. V., Brieland, J. K., and King, N. W.,** Evolution and natural history of colonic disease in cotton-top tamarins *(Saguinus oedipus), Dig. Dis. Sci.,* 30, 54S, 1985.
8. **Lushbaugh, C. C., Hamason, G. L., Swartzendruber, D. C., Richter, C. B., and Gengozian, N.,** Spontaneous colonic adenocarcinoma in marmosets, *Primates Med.,* 10, 119, 1978.
9. **Swartzendruber, D. C. and Richter, C. B.,** Mucous and argentaffin cells in colonic adenocarcinomas, *Lab. Invest.,* 43, 523, 1980.
10. **Richter, C. B., Lushbaugh, C. C., and Swartzendruber, D. C.,** Cancer of the colon in cotton-top tamarins, in *Comparative Pathology of Zoo Animals,* Montali, R. J. and Migaki, G., Eds., Smithsonian Institution Press, Washington, D.C., 1980, 567.
11. **Chalifoux, L. V. and Bronson, R. T.,** Colonic adenocarcinoma associated with chronic colitis in cotton-top marmosets, *(Saguinus oedipus), Gastroenterology,* 80, 942, 1981.
12. **Clapp, N. K., Henke, M. A., Halloway, E. C., and Tankersley, W. G.,** Carcinoma of the colon in the cotton-top tamarin: a radiographic study, *J. Am. Vet. Med. Assoc.,* 183, 1328, 1983.
13. **Lushbaugh, C. C., Humason, G., and Clapp, N.,** Histology of colon cancer in *Saguinus oedipus oedipus, Dig. Dis. Sci.,* 30, 119S, 1985.
14. The Committee on Diet, Nutrition, and Cancer of the National Academy of Science, Lipids (fats and cholesterol), in *Diet Nutrition, and Cancer,* National Academy Press, Washington, D.C., 1982, 73.
15. The Committee on Diet, Nutrition, and Cancer of the National Academy of Science, Dietary fiber, in *Diet, Nutrition, and Cancer,* National Academy Press, Washington, D.C., 1982, 130.

Chapter 6

AN ANTIGENIC PROFILE IN COTTON-TOP TAMARINS — *Saguinus oedipus* — A MODEL FOR HUMAN INFLAMMATORY BOWEL DISEASE AND COLORECTAL CANCER

Martin Tobi, Sreeniwas Chintalapani, Vijaya Kaila, Karel Kithier, Marsha A. Henke, and Neal K. Clapp

TABLE OF CONTENTS

0-8493-5363-7/93/$0.00 + $.50

I. INTRODUCTION

Of the many challenges facing Western medicine, few are more urgent than the need to reduce the mortality from colorectal cancer (CRC) and more confounding than the elucidation of the pathogenesis of idiopathic colitis. These two elusive goals are intertwined, in that a well-recognized predisposition to colorectal cancer exists in individuals with long-standing colitis.[1] Both of these problems could be addressed by the existence of a suitable naturally occurring animal model.

The cotton-top tamarin (CTT) seems to answer many of the requirements of such a model. The effort in maintaining the few existing research colonies is considerable but may be cost-effective when one considers the toll taken both in human lives lost and the deterioration of the quality thereof. The questions that urgently demand an answer are what the biological similarities of these two diseases between *Homo sapiens* and a lower-order primate, *Saguinus oedipus,* and may scientific research data in one be extrapolated to the other?

Tumor markers for the detection of gastrointestinal cancer and as adjunct to therapy have been described but they are far from ideal.[2] Some of these markers have been evaluated in the setting of human inflammatory bowel disease (IBD).[3-5] Few have been investigated in both humans and tamarins.[6-8] Immunologically defined markers are therefore a potential means to discover antigens shared by these two species and are the subject of this chapter.

Monoclonal antibody (MAb) technology[9] provides a specific means of determining antigenic expression. Immunohistochemistry (IHC) is a popular and convenient method for such studies but, used alone, does not provide information on native antigens, is difficult to quantify, and presents many analytic pitfalls.[10] The work presented does not rely solely on IHC but includes observations on fresh-frozen biopsy tissue from tamarins.

Recently, it has become evident that much useful information about gastrointestinal antigen expression can be gained by examining colonic washings. This method has been used to quantify secreted immunoglobulins.[11,12] Cells shed into this effluent can be examined both by Papanicolaou staining[13] and when combined with IHC, increases the sensitivity for the diagnosis of CRC.[14] Shed antigens[15] can also be evaluated both quantitatively[4,5,16] and qualitatively.[17,18] This method has not yet been applied to tamarins but may confer important information regarding the spectrum of shed gastrointestinal antigens in this model.

This pilot study of tumor antigen expression in the CTT, which exclusively develops CRC following colitis, sheds light on the similarities with humans and offers the means to select potentially useful markers to evaluate the utility of the model with respect to the study of human colonic disease.

II. MATERIALS AND METHODS

A. TAMARIN TISSUES

These were available in three forms:

1. **Paraffin-embedded fixed tissue sections** — post-mortem specimens taken from 15 animals dying of colitis, CRC, or unrelated disorders were formalin-fixed and full-thickness colonic 4-μm sections were cut from the paraffin blocks for IHC. All these animals had an ante-mortem colonoscopic biopsy-proven diagnosis of colitis. The features of CTT colitis have previously been described.[19]
2. **Colonoscopic pinch biopsies** — these were taken by biopsy-forceps and immediately frozen in physiologic buffer for processing to produce a membrane-enriched extract (MEE) as previously described.[17] Briefly, tissue was homogenized and clarified by low-speed (1500 × *g*) centrifugation. The supernatant was sonicated and subjected to a higher-speed centrifugation (10,000 × *g*) and the supernatant which constituted the MEE assayed for protein using the Lowry method.[20] Colonoscopy in tamarins has been described previously.[21]
3. **Post-mortem tissues** — these were taken at necropsy and frozen in physiological buffer. The MEEs were performed as described above. The results derived from these latter two methods were combined for convenience and reported together. Half these animals were deceased and in these, paraffin-embedded tissues were also available.

B. TAMARIN COLONIC WASHINGS

These were obtained precolonoscopically and frozen immediately. A Lowry protein assay was performed upon thawing after clarification by centrifugation to serve as a standard for the antigen determinations to follow. All animals had colitis, though they varied in degree and extent of disease. No other tissues were available in this group of animals, with one exception.

C. HUMAN COLONIC WASHINGS

These were collected precolonoscopically after the patients had been prepared using a semiliquid diet and cathartics.[17] Effluent samples were processed and protein content was determined as above. These were collected randomly from a substantial number of patients undergoing endoscopy for a variety of indications. For the purposes of this study, effluent material was selected from a group of patients with IBD and a group with no macroscopically evident lesions were considered "normal".

D. IMMUNOHISTOCHEMISTRY

All specimens were evaluated by routine histology and 4-μm sections stained with a variety of MAbs. The avidin-biotin-peroxidase complex (ABC) technique of Hsu et al.[22] was employed, using a kit purchased from Vector Laboratories (Burlingame, CA). The substrate was nickel-enhanced diaminobenzidine (DAB). Positive controls were taken from human tissue sections known to react positively with the MAb used. Negative controls constituted nonimmune mouse serum used in place of the primary MAb.

E. QUALITATIVE ENZYME-LINKED IMMUNOSORBENT ASSAY (ELISA)

Samples were incubated overnight at 5 μg protein per well in 96-well microtiter plates (Nunc, Denmark), washed, and then blocked by 5% bovine serum albumin (BSA) (Sigma, St. Louis, MO). The MAbs were applied at a concentration determined by titration to confer the best result. After further washing, the appropriate goat anti-mouse alkaline phosphatase conjugate was applied, and after a final washing step, a color reaction using *p*-nitrophenyl phosphate substrate (Sigma) was developed and read on an ELISA plate-reader (Dynatech) at 30 min. For each sample, the background was obtained by substituting nonimmune mouse immunoglobulins for the primary MAb and completing the assay as above. The final results were obtained by subtracting the mean background binding from the mean binding of the sample treated with the MAb of interest. All results are reported in A^{405}/5 μg protein. Both colonic washings and MEEs were assayed by this method.

F. MONOCLONAL ANTIBODIES AND QUANTITATIVE DETERMINATIONS

1. Carcinoembryonic Antigen (CEA)

CEA is the best studied of all the colonic antigens in man. It is a 180-kDa glycoprotein member of the immunoglobulin supergene family[23] and is anchored to the cell membrane via a glycosylphosphatidylinositol moiety thought to have an important function in intercellular adhesion.[24,25] In animals, CEA has been sought after but only cross-reactive CEA-like, related gene-family entities have been described,[26-28] the latter two in monkeys and great apes. For IHC, T84.66, a highly specific MAb was used (a kind gift of Drs. J. Shively and S. Hefta, Beckman Research Institute, Duarte, CA). In the ELISA, MAbs recognizing common nonspecific cross-reacting antigen (NCA) and CEA were used (also obtained from the Beckman Research Institute). To confirm binding and provide quantitative levels of CEA in tissues and washings, a number of quantitative kits were used. Three of these commercially available kits (Roche™, Abbott™, Tosoh Medics) were based on monoclonal antibodies, one of which (Roche™) actually uses the T84.66 MAb used here for IHC. For human washings a polyclonal kit (Pharmatope DPC, Sweden) was used. Previous work has shown a good correlation between mono- and polyclonal CEA kits,[29] but caution should always be applied when attempting to correlate CEA levels determined by different kits, regardless of antibodies used.[30] Therefore, the same samples and standards were tested with both the

Abbott™ and Roche™ kits as a preliminary measure before embarking on this study. The results showed an excellent correlation (r = 0.99).

2. SPan-1

This MAb, developed and kindly provided by the laboratory of Dr. Y. S. Kim (V.A. Medical Center, University of California at San Francisco), appears to react with sialylated antigenic determinants in mucin species of high molecular weight.[31] It is important to evaluate mucin antigens in that alterations in mucins have been described both in colitis and CRC.[32,33] Although the CA19-9 antigen has been more fully characterized than that defined by SPan-1 and shares biological properties with it,[34] we and others have not found CA19-9 helpful in the setting of IBD in man.[3,5] Furthermore, CA19-9 staining has been reported to be negative in both cancerous and normal tissues of CTTs.[8]

3. CaCo 3/61

It is appropriate to evaluate a marker known to occur in mammalian species. For this reason the carbohydrate antigens (fucosylated aminoproteoglycans) defined by this MAb was selected for study in that it is oncodevelopmental in nature in rats.[35] It was raised using the CaCo2 CRC cell line as immunogen. The antibody was kindly provided by Dr. A. Quaroni (SUNY, Ithaca, NY). This MAb shows reactivity with most human CRC cell lines against which it was tested. It typically stains the cell membranes of crypt cells of the jejunum in rats and man.

III. RESULTS

A. IMMUNOHISTOCHEMISTRY

Sections from 15 tamarins were stained and the data is summarized in Table 1. Approximately one third of the animals examined died as a direct result of CRC, consistent with the reported prevalence.[36] CEA staining with T84.66 MAb was negative in all specimens. SPan-1 staining was present in one fifth of sections, and was noted to be focal in nature, staining isolated goblet cells. Heterogeneous CaCo 3/61 staining was positive in 100% of tissues stained. It was focal (+) and limited in some of the specimens, but others stained strongly (+ + + to + + + +). This evaluation mainly applies to the normal-appearing mucosa. A representative CaCo 3/61 stained specimen is shown in Figure 1. The distribution of staining in the tissues was similar to the staining in human jejunal tissues.[35] No correlation was seen between tissue staining intensity in the normal-appearing mucosa and the presence of CRC in these animals (2/6 which stained maximally bore CRC elsewhere in the colon compared to 3/9 which stained to a lesser degree). However, when the degree of colitis is considered, that is, acute colitis, which has been

TABLE 1
Immunohistochemistry on Normal-Appearing Tamarin Tissue

Code	Clinical data	CEA[a]	SPan-1	CaCo 3/61
Mo 4692	Chronic colitis	−	−	+ +
Mo 5787	Died <1 year, chronic colitis	−	−	+ + + +
Mo 4984	Cancer, acute colitis	−	−	+ + + +
Mo 5820	Chronic colitis at death	−	−	+ focal
Mo 5240	Chronic colitis at death	−	+ + focal	+ +
Mo 4524	Acute colitis	−	−	+
Mo 3097	Chronic colitis	−	+	+ + + +
Mo 1668	Acute colitis	−	−	+ + + +
Mo 3060	Chronic colitis	−	−	+ + +
Mo 4408	Cancer, chronic colitis	−	−	+ focal
Mo 4615	Acute colitis	−	−	+ + + +
Mo 1666	Cancer, acute colitis	−	−	±
Fo 4418	Acute colitis	−	−	+ focal
Fo 5461	Cancer, acute colitis	−	+ focal	+ focal
Fo 3216	Cancer, acute colitis	−	−	+ + + +

[a] CEA, Carcinoembryonic antigen as stained for with monoclonal antibody T84.66.

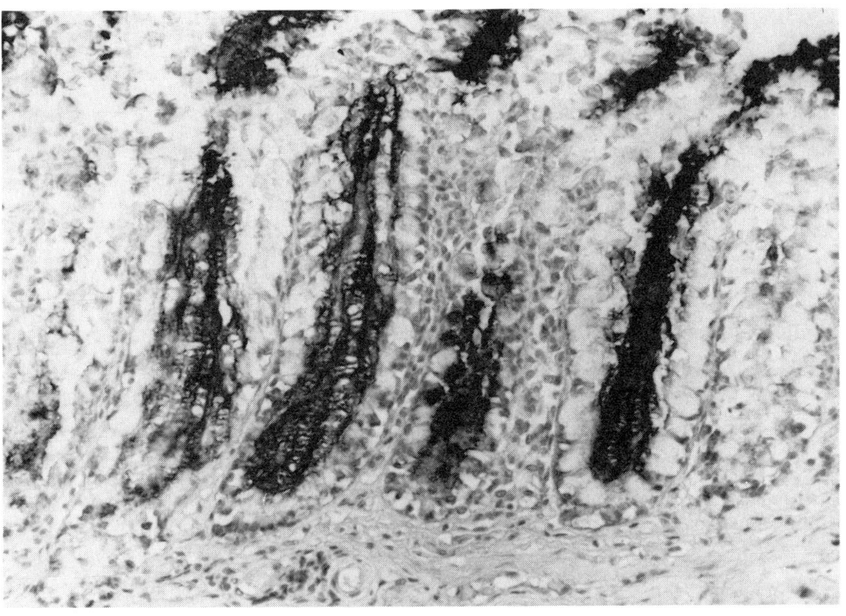

FIGURE 1. Immunohistochemistry in a cotton-top tamarin using CaCo 3/61 monoclonal antibody. Numerous glands in the normal-appearing epithelium show positive reaction by staining black with nickel-enhanced diaminobenzidine used as substrate. The distribution of the binding is mainly in the luminal cell surface and contents of colonic glands which may extend down, but are not necessarily limited, to the deepest regions of the crypt (magnification × 331).

TABLE 2
Antibody Binding in Tamarins and Man

Sample (*N*)	CEA	SPan-1	CaCo 3/61
Tamarin extract (9)	<1 ($N = 7$)	0.010 ± 0.016	0.416 ± 0.236
Tamarin IBD washing (11)	<1	0.091 ± 0.034	0.107 ± 0.056
Human IBD washing (12)	664 ± 924	0.054 ± 0.059	0.261 ± 0.181
Human Nl washing (14)	431 ± 449	0.150 ± 0.058	0.444 ± 0.658

Note: As quantified by both Abbott™ and Roche™ kits, all carcinoembryonic antigen (CEA) results are expressed in ng/ml and remainder of antibody binding in A^{405}/ 5 μg protein; *N*, number; IBD, inflammatory bowel disease; N1, normal.

associated with the development of CRC in these animals,[6] the staining in sections from CTTs with associated CRC showed maximal staining in 50% ($N = 4$).

B. QUALITATIVE ELISA IN TAMARIN TISSUE EXTRACTS AND WASHINGS

Extracts — The results are summarized in Table 2. Overall, binding of CEA in extracts was very poor as measured by anti-CEA or -NCA MAbs and, therefore, we resorted to measuring levels quantitatively in extracts and washings. SPan-1 binding was only minimally positive in 3/9 extracts from 8 animals, none of which were derived from cancerous tissues. One tamarin had cancer elsewhere in the colon, and the extract made from the corresponding cancerous tissue did not show binding. CaCo 3/61 binding was positive in all extracts. Binding levels were somewhat higher in cancer than in the normal extracts, suggesting a tendency for higher levels in cancer tissues, but the numbers are too small to allow for a definite conclusion.

Washings — Eleven samples from 10 tamarins with colitis and one with cancer were initially tested and showed little increase over the background when using anti-CEA antibodies. Hence, quantitative levels were determined (see below) and results are shown in Table 2. All washings showed moderate binding of SPan-1 overall which was somewhat higher in the washings from animals with acute as compared to chronic colitis. Greater numbers will be needed before confirming the suggestion of higher levels in the acute inflammatory state. Similar levels of binding were seen with CaCo 3/61 but no differences with disease activity were apparent.

C. QUANTITATIVE CEA LEVELS AND MAb BINDING IN HUMANS

As seen in Table 2, CEA levels were insubstantial in both tamarin extracts ($N = 7$) and washings ($N = 11$), when measured with Roche and Abbott Kits. These negative results correlate with IHC CEA staining. However, levels of >100 ng/ml were obtained when using the Tosoh Medics kit in all washings tested. CEA levels in extracts were not evaluated by the Tosoh Medics kit.

Levels in human washings from both "normal" and patients with IBD are also shown in Table 2, consistent with previously reported results,[4,16,18] with a somewhat broad range. For comparison, SPan-1 and CaCo 3/61 mean binding in human IBD washings are also shown. The wide variation here precludes an effective comparison, but CaCo 3/61 binding is lowest in tamarin washings. The higher levels seen in the "normal" human washings as compared to the IBD cases are probably a result of using protein as the standard and the mucin depletion usually seen in the colonic mucosa of IBD patients.[5]

IV. DISCUSSION

This study shows that an antigenic profile in the tamarin may differ from the human, depending upon the method of detection. However, aside from CEA, the expression of mucin and carbohydrate antigens tested compare favorably and may be used as biological markers. Quantitative CEA levels in tissues, circulating blood, and colonic washings tend to be higher in patients with IBD,[4] but are not useful in the diagnosis of the disease nor as a portent for CRC. Two commercially available kits show very low levels of CEA in tamarin tissue and colonic washings. However, one kit tested only with the colonic effluent shows substantial CEA levels. To resolve whether it is the 180-kDa species which is detected in these animals, Western blotting will need to be performed. This notwithstanding, if a CEA-like moiety shared by tamarins and man is detectable, this may provide a means of testing for its presence and hence enable us to elucidate its importance in the clinical setting of IBD and CRC in both species. The existence of such a species would not be surprising, since there is evidence for CEA-like antigens in great apes, lower-order Old World primates, rats, and mice.[26-28,37]

In the past, although important qualitative biochemical changes have been described in mucins from CRC and IBD patients with respect to the normal,[32,33] immunologic testing for mucin antigens has not been diagnostic.[3,5] CA19-9 has been the vanguard of mucin-associated antigens, but despite promise shown in the area of pancreatic cancer diagnosis and management,[38] is disappointing in the setting of IBD and CRC. CA19-9 staining (sialylated-Le^a) is negative in CTT tissues as well as that for the Le^x antigen, although staining for the Le^b antigen may be positive.[8] SPan-1 seems to share many features with CA19-9, but unlike CA19-9, can be detected in Le^a-Le^b- individuals. In this preliminary work, SPan-1 binding in tissue extracts did not correlate with the presence of CRC in the tamarin, but washings tended to show somewhat higher mean binding values in the presence of acute inflammation. Since alterations in mucin may be associated with the development of CRC in these animals, a mucin constituent such as SPan-1 may prove to be an important indicator of the premalignant state. That another cancer-derived tumor carbohydrate marker recognized by the CaCo 3/61 antibody did not show this tendency underscores the fact that SPan-1 and other mucin antigens may indeed fulfill an important role in the early detection of CRC in this setting. This is further supported by lectin binding in normal tamarin colonic tissue sections, which showed a significant correlation with the presence of CRC when using peanut agglutinin.[6] The reason for the lower binding of SPan-1 in the tissue extracts is not clear but may be related to the use of protein as a standard.[5] Another plausible explanation is that the SPan-1-defined antigen may percolate to the colon from an upper gastrointestinal source such as pancreatic secretions. Clearly, the SPan-1-defined antigen is shed into colonic washings in both tamarins and man, and lessons learned from its expression and shedding may be applicable to both.

Another antigen that appears to be common to the tamarin and man is defined by MAb CaCo 3/61. Since this carbohydrate antigen has been described developmentally in the rat and man,[35] it is not altogether surprising that it is found in the tissues and washings of the tamarin. Although it is tumor derived and clearly shared by these mammalian species, it has not proven to be useful in early detection of cancer or diagnosis of IBD.

Staining with CaCo 3/61 is positive in rat jejunal crypt cells and predominantly binds to membranes. In the colon, staining is present only in the fetal and neonatal stages. In dimethylhydrazine-induced rat tumors focal staining of variable location was described in half the tumors, mainly in the less-differentiated lesions. In humans, despite a majority of human colon cancer cell lines showing binding, human colonic mucosa (unlike normal jejunal tissue) did not show staining.[39] In diseased colonic tissues, focal staining was seen only in adenocarcinoma, a single polyp, and the transitional mucosa near a sigmoid adenocarcinoma. No staining was seen in four normal specimens, one case of ulcerative colitis, and two cases of Crohn's disease.[35] In contrast, all tamarin tissues had some degree of CaCo 3/61 staining. Clearly, it is difficult to make a direct comparison between these three species, as differing populations in each were assessed using different methods. In the CTT some staining was present in all animals, while overall maximal staining was present in 40% of all cases of acute and chronic colitis. Acute colitis was associated with the greatest number of CRC in this study (80%) but the proportion of intense CaCo 3/61 staining was similar (50% with vs. 40% without CRC). This data correlates well with those of CaCo 3/61 binding in washings. If we accept that colonic expression of CaCo 3/61 is oncodevelopmental for the tamarin and man, as it is for the rat, and at least one sample of transitional mucosa in man showed staining, then its presence in the tamarin is significant. In these animals, where better than one third will develop colon cancer, it may be speculated that CaCo 3/61 staining may be a marker reflecting the existence of a premalignant state.

Extracts derived from cancer tissues appear to have higher CaCo 3/61 binding in the tamarin, but further testing will be needed to confirm this. This antibody may also show binding in benign tissues and cancers of the small bowel in man.[35,40] The lower binding in the washings of tamarins as compared to the extracts may be explained by the fact that this MAb recognizes a crypt antigen which may not be as easily shed into the effluent as an antigen on the surface epithelium.

A broad selection of MAbs for the evaluation of shared tamarin and human colonic epitopes exists[10] and a judicious selection method may be necessary. Although no evidence for an infectious etiology for tamarin colitis has been found,[19,41] tamarins show aberrant responses to viral infections.[42] It may therefore be expedient to search for retroviral oncogene products or corresponding genetic polymorphisms implicated in human CRC[43] in these animals. Other examples of shared human and tamarin antigenic determinants already evaluated and found to be common to both species are a cross-reactive colonic ulcerative colitis antigen confined to the tamarin colon[7] and the CRC reactive MAb, BR 55.2.[44]

Finally, there are the categories of growth factors and differentiation antigens. While an exhaustive discussion of these is beyond the scope of this chapter, these are areas that should be researched. The relevance of gastrin to CRC and other hormones,[45] as well as epidermal growth factor and its receptor,[46] should be investigated in the CTT. Adnab-9 MAb recognizes a subpopulation of cells within benign colorectal adenomas that are absent in colorectal cancer.[47] The antigen recognized may be an early tumor marker, in that preliminary data suggest that it may be useful in the diagnosis of early-stage CRC in humans.[17] We are continuing our study using antibodies reactive with some of these antigens and hope to shed further light on the question of CTT colitis and cancer as a relevant model for the human disease.

ACKNOWLEDGMENTS

The authors wish to thank Drs. L. E. Nochomovitz and W. Sakr for reviewing histology, Drs. W. M. Steinberg, N. Trujillo, and D. O'Kieffe for clinical material, Greta van Heerden for providing immunologic reagents, E. Darmon and A. P. Spence for technical assistance and expertise. We are also grateful to Dr. M. Ehrinpreis for his comments in reviewing the manuscript and D. Farrah for expert typographical assistance.

REFERENCES

1. **Alpert, M. B. and Nochomovitz, L. E.,** Dysplasia and cancer surveillance in inflammatory bowel disease, *Gastroenterol. Clin. North Am.*, 18(1), 83, 1989.
2. **Solitzeanu, D.,** Human cancer-associated antigens: present status and implications for immunodiagnosis, *Adv. Cancer Res.*, 44, 1, 1985.
3. **Frykholm, G., Enblad, P., Pahlman, L., and Busch, C.,** Expression of the carcinoma-associated antigens CA19-9 and CA50 in inflammatory bowel disease, *Dis. Colon Rect.*, 30, 545, 1987.

4. **Vellacott, K. D., Groom, D., Balfour, T. W., Baldwin, R. W., and Hardcastle, J. D.,** Tumor associated products in colonic lavage fluid, *Clin. Oncol.*, 8, 61, 1982.
5. **Tobi, M., Steinberg, W., Henry, J., and Nochomovitz, L. E.,** Cancer associated antigen CA19-9 in colonic effluent of patients with neoplasia of the colon and inflammatory bowel disease, *Cancer Lett.*, 60, 19, 1991.
6. **Boland, C. R. and Clapp, N. K.,** Glycoconjugates in the colons of new world monkeys with spontaneous colitis: association between inflammation and neoplasia, *Gastroenterology,* 92, 625, 1987.
7. **Das, K. M., Vecchi, M., Sakamaki, S., and Clapp, N. K.,** Ulcerative colitis in humans and spontaneous colitis in tamarins: a common link through a crossreactive colonic antigen, *Gastroenterology,* 92, 1363, 1987.
8. **Steplewski, Z.,** Monclonal antibody-defined antigens detected in colonic tissues of cotton-top tamarin, Saguinus oedipus oedipus, *Dig. Dis. Sci.*, 30, 141S, 1985.
9. **Kohler, G. and Milstein, C.,** Continuous cultures of fused cells secreting antibodies of predetermined specificity, *Nature,* 256, 495, 1975.
10. **Arends, J. W., Bowman, F. T., and Hilgers, J.,** Tissue antigens in large bowel carcinoma, *Biochim. Biophys. Acta,* 780, 1, 1985.
11. **Gaspari, M. M., Brennan, P. T., Solomon, S. M., and Elson, C. O.,** A method of obtaining, processing, and analyzing human intestinal secretions for antibody content, *J. Immunol. Meth.*, 110, 85, 1988.
12. **O'Mahony, S., Barton, J. R., Crichton, S., and Ferguson, A.,** Appraisal of gut lavage in the study of intestinal humoral immunity, *Gut,* 31, 1341, 1990.
13. **Gordon, I. L., Rypins, E. B., and Wuerker, R. B.,** Cytologic detection of colorectal cancer after administration of oral gut lavage solution, *Cancer,* 68, 106, 1991.
14. **Rozen, P., Tobi, M., Darmon, E., and Kaufman, L.,** Colonic cytology: a simplified method of collection and initial results, *Acta Cytol.*, 34, 627, 1990.
15. **Black, P. H.,** Cell surface shedding, *Adv. Cancer Res.*, 32, 75, 1980.
16. **Winawer, S. J., Fleischer, M., Green, S. et al.,** Carcinoembryonic antigen in colonic lavage, *Gastroenterology,* 92, 719, 1977.
17. **Tobi, M., Darmon, E., Phillips, T. et al.,** Increased expression of a putative adenoma association antigen in precolonoscopic effluent of patients with colorectal cancer, *Cancer Lett.*, 50, 21, 1990.
18. **Darmon, E., Tobi, M., and Rozen, P.,** Newer tests, on the colonic effluent, for identifying persons with colorectal neoplasia, in *Advances in Large Bowel Cancer: Policy, Prevention and Treatment, Frontiers of Gastrointestinal Research,* Rozen, P., Reich, C. B., and Winawer, S. J., Eds., S. Karger, Basel, 1990, chap. 18.
19. **Lushbaugh, C. C., Humason, G. L., and Clapp, N. K.,** Histology of colon cancer in Saguinus oedipus oedipus, *Dig. Dis. Sci.*, 30, 119S, 1985.
20. **Lowry, O. H., Rosenbrough, N. J., Farr, A. L., and Randall, R. J.,** Protein measurements with folin phenol reagent, *J. Biol. Chem.*, 193, 265, 1951.
21. **Clapp, N. K., McArthur, A. H., Carson, R. L., Henke, M. A., Peck, O. C., and Wood, J. D.,** Visualization and biopsy of the colon in tamarins and marmosets by endoscopy: a promising technique, *Lab Anim. Sci.*, 27, 217, 1987.
22. **Hsu, S. M., Raine, L., and Fanger, V.,** Use of avidin-biotin-peroxidase complex (ABC) in immunoperoxidase techniques: a comparison between ABC and unlabeled antibody (PA) procedures, *J. Histochem.*, 21, 577, 1981.
23. **Paxton, R. J., Mooser, G., Rande, H., Lee, T. D., and Shively, J. E.,** Sequence analysis of carcinoembryonic antigen: identification of glycosylation sites and homology with the immunoglobulin supergene family, *Cancer Res.*, 84, 920, 1987.
24. **Benchimol, S., Fuks, A., Jothy, S., Beauchemin, N., Shirota, K., and Stanners, C. P.,** Carcinoembryonic antigen, a human tumor marker, functions as an intercellular adhesion molecule, *Cell,* 57, 327, 1989.

25. **Hefta, S., Hefta, L. J. F., Lee, T. D., Paxton, R. J., and Shively, J. E.,** Carcinoembryonic antigen is anchored to membranes by covalent attachment to a glycosylphophatidylinositol moiety: identification of the ethanolamine linkage site, *Proc. Natl. Acad. Sci. U.S.A.*, 85, 4648, 1988.
26. **Beauchemin, N., Turbide, C., Afar, D., Bell, J., Raymond, M., Stanners, C. P., and Fuks, A.,** A mouse analogue of human carcinoembryonic antigen, *Cancer Res.*, 49, 2017, 1989.
27. **Engvall, F., Vuento, M., and Rooslahti, E.,** A monkey antigen cross-reacting with carcinoembryonic antigen CEA, *Br. J. Cancer,* 34, 341, 1976.
28. **Haagensen, D. E., Jr., Metzgar, R. S., Swenson, B., Dilley, W. G., Cox, C. E., Davis, S., Murdoch, J., Zamcheck, N., and Wells, S. A.,** Carcinoembryonic antigen in nonhuman primates, *J. Natl. Cancer Inst.*, 69, 1073, 1982.
29. **Fleuren, H. and van Oers, R.,** Comparison of monoclonal and polyclonal enzyme immunoassays for carcinoembryonic antigen, *J. Clin. Chem. Clin. Biochem.*, 24, 741, 1986.
30. **von Kleist, S.,** Colorectal cancer, *Tumor Biol.*, 8, 78, 1987.
31. **Ho, S. B., Toribaraz, N. W., Bresalier, R. S., and Kim, Y. S.,** Biochemical and other markers of colon cancer, *Gastroenterol. Clin. North Am.*, 17, 811, 1988.
32. **Boland, C. R., Montgomery, C. K. and Kim, Y. S.,** Alterations in colonic mucin structure in differentiation and malignant transformation, *Proc. Natl. Acad. Sci. U.S.A.*, 79, 2051, 1982.
33. **Podolsky, D. K. and Isselbacher, K. J.,** Composition of human colonic mucin selective alteration in inflammatory bowel disease, *J. Clin. Invest.*, 72, 142, 1983.
34. **Schmiegel, W.,** Tumor markers in pancreatic cancer — current concepts, *Hepatogastroenterology,* 36, 446, 1989.
35. **Quaroni, A., Weiser, M. M., Lee, S., and Amodeo, D.,** Expression of developmentally regulated crypt cell antigens in human and rat intestinal tumors, *J. Natl. Cancer Inst.*, 77, 405, 1986.
36. **Clapp, N. K., Lushbaugh, C. C., Humason, G. L., Gangaware, B. L., and Henke, M. A.,** The marmoset as a model of ulcerative colitis and colon cancer, in *Colorectal Cancer and Its Precursors,* Ingalls, J. F. and Mastromarino, A., Eds., Allen R. Liss, New York, 1985, 247.
37. **Zimmerman, W. and Thompson, J.,** Recent developments concerning the carcinoembryonic antigen gene family and their clinical implications, *Tumor Biol.*, 11, 1, 1990.
38. **Steinberg, W., Gelfand, R., Anderson, K. A., Glenn, J., Kurtzman, S. H., Sindelar, W. F., and Toskes, P. P.,** Comparison of the sensitivity and specificity of the CA19-9 and carcinoembryonic antigen assays in detecting cancer of the pancreas, *Gastroenterology,* 90, 343, 1986.
39. **Quaroni, A.,** Crypt cell antigen in human colon tumor cell lines: analysis with a panel of monoclonal antibodies to CaCo-2 luminal membrane components, *J. Natl. Cancer Inst.*, 76, 571, 1986.
40. **Tobi, M. et al.,** An antigenic profile of adenocarcinoma of the small bowel: evidence for an adenoma-carcinoma sequence, *Am. Assoc. Cancer Res.*, 33, 96, 1992.
41. **Moore, R.,** Nonviral infectious agents and marmoset (Saguinus oedipus) colitis, *Dig. Dis. Sci.*, 30, 69S, 1985.
42. **Klein, E. and Musucci, M. G.,** Cell-mediated immunity against Epstein-Barr virus infected B lymphocytes, *Springer Semin. Immunopathol.*, 5, 63, 1982.
43. **Fearon, E. R. and Vogelstein, B.,** A genetic model for colorectal tumorigenesis, *Cell,* 61, 759, 1990.
44. **Lawless, B. D., Lee, Y. C., Fuhr, J. E., Clapp, N. K., and Crook, J. E.,** Colon cancer cells in peripheral blood of cancerous tamarins, *Clin. Immunol. Immunopathol.*, 48, 338, 1988.

45. **Morris, D. L., Watson, S. A., Durrant, L. G., and Harrison, J. D.,** Hormonal control of gastric and colorectal cancer in man, *Gut,* 30, 4254, 1989.
46. **Rodeck, U., Williams, N., Murthy, U., and Herlyn, M.,** Monoclonal antibody 425 inhibits growth stimulation of carcinoma cells by exogenous EGF and tumor-derived EGF/TGF-alpha, *J. Cell Biochem.,* 44, 69, 1990.
47. **Tobi, M., Maliakkal, B. J., Alousi, M. A., Voruganti, V., Shafiuddin, M., An, T., Fliegel, S. E. M., Yang, S., Gesell, M. S., Hatfield, J., Kaila, V., Goo, R., and Luk, G. D.,** Cellular distribution of a colonic adenoma-associated antigen as defined by monoclonal antibody adnab-9, *Scand. J. Gastroenterol.,* 27, 737, 1992.

Chapter 7

EXTRAINTESTINAL MANIFESTATIONS OF COTTON-TOP TAMARIN COLITIS

Bryan F. Warren, Marsha A. Henke, and Neal K. Clapp

TABLE OF CONTENTS

0-8493-5363-7/93/$0.00 + $.50

I. INTRODUCTION

Human idiopathic ulcerative colitis has many associated extraintestinal manifestations in the liver, blood, skin, bones and joints, and eyes, along with occasional bronchopulmonary, cardiovascular, and renal complications.[1] Study of these conditions has been severely hampered due to the lack of an animal model with both colitis and the extraintestinal manifestations.

The spontaneously occurring idiopathic colitis of the cotton-top tamarin bears close relationship to ulcerative colitis in man, clinically, endoscopically, histologically, and in its response to treatment. Finding such extraintestinal manifestations in the cotton-top tamarin (CTT) would strengthen its position as a model of human ulcerative colitis. The authors are not aware of any previous recognition or evaluation of these features in the cotton-top tamarin, nor are we aware of any demonstration of the extraintestinal manifestations of inflammatory bowel disease in any animal model system.

II. COMPLICATIONS BY ORGAN/SYSTEM IN MAN AND TAMARIN

A. LIVER

1. Human

The liver complications that may occur in human ulcerative colitis are found in about 5 to 6% of cases[2] and include a variety of histological features, incuding fatty liver, pericholangitis, sclerosing cholangitis, cholangiocarcinoma, hepatic abscesses, and cirrhosis.

Fatty liver is the most common and mildest hepatic abnormality found in inflammatory bowel disease (IBD) and, in one series, has been seen in up to 45% of patients coming to colectomy with ulcerative colitis and in association with mild periportal chronic inflammation or pericholangitis.[3-5] This early change may be related to the more serious condition of sclerosing cholangitis.[6] Cirrhosis is found very rarely (1 to 5%).

The most sinister liver manifestation of long-standing total ulcerative colitis in man is sclerosing cholangitis. There is a close association with IBD in that 70% of patients with sclerosing cholangitis will have ulcerative colitis.[1] This change occurs as a progressive sclerosis of both extra- and intrahepatic bile ducts for which no effective treatment has been found.

Sclerosing cholangitis is progressive periportal fibrosis of unknown cause in man, but its association with ulcerative colitis is very strong. It is found in 5% of most series of chronic ulcerative colitis. The abnormal findings in man are usually jaundice with greatly elevated alkaline phosphatase. Although the biopsy findings are not always specific, the radiological picture of multiple stricturing and dilatation of intra- and extrahepatic bile ducts is characteristic. The characteristic histological findings are of dense concentric submucosal fibrosis of bile ducts with enlargement of portal tracts, chronic inflammation, and bile duct proliferation. As the disease progresses, fibrosis becomes the predominant component with extension of tongues of connective tissue into the periportal liver parenchyma, and eventually fibrous septae may link portal tracts.

The suggested possible causes of sclerosing cholangitis have previously fallen into three main groups: chronic low-grade portal infection,[7] a reaction to toxic bile acids in the diseased colon,[8] or a possible previous infection.[9] Most recently, genetic susceptibility has been considered to be important in the pathogenesis of this condition. Evidence for this comes from family studies and from finding increased expression of the HLA-B8 and -DR3 in patients with sclerosing cholangitis. The finding of increased HLA expression and the presence of increased circulating immune complexes in the blood along with circulating autoantibodies against colonic epithelium support this concept.[9,10] A more balanced view is probably of a genetic susceptibility to an immune-mediated process which is triggered by an unknown environmental factor.

Other hepatic complications have included cholangiocarcinoma and hepatic abscesses.[11] Such abscesses are extremely rare, are seen in association with multiple intra-abdominal abscesses, and are usually fatal.[12] Granulomas and amyloidosis have also been observed.[1]

2. Tamarin

Post-mortem livers were examined from 100 cotton-top tamarins with severe total colitis. All livers were fixed in 10% buffered formalin solution within one hour of death. Tissues were processed routinely, sectioned at 2 μm, and stained with hematoxylin and eosin. These tamarins were considered to be pathogen-free, and their colons had a histological picture resembling human ulcerative colitis rather than infective colitis.

Sixty livers had pathological changes and 40 livers were histologically normal. The most interesting change was that of excessive periportal fibrosis in the presence of very little inflammation but with some abnormal small bile ducts at the edge of the portal tracts — a picture resembling human sclerosing cholangitis.

Mild periportal chronic inflammation (pericholangitis) was seen in 20 cases. Generalized steatosis was present in 16 cases; chronic active hepatitis was a feature in 4 cases. Massive hepatic abscesses involving most of the liver volume were found in 4 tamarins. Minor liver abnormalities not known to be associated with inflammatory bowel disease were present in 12 livers.

Both periportal and perivenous inflammation have been seen on review of post-mortem liver histology from cotton-top tamarins with long-standing total colitis who underwent necropsy within one hour of death. A histological appearance resembling cirrhosis in man was seen in only one cotton-top tamarin. A picture similar to sclerosing cholangitis with predominant periportal fibrosis was seen in 4 animals.

B. BONE AND JOINT

1. Human

Ulcerative colitis in man is often associated with a peripheral arthropathy (2 to 23%),[13] which usually parallels the gastrointestinal disease activity and affects knees, hips, ankles, wrists, and elbows. This disease usually presents as an arthralgia of insidious onset but occasionally may manifest itself as an acute arthropathy. Recurrence is common. A similar arthropathy is seen with increased frequency in Crohn's colitis.[13] There are only rarely radiological features of deformity or of bone destruction. Ankylosing spondylitis (2 to 6%) (20 to 30 times more often than in the general non-IBD population) is seen most commonly in patients who are HLA-B27 positive.[14]

2. Tamarin

Colonic barium enema examinations in the Oak Ridge CTT colony have provided an opportunity for extensive study of skeletal radiographs. A total of 217 cotton-top tamarins have been examined with a minimum of three films per examination (one film each: pre-barium, barium-filled, and post-evacuation of barium contrast medium). Some CTTs have had multiple procedures over several months to evaluate colitis and the development of colonic carcinoma.

The animals were anesthetized for the procedure. Most of the skeleton was readily visualized using one radiographic cassette, and only the feet and the end of the tail were not routinely visible. To date, no arthropathies have been diagnosed. This included observations on 162 films of 43 CTTs that were >10 years of age and that were approximately equivalent age-wise to >50-year-old humans. Recently, the synovia from 10 colitic CTTs that were asymptomatic for knee arthropathies were examined histologically; the knees had no evidence of synovitis and were considered normal.

3. Discussion

Treatment of human IBD will normally ameliorate the peripheral arthritis. However, unlike peripheral arthritis, ankylosing spondylitis bears no relationship to the activity or extent of IBD,[13] and neither bowel resection nor treatment changes the final outcome of the ankylosing spondylitis. Radiological study shows sacro-iliitis in 15% of cases[10] and in 68% if radionuclide scanning is used.[15] Another odd feature is that, although colitis-related ankylosing spondylitis is more common in females, noncolitic-associated ankylosing spondylitis is more common in males.[16]

C. HEMATOPOIETIC SYSTEM

Iron deficiency anemia is the most common human complication in IBD. A raised erythrocyte sedimentation rate (ESR) is a useful monitor of disease activity in man.

Iron deficiency anemia has been seen in some cotton-top tamarins with very severe colitis. In a survey of repeated blood samples from very sick tamarins before and after treatment, ESR has not been helpful as an indicator of the disease activity. Other associated blood dyscrasias have not been found.

D. EYE

Simultaneous skin and eye manifestations are seen in 50% of human patients with peripheral arthritis.[17] Human patients with IBD may develop episcleritis (3 to 4%),[12] iritis (0.5 to 3.0%),[18] or conjunctivitis. Conjunctivitis is much more common, but of uncertain relationship to IBD. Eye afflictions are more common in patients who are HLA-B27 positive. The severity of eye complications seems to be related to disease activity but bears no relationship to the length of colon involved or the severity of the inflammation. Like the joint processes, these changes are more common in Crohn's colitis.

Clinical eye complications have not been observed in the cotton-top tamarin, but extensive post-mortem studies are ongoing. A pilot study looking for eye changes in CTTs with colitis is in progress.

E. SKIN

Pyoderma gangrenosum is classically associated with long-standing total ulcerative colitis in man. This is a large ulcerated skin lesion with a rolled edge and is common on the lower limbs or trunk.

Although subtle skin manifestations may be masked by the animals' fur, all observed skin lesions have been readily attributable to attacks by other cotton-tops in the family groups.

III. SUMMARY

Extraintestinal manifestations of human ulcerative colitis are well-recognized features of the disease. Finding such extraintestinal manifestations in the cotton-top tamarin would strengthen its position as a useful model of human ulcerative colitis.

Although evidence of joint disease is lacking, the associated liver conditions, in particular the rare cases that resemble sclerosing cholangitis in humans, are important in establishing the cotton-top tamarin as the only spontaneously occurring model of human ulcerative colitis which develops at least some of the extraintestinal manifestations of the disease.

Elucidation of the mechanism(s) of extraintestinal manifestations of IBD in cotton-top tamarins, whether they arise by genetic, immunological, endotoxic, or other means, may shed some light on their pathogenesis in human IBD.

ACKNOWLEDGMENTS

This research was conducted in ORAU's AAALAC-accredited Marmoset Research Center at Oak Ridge (MARCOR) and was approved and monitored by ORAU's Animal Care Standards Committee. Research was supported, in part, by the ORAU Corporation. The authors acknowledge the manuscript preparation by S. Womble.

REFERENCES

1. **Chapman, R. W.,** Hepatobiliary disease, in *Inflammatory Bowel Diseases,* Allan, R. N., Keighley, M. R. B., Alexander-Williams, J., and Hawkins, C., Eds., Churchill Livingstone, London, 1990, 513.
2. **Perett, A. D., Higgins, G., Johnston, H. H., Massarella, G., Truelove, J. C., and Wright, R.,** The liver in ulceratative colitis, *Q. J. Med.,* 40, 211, 1971.
3. **Mistilis, S. P.,** Pericholangitis and ulcerative colitis: pathology, aetiology and pathogenesis, *Ann. Int. Med.,* 63, 1, 1965.
4. **Mistilis, S. P., Skyring, A. P., and Goulston, S. J. M.,** Pericholangitis and ulcerative colitis. II. Clinical aspects, *Ann. Int. Med.,* 63, 17, 1965.
5. **Thomas, C. H.,** Ulceration of the colon with a much enlarged fatty liver, *Trans. Pathol. Soc. Philadelphia,* 4, 87, 1974.
6. **Blackstone, M. O. and Nemchausky, B. A.,** Cholangiographic abnormalities in UC associated pericholangitis which resemble sclerosing cholangitis, *Dig. Dis. Sci.,* 23, 5769, 1978.
7. **Warren, W., Athanassiales, S., and Monge, J. I.,** Primary sclerosing cholangitis, *Am. J. Surg.,* 111, 23, 1966.
8. **Carey, J. R.,** Bile acids, cirrhosis and human evolution, *Gastroenterology,* 46, 490, 1964.
9. **Chapman, R. W., Varghese, Z., Gaul, R., Patel, G., Kokinon, N., and Sherlock, S.,** Association of primary sclerosing cholangitis with HLA B8, *Gut,* 24, 38, 1983.
10. **Chapman, R. W., Cottone, M., Selby, W. J., and Jewell, D. P.,** Serum autoantibodies ulcerative colitis, and primary sclerosing cholangitis, *Gut,* 27, 86, 1986.
11. **Mir-Madjlessi, S. H., Farmer, R. G., and Sivak, M. V.,** Bile duct carcinoma in patients with ulcerative colitis, *Dig. Dis. Sci.,* 32, 145, 1987.
12. **Greenstein, A. J., Janowitz, H. D., and Sachar, D. B.,** The extraintestinal complications of Crohn's disease and ulcerative colitis: a study of 700 patients, *Medicine,* 55, 401, 1976.
13. **Mayer, L. and Janowitz, H. D.,** Extraintestinal manifestations, in *Inflammatory Bowel Diseases,* Allan, R. N., Keighley, M. R. B., Alexander-Williams, J., and Hawkins, C., Eds., Churchill Livingstone, London, 1990, 501.
14. **McEwen, C., Ling, C., and Kirsner, J. B.,** Arthritis accompanying ulcerative colitis, *Am. J. Med.,* 33, 923, 1962.
15. **Wright, V. and Watkinson, G.,** Sacroiliitis and ulcerative colitis, *Br. Med. J.,* 2, 675, 1965.
16. **Palumbo, P. J., Ward, L. E., Sauer, W. G., and Scudamore, H. H.,** Musculoskeletal manifestations of chronic ulcerative colitis, *Mayo Clin. Proc.,* 48, 411, 1973.
17. **Goldgraber, M. B. and Kirsner, J. B.,** Gangrenous skin lesions associated with chronic ulcerative colitis, *Gastroenterology,* 39, 94, 1969.
18. **Hopkins, D. J., Homer, E., Bourtin, L., Clamp, S. E., De Dombal, F. T., and Goligher, J. C.,** Ocular disorders in a series of 332 patients with Crohn's disease, *Br. J. Ophthalmol.,* 58, 733, 1974.

Chapter 8

A PROTOCOL TO EVALUATE THE EFFICACY OF ANTICOLITIC AGENTS AGAINST ULCERATIVE COLITIS IN COTTON-TOP TAMARINS

Neal K. Clapp, Marsha A. Henke, Robert M. Hansard, and Robert L. Carson

TABLE OF CONTENTS

0-8493-5363-7/93/$0.00 + $.50

I. INTRODUCTION

The development of new therapeutic agents is dependent, not only on the medicinal chemistry laboratory to produce chemical configurations that are effective, but also on the ability of the biologist/pharmacologist to be able to evaluate accurately the therapeutic efficacy of the agent first in animals and then ultimately in humans. Every effort is made to maximize the desired therapeutic effect while minimizing deleterious side effects. Compounds are only approved for human use after extensive testing of biological activities both *in vitro* and *in vivo* in a manner regulated by the Food and Drug Administration (FDA). Prior to a compound being entered in human clinical trials, exhaustive toxicological and pathological data are obtained in FDA-recognized experimental models that strongly suggest (1) that the compound has demonstrated one or more desired biological activities and (2) that there is reasonable assurance that no harmful effects will occur in prescribed human treatment that was first used in healthy volunteers.

One concern that surfaces in this procedure is that the data (both efficacy and toxicological) obtained in experimental models may not approximate either efficacy or toxicity in humans. A simple question remains, how well can rodent and/or other animal model efficacy or toxicity data be extrapolated to humans? Are the animal models so close in pathogenesis of and response to the human disease in question that the producers (and regulating personnel) can be reasonably assured that the compound will behave identically in humans? Could another logical step be interjected in this elaborate and well-designed system that would provide a more accurate evaluation upon which production and further developmental decisions can be based?

Studies in rodent models are relatively inexpensive to conduct and the limitations are relatively well known. In contrast, in at least some situations, primate models may more closely approximate the human disease(s), but they are more costly and animal numbers available often create a somewhat limited supply. In addition, most animal models are induced systems where an animal is given an agent, i.e., bacterial, physical, or chemical, which is usually a toxin that produces directly or indirectly a diseased condition that can be evaluated both quantitatively and qualitatively. Few spontaneous animal diseases occur that would be suitable for such evaluations. A further complication in selecting an animal model is that some induced systems have little resemblance to the natural course of the human disease; therefore, their relevance as a model may be open to question. A biochemical product that is found in the human disease may be induced in animals and then be measured with the results used as indirect evidence of therapeutic efficacy. For example, reductions in levels of inflammatory mediators induced by a toxin are often cited as evidence of a compound's anti-inflammatory efficacy.[1]

The occurrence of spontaneous idiopathic colitis in cotton-top tamarins (CTT) (*Saguinus oedipus*) offers a primate model that closely duplicates the human disease, an advantage of using this model.[2] If an anticolitic test compound is efficacious in this primate model, the probability is reasonable that the compound will also be effective in humans. The spontaneous nature of the CTT disease requires careful selection of the population to be tested to avoid including those that may enter into spontaneous remissions and result in a false-positive effect attributed to the compound. Use of the CTT model of colitis for evaluating efficacy could be of considerable financial benefit while providing "more accurate" data if the protocol is found to be reliable and predictive of future results in humans. Realistically, the CTT model probably should be used as an adjunct and not as a sole method for evaluating a compound for FDA approval.

The protocol described in this chapter has been used to evaluate several compounds that were either ready to enter Phase I human clinical trials or that were already in them. Those compounds in clinical trials were evaluated primarily to test the predictability of the model and to see if accurate projections could be obtained in a shorter time frame than was possible in humans. Some interesting results of using this model are presented in this chapter, while confidentiality of those who developed the agents is maintained throughout.

II. METHODS

A. PHARMACODYNAMICS AND DOSE TOLERANCE

Animal selection — For this phase of the study, healthy young adult surrogate saddle-back tamarins (*Saguinus fuscicollis*) or common marmosets (*Callithrix jacchus*) are used rather than the endangered CTTs that are used in efficacy studies. Use of surrogate species avoids endangering cotton-top tamarins while identifying an acceptable dose level for the 8-week treatment regimen for determining therapeutic efficacy. Usually, two animals are used at each projected dose level.

Dose determination — Dose levels (usually "X" and 0.5 "X") are determined from the rodent toxicity studies; these data suggest doses with a reasonable margin of safety as well as an anticipated efficacious level.

Hematology and clinical chemistry — Pre- and post-treatment CBCs and clinical chemistry blood levels are obtained (i.e., Panel 19). Each animal serves as its own control for these studies. Changes due to treatment that vary from accepted normal ranges will detect species-to-species variations and/or susceptibilities.

Treatment — Two healthy animals are gavaged, usually BID (other routes of administration can be used), for 7 d. On occasion, we have been able to "hide" the compound in a vehicle such as flavored corn syrup and give the compound without having to catch and restrain the animal. Unfortunately, highly selective feeding habits of callitrichids often create an inconsistent consumption; thus, this approach may not always be the best choice for administration.

Pharmacodynamics — Plasma samples are usually drawn at 0, 1, 2, 4, 8, 24, and 72 h to determine blood levels in these animals. The animal is restrained on a mylar bleeding board, and venipuncture is made in the femoral vein. Minimal blood volumes (<0.5 ml) are taken, and animals have no deleterious effects. (Note: A limit of ~3 ml whole blood may be drawn each week). We also recognize that blood levels may not always accurately reflect the level of compound delivered at the targeted site.

Dose selection for efficacy study — From these data the dose is selected for the anticolitis study. Use is made of both rodent data and the tamarin pharmacodynamic and tolerance study to select the dose that should produce the desired therapeutic effect with the least toxicity.

B. ANTICOLITIS EVALUATION

Animal selection — Cotton-top tamarins with a persistent active colitis are relatively uncommon in the UT/Marmoset Research Center at Oak Ridge (MARCOR) colony (≤10%); thus, each animal was used as its own control by using pre- and post-treatment observations. At least two consecutive colonic mucosal biopsies were graded as active histologically before the animal was included in the treatment group. Alternatively, a CTT that had been treated previously for colitis could be included in the study if it had been through at least 4 weeks "wash out" time and mucosal biopsy indicated no change in inflammatory condition.

Treatment procedure — After the pharmacodynamic and tolerance studies were completed on surrogates, the dose of the compound to be given to the test group was determined through discussions with the project officer. Treatment was usually by gavage BID for 8 weeks. Other routes of administration could be used if appropriate and requested but would most often follow expected routes of administration in humans.

Colonoscopy, body weights, and stool condition — Other end-points that were scored and used as parameters in evaluating the colitic state were colonoscopy observations that were recorded on video tape, body weights that were obtained pre-, mid-, and post-treatment, and stool condition which was determined daily. Colonoscopy procedure details have been described elsewhere; they are performed under anesthesia using a 5.0-mm fiberoptic pediatric bronchoscope (Fujinon BR-YP_2 with EPX-301-A endoscopy processor).[2] Stool conditions were obtained daily and were described as firm, loose, puddly, or diarrhea.[2] Data were recorded and correlations were attempted.

Mucosal evaluation (histologic criteria) — Colonic mucosal biopsies were taken pre-, mid-, and post-treatment, routinely at 5 and 15 cm from the anus; these sampling points provided a very good representation of the overall colitic state as previously described.[2] In addition, any mucosal abnormality was also biopsied for histological evaluation. The criteria used for evaluating the colitis (grading was from 1 to 5) is shown in Table 1. Using five levels to grade active (acute) colitis rather than the previous grading system of either mild

TABLE 1
Criteria Used for Evaluating Colitis

Status	Description
Inactive (chronic)	Increase in mononuclear cells (e.g., lymphocytes, monocytes, plasma cells, etc.). No evidence of increased PMNs in lamina propria (LP), crypt epithelium, or in the crypt lumen; regeneration and repair of colonic mucosa is also evident.
Active (acute)	
Mild (1)	Increase of a few PMNs, usually in lamina propria
Moderate (3)	PMNs increased in at least two of the areas (LP, epithelium, and some crypt abscesses).
Severe (5)	PMNs heavily infiltrated throughout mucosa and lamina propria with abscesses in most crypts.

Note: PMNs, Polymorphonuclear leukocytes.

(A1) or severe (A2) acute colitis was extremely helpful in evaluating subtle changes; this method allowed a more accurate assessment of the colonic changes.

Hematology and clinical chemistry — Data were summarized and tabulated for convenience of recording and for evaluating any changes associated with treatment (e.g., Table 2).

Inflammatory mediators — Three sampling methods (circulating blood, mucosal biopsies, and rectal dialysate) were used to determine quantitatively the presence of inflammatory mediators that have been demonstrated in human and experimental colitis.[3] Blood samples and biopsy tissues have some limitations and difficulty in interpretation of data. Plasma samples only identify those mediators present in the circulating blood and may not correctly reflect activity in the colonic mucosa. Mucosal biopsies are less than 2 mm in diameter, which limits the number and kinds of assays that can be run.

Another protocol that identifies and evaluates inflammatory mediators in the colonic lumen is the use of a rectal dialysate. Dialysis bags were placed in the rectum and descending colon for 1½ hours under pentobarbital sodium anesthesia (0.15 to 0.25 mg/kg); during the procedure, animals were maintained on a warm-water blanket. The dialysate solution was prepared after Zipser's formulation[4] and included sodium chloride, potassium bicarbonate, and fatty acid-free bovine serum albumin with pH adjusted to 7.1 by NaOH. Upon removal, the dialysate was frozen (−70°C) and later analyzed by radioimmunoassays.[3] This method more accurately reflected the total inflammatory mediator status in the colonic microenvironment. After the procedure is completed, the anesthetized animal is then wrapped with a warmed water bottle (slightly above body temperature) and placed in a recovery cage where it is closely observed during the recovery period.

TABLE 2
Example of Hematological and Clinical Chemistry Information Obtained on MO-1743

Project	MO-1743	Laboratory analysis		
		Report date	Report date	Report date
CBC		1/17/92	6/28/91	7/29/91
WBC	Thous/mm³	15	14.6	8.5
RBC	Mill/mm³	5.48	5.81	5.84
HGB	gm/dl	14	14.1	13.6
HCT	%	45	45.3	45.0
MCV	UUU3	82.1	78	77.1
MCH	pg			
MCHC	g/dl			
THROMBO	Thous			
DIFF				
Segs	%	59	66	57
Bands	%	7		1
Lymphs	%	28	32	37
Monos	%	6	2	3
Eosinophil	%			2
Hypochromia	%			
Polychromasia	%	Slight		
Ansio	%			
Platelets		Adequate	Adequate	Adequate
Chemistry panel				
Calcium	mg/dl	9.6	9.2	9.3
Phosphorus	mg/dl	3.4	3.6	4.2
Glucose	mg/dl	133	150	173
Bun	mg/dl	20	24	29
Creatinine	mg/dl	0.7	0.5	0.7
Cholesterol	mg/dl	115	113	104
Total prot.	g/dl	7.5	7.2	7.3
Albumin	g/dl	3.9	3.6	4.1
A/G Ratio	Ratio	1.1	1.0	1.3
Globulin	g/dl	3.6	3.6	3.2
Bilir. Total	mg/dl	0.1	0.1	0.2
Alk. phos.	U/l	124	402	330
LDH	U/l	205	353	403
SGPT (ALT)	U/l	24	40	89
SGOT (AST)	U/l	169	234	321
CPK	U/l			
Sodium	mEq/l	154	154	154
Potassium	mEq/l	4.3	5.5	5.1
Chloride	mEq/l	102	106	103
Bun/creat ratio	Ratio	28.6	48	41.4
Weight		430	440	420
Stool condition		Puddly	Puddly	Puddly

III. RESULTS

Some typical results from an experiment are summarized in Table 3. In this particular experiment, inflammatory mediators arising from arachidonic acid metabolites (e.g., LTB_4, PGE_2) were measured in four animals by rectal dialysate at pre-, mid-, and post-treatment times. In Table 2 is an example of a typical presentation of the hematology and clinical chemistry results obtained from a treated animal. For comparison, Table 4 contains the normal ranges for these parameters as compiled by Dr. James V. Hawkins, MARCOR primate veterinarian.

Grading of colitis has been described in detail in this volume.[2] A score is recorded for each colonic segment that is biopsied, and the most serious grade in the histologic sections is assigned. For example, a CTT that had diffuse grade 4 active colitis pretreatment but then post-treatment had focal severe active colitis of grade 4 in one segment but grade 1 (mild active) elsewhere in the colon would both be scored as grade 4; obviously, these two examples of grade 4 have a very different meaning that must be factored into interpretation of the data. From a table similar to Table 3, one can determine the number of animals that improved, worsened, or were unchanged. Endoscopic evaluations are currently not as easily and consistently quantified as are the cellular counts observed histologically; in part, this may be due to sampling error that could accompany the very small biopsy volume obtained (<0.2 mm).

Attempts are made to provide as many conclusions as possible from the information, but caution must be exerted not to overinterpret the data. Some of the questions that usually arise are

1. Was the treatment level well tolerated? Any drug-related deaths?
2. Was there any evidence of therapeutic efficacy? Can it be quantitated?
3. These are colitic animals that have been subjected to repeated catching and treatment, anesthesia, and handling. Were any deleterious effects seen?
4. Did changes in types and quantity of inflammatory mediators offer any information about mechanisms in tamarin colitis pathogenesis?
5. Circulating blood levels of drug may not accurately reflect therapeutic delivery or efficacy to a particular target organ.

IV. DISCUSSION

While some species differences exist between human and CTT ulcerative colitis, remarkable similarities are also present; these further support the idea that information that is not available from other models can be obtained through appropriate use of this model. As in any model, the more that is known about the particular model, the more valuable it becomes.

TABLE 3
Example of Results from an Efficacy Study

Pretreatment						Treatment							Post-treatment			
								Stool Consistency								
Animal No.	Fasting wt (g)	Colon biopsy	Stool consistency	Hematology	Compound	Nonfasting wt (g)	Colon biopsy	Wks 0–2	Wks 2–4	Wks 4–6	Wks 6–8	Hematology (4 weeks)	Fasting wt (g)	Colon biopsy	Stool consistency	Hematology
MO-1743	400	A_2	P	Table 2	—	450	A_2	P	P	P	P	Table 2	420	A_1	P	Table 2
FO-4290	430	A_3	P	Table 3	—	440	A_3	P	P	P	P	Table 3	420	A_3	P	Table 3
MO-4502	450	A_1	F	Table 4	—	440	Dial[a]	P	P	P	P	Table 4	430	A_1	P	Table 4
FO-4701	450	A_3	L–P	Table 5	—	460	A_3	P	P	P	P	Table 5	440	A_1	P	Table 5
MO-4776	500	A_3	P	Table 6	—	520	Dial	P	P	P	P	Table 6	470	A_4	P	Table 6
MO-5131	450	A_2	P	Table 7	—	470	Dial	P	P	P	P	Table 7	470	A_1	P	Table 7
FO-5456	410	A_3	P	Table 8	—	500	Dial	P	P	P	P	Table 8	440	A_1	P	Table 8
MO-1668	370	A_1	P	Table 9	—	450	Sick	P	P	Died (44 days into expt.)						

Code for colon biopsy: C, chronic; A_1, mild active; A_3, moderate active; A_5, severe active. Code for stool consistency: F, firm; L, loose; P, puddly; D, diarrhea.

[a] Dialysate determinations.

Inflammatory Mediators

	Pretreatment		Treatment (after 4 weeks of treatment)		Post-treatment	
	LTB_4	PGE_2	LTB_4	PGE_2	LTB_4	PGE_2
MO-4502	1.63	17.7	1.58	12.1	2.72	21.4
MO-4776	3.88	22.95	0.14	39.49	2.37	115.29
MO-5131	8.59	45.12	0.32	149.43	2.10	250.0
FO-5456	5.36	12.5	3.95	0.75	2.60	0.30

TABLE 4
Normal Hematological and Clinical Chemistry Blood Values for *Saguinus oedipus* and *Callithrix jacchus*

	C. jacchus	*S. oedipus*	
WBC	4.2–22.6	4.1–20.3 (mm^3)	
RBC	5.7–7.3	4.9–7.4 (mm^3)	
Hemoglobin	13–17	10.6–18.7 (g/dl)	
Hematocrit	36–50	36–63 (%)	
MCV	61–71	59–91 (U^3)	
Neutrophils	59–79 (%)	58–73 (%)	2,100–8,680
Lymphocytes	16–46 (%)	15–45 (%)	910–4,280
Monocytes	0.5–6.9 (%)	0–2.8 (%)	0–340
Eosinophils	0.4–0.6 (%)	0–2.3 (%)	0–300
Basophils	0–1.5 (%)	0–1.9 (%)	0–260
Calcium	9–12	9–11	mg/dl
Phosphorus	4–8	4–7	mg/dl
Glucose	169–287	125–188	mg/dl
BUN	<25	<25	mg/dl
Creatinine	0.4–1.9	0.4–1.9	mg/dl
Total protein	5.7–8.7	6.2–8.6	g/dl
Globulin	2.3–5.8	2.5–6.1	g/dl
Albumin	2.8–4.4	2.9–4.1	g/dl
Bilirubin	0.0–2.0	0.0–2.0	mg/dl
Alk. Phos.	11.7–75.9	3.6–39.9	U/l
LDH	<180	<180	U/l
SGOT (AST)	<100	<100	U/l
SGPT (ALT)	<50	<50	U/l
Sodium	160–178	155–166	mEq/l
Potassium	4.8–6.6	4.7–7.3	mEq/l
Chloride	108–120	103–113	mEq/l

Data from personal observations and References 5–8. Compiled by J. V. Hawkins.

Selection of the animals for inclusion in any study is extremely important. The investigator must carefully select animals, with the assurance that the active colitis that is being treated is persistent and not going through spontaneous exacerbations and remissions that could make evaluation of therapeutic efficacy very difficult if not impossible to interpret.

A part of the drug tolerance and pharmacodynamics protocol is now being used to select which of three compounds should be used as most promising in the CTT efficacy study. By treating surrogates with the three compounds for one week and collecting CBCs and clinical chemistry, one may eliminate a compound that might, for example, induce liver enzymes or produce other serious toxic changes that might eliminate any chance of it being used in humans.

An observation was made during the pharmacodynamic phase of one study that was of interest. When we received data on the blood levels for the compound which had been given (pharmacodynamics), the 4-h levels had returned to baseline (zero). During some follow-up phone calls, we discovered that the levels of the compound persisted for 8 to 12 h in rodents; however, the CTT data that showed an ~2-h half-life was almost identical with that in humans. Thus, our experimental data correctly predicted that physiological data in humans were very close to those of tamarins and extrapolation of rodent data to man was misleading.

V. SUMMARY

A technique has been developed that allows the anticolitic efficacy of a compound to be tested in colitic cotton-top tamarins. A preliminary pharmacodynamic and drug tolerance study is completed in surrogate tamarins to assess any detectable toxicity and the appropriateness of using the tamarin model. The compound is then given to highly selected CTTs that have well-documented persistent active colitis; because of the limited numbers of these afflicted animals available, each serves as its own control. Selecting CTTs with persistent colitis avoids difficulty in interpreting results from undetected spontaneous remissions of a tamarin with a nonpersistent colitis giving a false-positive result. Mucosal biopsy grading of colitis is combined with colonoscopy observations, body weight, stool condition, and inflammatory mediator to assess the impact of the compound on the disease state. To date, this procedure has been used to evaluate five compounds for anticolitic efficacy and has been reliable in its results. In fact, data from tamarins have been shown to more accurately predict a compound's bioavailability in humans than similar experimental data in rodents.

ACKNOWLEDGMENTS

This research was conducted in ORAU's AAALAC-accredited Marmoset Research Center at Oak Ridge (MARCOR) and was approved and monitored by ORAU's Animal Care Standards Committee. Research was supported, in part, by the ORAU Corporation.

The authors acknowledge the excellent manuscript review by D. Fretland, S. Tardif, and R. Damian, and manuscript preparation by Sandy Womble.

REFERENCES

1. **Fretland, D. J., Djuric, J. W., and Gaginella, T. S.,** Eicosanoids and inflammatory bowel disease, *Prostaglandins, Leukotrienes, Essential Fatty Acids,* 41, 215, 1990.
2. **Clapp, N. K., Henke, M. A., Hansard, R. M., Carson, R. L., Adams, L. E., and Nardi, R. V.,** Natural history, time course, and pathogenesis of idiopathic colitis in cotton-top tamarins *(Saguinus oedipus),* This volume, Chapter 4.
3. **Clapp, N. K., Henke, M. A., Hansard, R. M., Walsh, R. E., Widomski, D. L., Anglin, C. P., Fretland, D. J., and Gaginella, T. S.,** Inflammatory mediators in cotton-top tamarins (CTT) with acute and chronic colitis, *Agents Actions,* 34, 1/2, 1991.
4. **Zipser, R. D.,** personal communication.
5. **McNees, D. W., Ponzio, B. J., Lewis, R. W., Stein, F. J., and Sis, R. F.,** Hematology of common marmosets *(Callithrix jacchus), Primates,* 23, 145, 1982.
6. **Holmes, A. W., Mitchell, P., and Capps, R. B.,** Marmosets as laboratory animals. III. Blood chemistry of laboratory-kept marmosets with particular attention to liver function and structure, *Lab. Anim. Care,* 17, 41, 1967.
7. **Hawkey, C. M., Hart, M. G., Knight, J. A., Fitzgerald, A. K., and Jones, D. M.,** Cotton-top tamarins *(Saguinus oedipus oedipus)*: hematologic reference values and hemopathologic responses, *Am. J. Primatol.,* 5, 231, 1983.
8. **Loeb, W. F.,** The nonhuman primate, in *The Clinical Chemistry of Laboratory Animals,* Loeb, W. F. and Quimby, F. W., Eds., Pergamon Press, Oxford, England, 1989, 59.

Chapter 9

CORONAVIRUSES IN TAMARIN AND MARMOSET COLITIS

David A. Brian and Linda J. Shockley

TABLE OF CONTENTS

0-8493-5363-7/93/$0.00 + $.50

I. INTRODUCTION

We hypothesize that coronaviruses cause acute and chronic colitis in tamarins and marmosets. To date, the data are few that support this hypothesis, but there exist precedents for coronavirus-induced acute and chronic colitis in other animal species. We review the data that support coronavirus involvement in cases of colitis in these primate species and propose approaches that would more firmly establish their role in this disease.

II. BACKGROUND ON CORONAVIRUSES AND THEIR ROLE IN GASTROENTERITIS AND COLITIS IN SPECIES OTHER THAN TAMARINS AND MARMOSETS

Coronaviruses are 1 of 15 families of animal RNA viruses[1,2] and as a family they are unique in both their electron microscopic appearance and in their molecular strategy for replication (for reviews, see References 3 and 4). Morphologically they are medium-sized (80 to 100 nm diameter), enveloped viruses with knobby surface projections (peplomers) that extend 12 to 20 nm from the envelope surface, giving them the striking appearance of having a "corona". They are positive-stranded RNA viruses with an infectious single-stranded RNA genome of 28 to 30 kilobases that has a 5′ methylated cap structure and a 3′ polyadenylic acid. The genome is the largest for any single-stranded RNA virus known and it encodes three or four structural proteins (depending on the species of coronavirus) and an estimated five or six non-structural proteins, incuding the RNA-dependent RNA polymerase. The major unique aspect of coronavirus replication is that, unlike other known RNA viruses, transcription (generation of the mRNA molecules) is apparently initiated (primed) by a 72 base leader-primer that binds to various sites along the full-length minus-strand copy of the genome.[5] The leader sequence is identical to the very 5′ end of the genome[6] and the resulting messengers RNAs form a 3′ coterminal nested set.[3] The open reading frame at the 5′ end of each messenger RNA molecule is usually the only one translated, making most mRNAs functionally "monocistronic".[7,8] The genes for the virion structural proteins reside at the 3′ end of the genome, and recently the nucleotide sequence for several of the structural protein genes in the avian infectious bronchitis virus (IBV),[9-11] the mouse hepatitis virus (MHV) strains A59 and JHM,[12-14] the bovine enteric coronavirus (BCV),[15] and the porcine transmissible gastroenteritis coronavirus (TGEV)[16-18] have been reported. In addition, the nucleotide sequence for the entire 27.8-k genome of IBV has been determined,[19] and the sequence reveals a very large RNA-dependent RNA polymerase molecule or molecules residing at the 5′ end of the genome.

The coronavirus family is currently comprised of 16 members and each belongs to one of four antigenic subgroups.[4,20] Coronaviruses show many tissue tropisms but they cause primarily diseases of the respiratory and gastrointestinal systems. The prototype coronavirus, the avian infectious bronchitis virus, causes a severe respiratory disease in chickens. The best documented human coronaviruses, those related to human coronavirus OC43 (HCV OC43) or human coronavirus 229E (HCV 229E), cause an estimated 20% of all upper respiratory disease suffered by humans.[21,22] Coronaviruses known to cause gastroenteritis in animals and humans are listed in Table 1. Viruses that cause gastroenteritis and are potential members of the coronavirus family on the basis of electron microscopic structure are also listed. These include the virus of epizootic diarrhea in pigs,[38] and the virus of necrotizing enterocolitis in humans.[31]

III. CORONAVIRUSES READILY CAUSE PERSISTENT INFECTIONS IN CELL CULTURES AND IN SOME ANIMALS

One property that has been noted for many, if not all, culturable coronaviruses is that they readily establish persistent infections in cell culture without requiring special manipulation such as coinfection with defective interfering particles. That is, most coronaviruses are not completely cytocidal in cell culture even when multiplicities of 10 or greater are used, and cells surviving acute infection are persistently infected. In some cases (e.g., with TGEV), the number of surviving cells is less than 10%, in others (e.g., with BCV), the number of surviving cells is far greater than 50%. Surviving cells are most difficult to obtain with viruses that cause cell fusion, such as MHV. Surviving cells that are refed will grow to confluency, albeit much more slowly than uninfected cells, and usually with a more grainy and ragged appearance. They can be serially passaged indefinitely. Interferon appears not to be important for the maintenance of coronavirus persistent infections *in vitro,* since no interferon can be measured, and persistently infected cells are susceptible to superinfection by a virus from another family.[42,43] In most cases studied, virus continues to be shed and progeny virions are infectious, causing a cytopathic effect on new cells.[44] In some cases, recovery of coronaviruses from persistently infected cells required cocultivation with new susceptible cells.[45] Persistently infected cells appear ''resistant'' to infections by wild-type virus of the parental type, at least by the criterion of cytopathic effect. It is not known whether all cells are infected and continue to shed virus. The mechanisms by which coronaviruses readily persist in cell culture, that is, the mechanisms by which the cell escapes death from the replicating virus, are not known. Certainly MHV is known to cause defective RNA species that may reflect the development of defective interfering viruses,[46] a phenomenon that has been used to explain the persistence of many RNA viruses.[47] If generation of defective interfering particles is the only mechanism by which coronaviruses persist, then the defective interfering particles must

TABLE 1
Enteric Coronaviruses and their Involvement in Colitis

Common name	Abbreviation	Natural host	Disease	Colitis?	Ref.
Bovine enteric coronavirus	BCV	Calf	Enteritis, colitis	Yes	23, 24
Canine coronavirus	CCV	Dog	Gastroenteritis	Slight in young dogs	25
Equine coronavirus	ECV	Foal	Enteritis	?	26
Feline enteric coronavirus	FECV	Cat	Mild gastroenteritis	?	27
Hemagglutinating encephalo-myelitis virus	HEV	Pig	Vomiting and wasting, encephalomyelitis	No	28
Human enteric coronavirus	HEV	Human	Gastroenteritis	?	29, 30
Human necrotizing enterocolitis virus[a]	?	Human	Necrotizing enterocolitis	Yes	31
Mouse hepatitis virus	MHV-LIVM	Mouse	Gastroenteritis	?	32
Lethal intestinal virus of in-fant mice (other similar strains include MHV-D, DVIM, MHV-S/CDC)					33 34 35 36
Yale strain	MHV-Y	Mouse	Typlocolitis	Yes	37
Porcine epizootic diarrhea virus[a]	?	Pig	Gastroenteritis	?	38
Porcine transmissible gastro-enteritis virus	TGEV	Pig	Gastroenteritis	No	39
Rabbit enteric coronavirus	RbECV	Rabbit	Gastroenteritis	?	40
Turkey coronavirus	TCV	Turkey	Gastroenteritis	Yes (cecum)	41

[a] These viruses are tentatively classified as coronaviruses. For these, no antigenic cross-reactivity with other coronavirus has been demonstrated, nor has a 3′ coterminal nested set pattern for multiple mRNAs been described.

arise extremely rapidly, since TGEV can establish a persistent infection with the use of stock virus that is only three passages beyond plaque purification. In this case, plaque purification was done using infectious RNA, so there is little chance that a defective interfering RNA species coinfected the cell along with the full-length genome.

To what extent coronaviruses establish long-term persistent infection in animals has been more difficult to establish. Enzootic infections of MHV in mouse colonies have long been proposed to be caused by persistently infected individuals that continuously shed virus and perpetuate the infection.[48] A number of recent experiments under controlled conditions, however, demonstrate that, for the several strains of MHV that have been tested, infection, when obtained through the natural route (oropharynx), as a rule, is limited to 2–3 weeks in duration.[49,50] MHV shedding cannot be demonstrated beyond this time. Furthermore, offspring of recovered animals are virus-free as determined by virus shedding and susceptibility to subsequent virus challenge.[51] Exceptions to this rule exist, however. (1) Athymic nude mice infected by the natural route readily acquire a life-long persistent infection with MHV.[52] Many of these mice die from a ''wasting'' syndrome. (2) Many mice experimentally infected by artificial routes, for example by intracerebral or intraperitoneal inoculation, become persistently infected for weeks or even months.[53-58] Persistence in these cases ranges from detection of viral RNA or proteins in the brain to shedding of infectious virus. Since recovery from infection in mice requires an intact cellular (T cell) immune system, one could postulate that persistent infections might arise in immunocompromised mice when infected by the natural route.

Enteric coronaviruses from other species may, however, behave differently and establish long-term, even life-long, persistent infections. TGEV has been isolated from pigs for up to 100 days following initial infections,[59] suggesting that long-term persistent infection is established in some animals and this may perpetuate enzootic TGEV infections. Cats suffering from the immunosuppressive feline leukemia virus infection have been shown to shed feline infectious peritonitis coronavirus in approximately one third of the cases and this is apparently a reactivation of a virus persisting in the animal.[60] Chronic shedding of enteric coronavirus-like particles are reported in humans with an immunosuppressive sprue condition.[61]

The site(s) of persistent coronavirus infection in animals remains to be established. In the case of chronic intestinal disease, it may be a persistent infection of the enterocytes, as is apparently the case in certain immunosuppressed humans,[61] or it may be a persistent infection of adjacent tissues, including such tissues as parasympathetic nerves. Certainly the lesions observed in marmoset chronic colitis, that is, interstitial infiltration of lymphocytes in the submucosa of the colon, are consistent with a long-term infection by a virus.[62,63]

Clearly more studies are needed to document the sites, degree, and mechanism of coronavirus persistence in animals.

IV. WORKING HYPOTHESIS: CORONAVIRUSES CAUSE COLITIS IN TAMARINS AND MARMOSETS

Evidence to support our hypothesis so far is slim, and entirely the result of retrospective studies. During a recent series of outbreaks of diarrhea in the colony of tamarins and marmosets located at the Oak Ridge Associated Universities, Oak Ridge, TN, coronavirus-like particles were found in feces of animals with acute diarrhea (Figure 1).[64] Coronavirus-like particles were also observed in several animals displaying lesions of subacute and chronic colitis, a condition that is common in the Oak Ridge marmosets (Table 2)[63] as well as marmosets in other colonies.[65,66] To date, only a loose association can be made between the virus particles and the diarrhea and colitis, and no attempt has yet been made to make a correlation between the coronavirus-like particles and diseased animals as compared to healthy animals. Clearly a correlative study is required, especially in light of the fact that coronavirus-like particles have been observed in the stools of both healthy and diseased primates.[65,66]

Our attempts to culture the coronavirus-like particles from tamarins and marmosets in several cell lines have been unsuccessful so far. Because all characterized mammalian coronaviruses clearly fall into one of two antigenic subgroups, we reasoned that marmoset serum from diseased animals might react with representatives of one of the two antigenic subgroups. When serum from the tamarins and marmosets was tested by Western blotting against the virion proteins of TGEV and BCV, each a representative of one of the two major antigenic mammalian coronavirus subgroups, reactivity in some animals was found against BCV.[64] Antiserum from three diseased animals identified the nucleocapsid and matrix protein of BCV, two proteins of highly conserved amino acid sequence within the antigenic subgroups.[15] This led us to believe that the coronavirus-like particle might be BCV-related.

To investigate this further, we have used a dot blot hybridization assay to examine the identity of putative coronaviruses in tamarin and marmoset feces. We used probes of known sequence, cDNA clones derived from the TGEV and BCV genomes, that both specifically and sensitively distinguish TGEV and related viruses from BCV and related viruses in fecal specimens.[67] Two of twelve samples reacted strongly with the BCV probe (giving a single that is $\geq 10^{10}$ virus particles/ml), further suggesting a relatedness with BCV (Figure 2). Some samples also reacted weakly with the TGEV-specific probe, suggesting for the first time that a TGEV-related coronavirus may also be present.

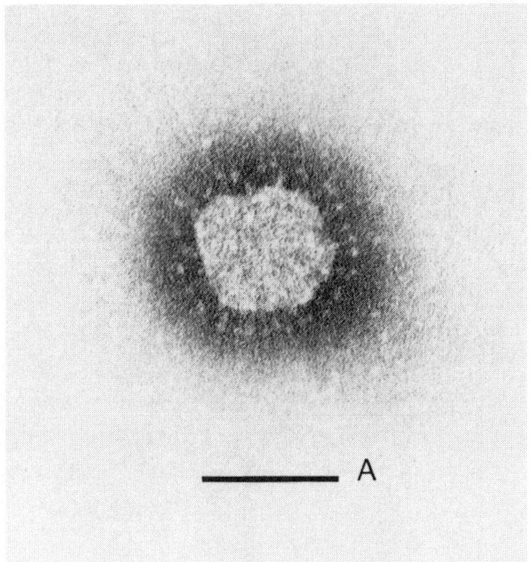

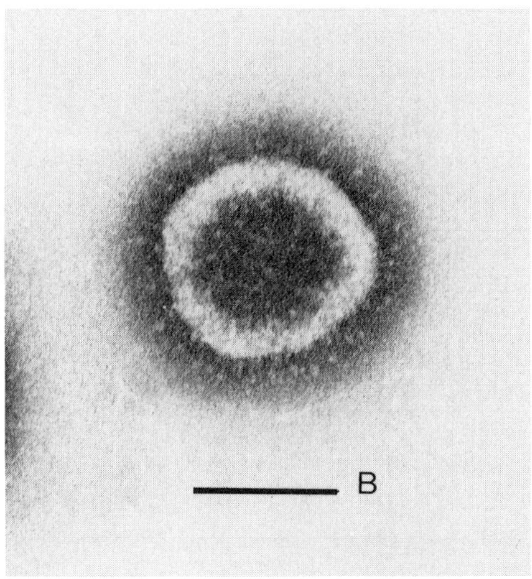

FIGURE 1. Coronavirus-like particles in marmoset diarrheic feces negatively stained with phosphotungstic acid. (A) Spherical particle showing petal-shaped projections. (B) A particle apparently devoid of a nucleocapsid. The bar represents 100 nm. (From Russell, R. G. et al., *Digest. Dis. Sci.*, 30, 725, 1985. With permission.)

TABLE 2
Colitis in Marmosets Having Coronavirus-Like Particles in Feces[a]

Animal no.	Species	Age	Clinical condition	Pathology		Coronavirus by EM[c]	Immunoblot[d]		Dot blot hybridization[e]	
				Colitis[b]	Other		BCV protein	TGEV protein	BCV probe	TGEV probe
1364	*S. oed.*	>14 years	Loose diarrhea			+	+	–	ND	ND
1379	*S. oed.*	>12 years	Loose diarrhea	Acute		ND	+	–	ND	ND
1544	*S. oed.*	7 years	Chronic diarrhea	Acute	Colon adenocar-cinoma	+	+	–	ND	ND
1558	*S. fusc.*	9 years	Diarrhea, wasting, spontaneous death	Chronic		+ +	ND	ND	ND	ND
1586	*S. oed.*	>9 years	Loose diarrhea			+	ND	ND	–	–
1588	*S. fusc.*	9 years	Wasting	Chronic		+	ND	ND	–	–
1624	*S. oed.*	>10 years	Loose diarrhea	Chronic		+ +	ND	ND	+	+
1662	*S. oed.*	Adult	Wasting, sponta-neous death	Subacute	Lymphosarcoma	+	ND	ND	–	–
1675	*S. oed.*	8 years	Diarrhea, wasting, spontaneous death	Subacute	Intussusception	+	ND	ND	–	–

1719	*S. oed.*	8 years	Wasting, spontaneous death		Colon adenocarcinoma	+ +	ND	ND	–	–
1723	*S. oed.*	8 years	Loose diarrhea	Acute	Colon adenocarcinoma	+	ND	ND	–	–
1739	*S. oed.*	8 years	Loose diarrhea	Chronic	Colon adenocarcinoma	+	+	–	–	+ –
2683	*S. fusc.*	8 years	Sudden-onset weakness, dehydration	Subacute	Bronchopneumonia, nephritis	+	ND	ND	ND	ND
3210	*S. oed.*	7 years	Loose diarrhea	Chronic		+	+	–	+ + +	–
3842	*C. jacc.*	7 years	Loose diarrhea	Chronic		+	ND	ND	–	–
3873	*S. oed.*	7 years	Loose diarrhea	Acute	Colon adenocarcinoma	+	ND	ND	–	–
3878	*S. oed.*	7 years	Bloody, loose diarrhea	Chronic		+	ND	ND	+ + +	–
4459	*C. jacc.*	9 months	Repeated diarrhea	Subacute		+	ND	ND	ND	ND

[a] 18 animals (*Saguinus oedipus, Sanguinus fuscicollis,* or *Callithrix jacchus*) having coronavirus-like particles in their feces and also having biopsy or necropsy hsitopathological examination of the colon are listed. Animals having fecal coronavirus-like particles, but not examined histopathologically (approximately 10) were not included, nor were animals having colitis and no coronavirus-like particles by electron microscopy (approximately 50).

[b] Colitis was diagnosed according to lesions described by Lushbaugh et al.[63]

[c,d] For experimental details, see Russell et al.[64]

[e] For experimental details, see Shockly et al.[67]

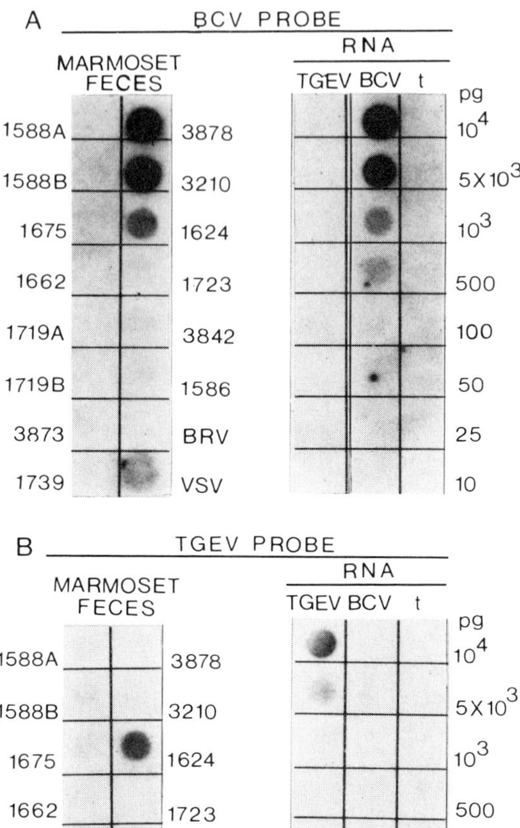

FIGURE 2. Dot blot hybridization detection of coronavirus in feces of tamarins and marmosets. Cloned cDNA of the 3′ end of the BCV genome (clone pMN3, the BCV probe) and of the 3′ end of the TGEV genome (clone pFG5, the TGEV probe) were purified away from the pUC9 vector DNA, nick translated so as to be labeled with ^{32}P, and hybridized to fecal samples treated with detergent NP40 and formaldehyde and immobilized on nitrocellulose. (For experimental details, see Shockley et al., Reference 67). Fecal specimens collected by saturating a cotton swab were suspended in 1 ml of sterile Earle's balanced salt solution, vortexed, clarified, and 25 μl of clarified supernatant was mixed with 25 μl of 1% NP40 solution and 50 μl formaldehyde-200X SCC solution, and the entire 100-μl volume used to prepare 1 dot. Known quantities of purified BCV and TGEV genomic RNA likewise immobilized served as standards for quantitation. 500 pg of virion RNA is equivalent to 4×10^7 virions. Animal numbers correspond with those listed in Table 2. BRV dot represents approximately 10^8 infectious particles of bovine rotavirus and VSV dot represents approximately 10^9 infectious particles of vesicular stomatitis virus; t represents transfer RNA.

Clearly, much work needs yet to be done to establish, first, that the coronavirus-like particles from the feces of tamarins and marmosets are indeed coronaviruses, and, second, that there is a causal relationship between the coronavirus-like particles and the diarrhea (potentially acute colitis) and the subacute or chronic colitic conditions.

V. STEPS NEEDED TO ESTABLISH A CORONAVIRUS ETIOLOGY FOR COLITIS IN TAMARINS AND MARMOSETS

1. Establish that the coronavirus-like particle is a coronavirus by growing it in cell culture and (a) demonstrating that it is related antigenically to another known coronavirus, or (b) demonstrating that it replicates by using multiple subgenomic mRNAs having a 3′ coterminal nested set pattern, in the event that it is not antigenically related to any other known coronavirus. Once isolated, Koch's postulates can be applied. That is, young virus-free animals can be infected with the plaque-purified, cell-culture-grown virus, and development of disease can be observed.
2. Establish that coronavirus proteins are present in chronically diseased colon tissue or in nearby tissue. This can be done using hyperimmune serum prepared against the primate coronavirus (if grown) or against a close relative, such as the bovine coronavirus if this turns out to be the case, and immunofluorescence. An enzyme-linked immunosorbent assay (ELISA) could be developed to examine the virus if shed, or immunocytochemistry could be employed on formalin-fixed gut tissues. Because formalin-fixed tissues can be used, retrospective studies can be done on stored specimens.
3. Establish that coronavirus nucleic acids are present in chronically infected colon cells. We have established that cloned cDNA to the bovine enteric coronavirus can recognize material in the feces of tamarins and marmosets. Assuming this can be firmly established as being the result of the marmoset coronavirus-like particle, then both shed virus particles and *in situ* hybridization of diseased tissues can be monitored by hybridization tests. With this approach, it may be useful to employ a variation of the recently developed DNA polymerase chain reaction which has the ability to greatly amplify sequence present in numbers as low as 1 in 10^5 cells.[68]

It should be noted that if the coronavirus from tamarins or marmosets cannot be isolated and grown, then Koch's postulates cannot be applied and a different set of criteria will need to be applied.[69] The coronavirus-like particle, or its antigens or nucleic acid, will need to be regularly associated with the disease. The coronavirus-like particle, free of other agents, must be able to transmit the colitis to susceptible animals and induce an immune response. The absence of antibody should correlate with susceptibility, but its presence may not necessarily correlate with protection from infection since, for many culturable coronaviruses, infection does not establish a protective immunity. Some studies with the feline infectious peritonitis virus suggest there may even be an immune enhancement of the disease.[60]

The association of coronavirus-like particles with colitis in tamarins and marmosets and the established role of coronaviruses as enteric pathogens in many animal species suggest the possibility that they are the cause of chronic intestinal disease in these and other primates, and in humans. With the advent of cloned coronavirus nucleic acid sequences, sensitive analytical approaches can now be employed to investigate the role of coronaviruses in persistent infection and chronic diseases of the gut and other organ systems.

REFERENCES

1. **Fenner, F., Bachmann, P. A., Gibbs, E. P. J., Murphy, F. A., Studdert, M. J., and White, D. O.,** *Veterinary Virology,* Academic Press, New York, 1987, 15.
2. **Cavanagh, D., Brian, D. A., Eujuanes, L., Holmes, K. V., Lai, M. M. C., Laude, H., Siddell, S. G., Spaan, W., Taguchi, F., and Talbot, P. J.,** Coronaviridae: Fifth Report of the Coronavirus Study Group, Vertebrate Virus Subcommittee on Taxonomy of Viruses, *Intervirology,* 2 (Suppl.), 234, 1990.
3. **Siddell, S., Wege, H., and ter Meulen, V.,** The structure and replication of coronavirus, *Curr. Top. Microbiol. Immunol.,* 99, 131, 1982.
4. **Sturman, L. S. and Holmes, K. V.,** The molecular biology of coronaviruses, *Adv. Virus Res.,* 28, 35, 1983.
5. **Lai, M. M. C., Baric, R. S., Brayton, P. R., and Stohlman, S. A.,** Characterization of leader RNA sequences on the virion and mRNAs of mouse hepatitis virus, a cytoplasmic RNA virus, *Proc. Natl. Acad. Sci. U.S.A.,* 81, 3626, 1984.
6. **Shieh, C. K., Soe, L. H., Makino, S., Chang, M. F., Stohlman, S. A., and Lai, M. M. C.,** The 5′-end sequence of the murine coronavirus genome: implications for multiple fusion sites in leader-primer transcription, *Virology,* 156, 321, 1987.
7. **Leibowitz, J. L., Weiss, S. R., Paavola, E., and Bond, C. W.,** Cell-free translation of murine coronavirus RNA, *J. Virol.,* 43, 905, 1982.
8. **Rottier, P. J. M., Spaan, W. J. M., Horzinek, M. C., and Van Der Zeijst, B. A. M.,** Translation of the three mouse hepatitis virus strain A59 subgenomic RNAs in Xenopus laevis oocytes, *J. Virol.,* 38, 20, 1981.
9. **Boursnell, M. E. G., Binns, M. M., Foulds, I. J., and Brown, T. D. K.,** Sequences of the nucleocapsid genes from two strains of avian infectious bronchitis virus, *J. Gen. Virol.,* 66, 573, 1985.
10. **Boursnell, M. E. G., Brown, T. D. K., and Binns, M. M.,** Sequence of the membrane protein gene form avian coronavirus IBV, *Virus Res.,* 1, 303, 1984.
11. **Binns, M. M., Boursnell, M. E. G., Cavanagh, D., Pappin, D. J. C., and Brown, T. D. K.,** Cloning and sequencing of the gene encoding the spike of the coronavirus IBV, *J. Gen. Virol.,* 66, 719, 1985.
12. **Armstrong, J., Smeekens, S., and Rottier, P.,** Sequence of the nucleocapsid gene from murine coronavirus MHV-A59, *Nucleic Acids Res.,* 11, 833, 1983.

13. **Armstrong, J., Niemann, H., Smeekens, S., Rottier, P., and Warren, G.,** Sequence and topology of a model intracellular membrane protein, E1 glycoprotein, from a coronavirus, *Nature (London),* 308, 751, 1984.
14. **Schmidt, J., Skinner, M., and Siddell, S.,** Nucleotide sequence of the gene encoding the surface projection glycoprotein of coronavirus MHV-JHM, *J. Gen. Virol.,* 68, 47, 1987.
15. **Lapps, W., Hogue, B. G., and Brian, D. A.,** Sequence analysis of the bovine coronavirus nucleocapsid and matrix protein genes, *Virology,* 157, 47, 1987.
16. **Kapke, P. A. and Brian, D. A.,** Sequence analysis of the porcine transmissible gastroenteritis coronavirus nucleocapsid protein gene, *Virology,* 151, 41, 1986.
17. **Kapke, P. A., Tung, F. Y. T., Brian, D. A., Woods, R. D., and Wesley, R. D.,** The amino terminal signal peptide on the porcine transmissible gastroenteritis coronavirus matrix protein is not an absolute requirement for membrane translocation and glycosylation, *Virology,* 165, 367, 1988.
18. **Rasschaert, D. and Laude, H.,** The predicted primary structure of the peplomer protein E2 of the porcine coronavirus transmissible gastroenteritis virus, *J. Gen. Virol.,* 68, 1883, 1987.
19. **Boursnell, M. E. G., Brown, T. D. K., Foulds, I. J., Green, P. F., Tomley, F. M., and Bins, M. M.,** Completion of the sequence of the genome of the coronavirus avian infectious bronchitis virus, *J. Gen. Virol.,* 68, 57, 1987.
20. **Wege, H., Siddell, S., and ter Meulen, B.,** The virology and pathogenesis of coronaviruses, *Curr. Top. Microbiol. Immunol.,* 99, 165, 1982.
21. **Hierholzer, J. C. and Tannock, G. A.,** Coronaviridae, *Lab. Diagn. Infect. Dis.,* 2, 451, 1988.
22. **McIntosh, K.,** Coronaviruses, in *Virology,* Fields, B. N., Ed., Raven Press, New York, 1985, chap. 56.
23. **Mebus, C. A., Newman, L. E., and Stair, L. E.,** Scanning electron, light and immunofluorescent microscopy of intestine of gnotobiotic calf with calf diarrheal coronavirus, *Am. J. Vet. Res.,* 36, 1719, 1975.
24. **Storz, J., Dougri, A. M., and Hajer, I.,** Coronaviral morphogenesis and ultrastructural changes in intestinal infections of calves, *J. Am. Vet. Med. Assoc.,* 173, 633, 1978.
25. **Keenan,K. P., Jervis, H. R., Marchwicki, R. H., and Binn, L. N.,** Intestinal infection of neonatal dogs with canine coronavirus 1-71: studies by virologic, histologic, histochemical, and immunofluorescent techniques, *Am. J. Vet. Res.,* 37, 247, 1976.
26. **Bass, E. P. and Sharpee, R. L.,** Coronavirus and gastroenteritis in foals, *Lancet,* 2, 822, 1975.
27. **Pedersen, N. C., Boyle, J. F., Floyd, K., Fudge, A., and Barker, J.,** An enteric coronavirus infection of cats and its relationship to feline infectious peritonitis, *Am. J. Vet. Res.,* 42, 368, 1981.
28. **Andries, K. and Pensaert, M. B.,** Immunofluorescence studies on the pathogenesis of hemagglutinating encephalomyelitis virus in pigs after oronasal inoculation, *Am. J. Vet. Res.,* 41, 1372, 1980.
29. **Caul, E. O. and Clarke, S. K. R.,** Coronavirus propagated from patients with non-bacterial gastroenteritis, *Lancet,* 2, 953, 1975.
30. **Caul, E. O. and Egglestone, S. I.,** Further studies on human enteric coronavirus, *Arch. Virol.,* 54, 107, 1977.
31. **Resta, S., Luby, J. P., Rosenfeld, C. R., and Siegel, J. D.,** Isolation and propagation of a human enteric coronavirus, *Science,* 229, 978, 1985.
32. **Biggers, D. C., Kraft, L. M., and Sprinz, H.,** Lethal intestinal virus infection of mice (LIVM): an important new model for study of the response of the intestinal mucosa to injury, *Am. J. Pathol.,* 45, 413, 1964.
33. **Hierholzer, J. C., Broderson, J. R., and Murphy, F. A.,** New strain of mouse hepatitis virus as the cause of lethal enteritis in infant mice, *Infect. Immun.,* 24, 508, 1979.

34. **Ishida, T. and Fujiwara, K.,** Pathology of diarrhea due to mouse hepatitis virus in the infant mouse, *Jpn. J. Exp. Med.,* 49, 33, 1979.
35. **Kraft, L. M.,** Epizootic diarrhea of infant mice and lethal intestinal virus infection of infant mice, *Natl. Cancer Inst. Monogr.,* 20, 55, 1966.
36. **Sugiyama, K. and Amano, Y.,** Morphological and biological properties of a new coronavirus associated with diarrhea in infant mice, *Arch. Virol.,* 67, 241, 1981.
37. **Barthold, S. W., Smith, A. L., Lord, P. F. S., Bhatt, P. N., Jacoby, R. O., and Main, A. J.,** Epizootic coronaviral typhlocolitis in suckling mice, *Lab. Anim. Sci.,* 32, 376, 1982.
38. **Pensaert, M. B. and de Bouck, P.,** A new coronavirus-like particle associated with diarrhea in swine, *Arch. Virol.,* 58, 243, 1978.
39. **Olson, D. P., Waxler, G. L., and Roberts, A. W.,** Small intestinal lesions of transmissible gastroenteritis in gnotobiotic pigs: a scanning electron microscopic study, *Am. J. Vet. Res.,* 34, 1239, 1973.
40. **Lapierre, J., Marsolais, G., Pilon, P., and Descoteaux, J. P.,** Preliminary report on the observation of a coronavirus in the intestine of the laboratory rabbit, *Can. J. Microbiol.,* 26, 1204, 1980.
41. **Ritchie, A. E., Deshmukh, D. R., Larsen, C. T., and Pomeroy, B. S.,** Electron microscopy of coronavirus-like particles characteristic of turkey bluecomb disease, *Avian Dis.,* 17, 546, 1973.
42. **Coulter-Mackie, M., Adler, R., Wilson, G., and Dales, S.,** In vivo and in vitro models of demyelinating diseases XII: persistence and expression of corona JHM virus functions in RN2-2 Schwannoma cells during latency, *Virus Res.,* 3, 245, 1985.
43. **Dupuy, J. M. and Lamontagne, L.,** Genetically-determined sensitivity to MHV3 infections is expressed in vitro in lymphoid cells and macrophages, *Adv. Exp. Med. Biol.,* 218, 455, 1987.
44. **Chaloner-Larsson, G. and Johnson-Lussenburg, C. M.,** Characteristics of a long term in vitro persistent infection with human coronavirus 229E, *Adv. Exp. Med. Biol.,* 142, 309, 1981.
45. **Stohlman, S. A. and Weiner, L. P.,** Chronic central nervous system demyelination in mice after JHM virus infection, *Neurology,* 31, 38, 1981.
46. **Makino, S., Shieh, C. K., Keck, J. G., and Lai, M. M. C.,** Defective-interfering particles of murine coronavirus: mechanism of synthesis of defective viral RNAs, *Virology,* 163, 104, 1988.
47. **Holland, J. J.,** Generation and replication of defective viral genomes, in *Virology,* Fields, B. N., Ed., Raven Press, New York, 1985, chap. 6.
48. **Rowe, W. P., Harley, J. W., and Capps, W. I.,** Mouse hepatitis virus infection as a highly contagious, prevalent, enteric infection of mice, *Proc. Soc. Exp. Biol. Med.,* 112, 161, 1963.
49. **Barthold, S. W.,** Mouse hapatitis virus biology and epizoobiology, in *Viral and Mycoplasmal Infections of Laboratory Rodents,* Bhatt, P. N., Jacoby, R. O., Morse, H. C. III, and New, A. E., Eds., Academic Press, New York, 1986, 571.
50. **Barthold, S. W. and Smith, A. L.,** Mouse hepatitis virus S in weanling Swiss mice following intranasal inoculation, *Lab Anim. Sci.,* 33, 355, 1983.
51. **Weir, E. C., Bhatt, P. N., Barthold, S. W., Cameron, G. A., and Simack, P. A.,** Elimination of mouse hepatitis virus from a breeding colony by temporary cessation of breeding, *Lab. Anim. Sci.,* 34, 455, 1987.
52. **Barthold, S. W., Smith, A. L., and Povar, M. L.,** Enterotropic mouse hepatitis virus infection in nude mice, *Lab. Anim. Sci.,* 35, 613, 1984.
53. **Knobler, R. L., Lampert, P. W., and Oldstone, M. B. A.,** Virus persistence and recurrent demyelination produced by a temperature-sensitive mutant of mouse hepatitis virus, *Nature,* 298, 279, 1982.

54. **Lavi, E., Gilden, D. H., Highkin, M. K., and Weiss, S. R.,** Persistence of mouse hepatitis virus A59 in a slow virus demyelinating infection in mice as detected by in situ hybridization, *J. Virol.,* 51, 563, 1984.
55. **Suzumura, A., Lavi, E., Weiss, S. R., and Silberberg, D. H.,** Coronavirus infection induces H-2 antigen expression of oligodendrocytes and astrocytes, *Science,* 232, 991, 1986.
56. **Taguchi, F., Siddell, S. G., Wege, H., and ter Meulen, V.,** Characterization of a variant virus selected in rat brains after infection by coronavirus mouse hepatitis virus JHM, *J. Virol.,* 54, 429, 1985.
57. **Virelizier, J. L., Dayan, A. D., and Allison, A. C.,** Neuropathological effects of persistent infection of mice by mouse hepatitis virus, *Infect. Immun.,* 12, 1127, 1975.
58. **Wege, H., Watanabe, R., and ter Meulen, V.,** Relapsing subacute demyelinating encephalomyelitis in rats in the course of coronavirus JHM infection, *J. Neuroimmunol.,* 6, 325, 1984.
59. **Underdahl, N. R., Mebus, C. A., and Torres-Medina, A.,** Recovery of transmissible gastroenteritis virus from chronically infected experimental pigs, *Am. J. Vet. Res.,* 36, 1473, 1975.
60. **Pedersen, N. C.,** Virologic and immunologic aspects of feline infectious peritonitis virus infection, *Adv. Exp. Med. Biol.,* 218, 529, 1987.
61. **Baker, S. J., Mathan, M., Mathan, V. I., Jesudess, S., and Swaminathan, S. P.,** Chronic enterocyte infection with coronavirus: one possible cause of the syndrome of tropical sprue?, *Digest. Dis. Sci.,* 27, 1039, 1982.
62. **Chalifoux, L. V., Brieland, J. K., and King, N. W.,** Evolution and natural history of colonic disease in cotton top tamarins (Saguinus oedipus), *Digest. Dis. Sci.,* 30, 54S, 1985.
63. **Lushbaugh, C., Humason, G., and Clapp, N.,** Histology of colitis: Saguinus oedipus and other marmosets, *Digest. Dis. Sci.,* 30, 45S, 1985.
64. **Russell, R. G., Brian, D. A., Lenhard, A., Potgieter, L. N. D., Gillespie, D., and Clapp, N. K.,** Coronavirus-like particles and Campylobacter in marmosets with diarrhea and colitis, *Digest. Dis. Sci.,* 30, 72S, 1985.
65. **Caul, E. O. and Egglestone, S. I.,** Coronavirus-like particles present in simian feces, *Vet. Rec.,* 104, 168, 1979.
66. **Smith, G. C., Lester, T. L., Heberling, R. L., and Kalter, S. S.,** Coronavirus-like particles in nonhuman primate feces, *Arch. Virol.,* 72, 105, 1982.
67. **Shockley, L., Kapke, P. A., Lapps, W., Brian, D. A., Potgieter, L., and Woods, R.,** Diagnosis of porcine and bovine enteric coronavirus infections using cloned cDNA probes, *J. Clin. Microbiol.,* 25, 1591, 1987.
68. **Saiki, R. K., Gelfand, D. H., Stoffel, S., Scharf, S. J., Higuchi, R., Horn, G. T., Mullis, K. B., and Erlich, H. A.,** Primer-directed enzymatic amplification of DNA with a thermostable DNA polymerase, *Science,* 239, 487, 1988.
69. **Estes, M. K.,** Evaluating viral agents in marmoset colitis, *Digest. Dis. Sci.,* 30, 80S, 1985.

Chapter 10

DO REPEATED COLONIC MUCOSAL BIOPSIES IMPACT MORTALITY IN COTTON-TOP TAMARINS?

Neal K. Clapp, Marsha A. Henke, Robert M. Hansard, Robert L. Carson, and Ronald V. Nardi

TABLE OF CONTENTS

0-8493-5363-7/93/$0.00 + $.50

I. INTRODUCTION

The importance of understanding the pathogenesis of a disease is well recognized as a basic need to conduct productive biomedical research. However, it is not always possible to exhaustively study pathogenesis of the human condition. Researchers are often not able to obtain the necessary repeated samplings. Very simple procedures (e.g., urine or blood samples) meet some patient resistance, and more invasive or more ambitious evaluations (e.g., endoscopy) will have even lower acceptance. Costs also enter into such an endeavor; medical insurance companies do not pay for repeated elective procedures such as colonoscopies, nor is it considered good medical practice to request such without sufficient clinical justification.

An animal model provides not only a surrogate of the human condition but also the opportunity to study the disease model exhaustively so that extrapolation can be made more accurately to the human situation. Researchers can justify the intense study of a disease process in an experimental animal that could not be considered in the human population. The fact that most disease processes in animals, induced or spontaneous, will usually occur in a much shorter time frame than in humans also makes animal studies attractive. Thus, reliable experimental animal data can be obtained and results exploited long before the research could be completed in man.

The study of idiopathic ulcerative colitis provides an excellent example of such a situation. Long-standing (>10 to 15 years) ulcerative colitis in man predisposes the patient to develop colonic carcinoma which adds several years of observation to acquire experimental data in a prospective study. In the cotton-top tamarin (CTT), *Saguinus oedipus,* spontaneous idiopathic colitis occurs relatively early in life (ages of 1 to 2 years) and increases in severity and frequency of exacerbations through 3 to 5 years of age.[1,2] This disease may well predispose the CTTs to develop colon cancer in high incidences (~35% of adults), the most important cause of death in adult CTTs.[1,3,4] Repeated colonic mucosal biopsies have been performed on adult CTTs for 6 years to determine the pathogenesis and time course of the disease and if the patterns mimic the human disease.[1,5,6] However, a serious experimental question arises: "Do the repeated colonic biopsies affect (in particular, increase) mortality in these valuable animals?"[7] Answering this important question is the subject of this chapter.

II. METHODS

Colonscopies were performed and colonic mucosal biopsies obtained at 3-month intervals for 5 years (1985 to 1990) in a group of 38 cotton-top tamarins.[2-4] These animals (cohort I) were selected because they had first-degree relatives that died with colon cancer, and they were in high-risk ages (2.7 to 6.5 years) to develop ulcerative colitis and colonic carcinoma.[2,4] These animals had large numbers of multiple biopsies (~20) if they survived the entire 5-year period.

Three other cohorts of age-matched cotton-tops were examined only occasionally, if ever, by colonoscopy and mucosal biopsy; two cohorts (II and III) lived concurrently with cohort I and another cohort (IV) lived in the preceding 5 years (1980 to 1985). Cohort III was transferred to the Marmoset Research Center at Oak Ridge (MARCOR) in 1982 from Rush Presbyterian-St. Luke's Medical Center in Chicago under National Cancer Institute (NCI) Contract NO1 CP21004, while I, II, and IV have lived only in MARCOR. Cumulative mortality at the end of the 5-year period was determined for each cohort.

III. RESULTS

The comparison of cumulative mortality and colonic biopsy data in the four cohorts of age-matched cotton-top tamarins is shown in Table 1. The age ranges and the mean age of the four cohorts were almost identical. Cohort II ($N = 58$) was composed of two subgroups of CTTs; some ($N = 31$) were breeding animals and were housed in MARCOR's spacious breeding cages, whereas others ($N = 27$) were housed only in individual cages in the research or animal holding rooms. Data for these subsets are shown separately and also collectively. Mean numbers of colonic biopsies for cohort I were 14.6 (range: 1 to 23) and the other cohorts and subgroups had ~1.0 (range: 0 to 7) biopsies.

Percentages of cumulative mortality during the 5-year periods for the various cohorts were I (44.7%), II (63.8%), III (70.0%), and IV (72.2%); mortality in cohorts I and II were significantly different, $p < .005$). Thus, mortality was *not increased, but actually lowered,* in the cohort with large numbers of colonic biopsies over those cohorts with few to no biopsies. Cumulative mortality was not different between CTTs in cohort II that were housed for the entire experimental period in the breeding facility and those that were housed entirely in individual housing. There was no difference in cumulative mortality between cohorts that lived in 1980 to 1985 and 1985 to 1990.

IV. DISCUSSION

The initial question was whether repeated colonic biopsies, e.g., 15 to 20 over a 5-year period, would increase mortality in the cotton-top tamarins so examined. Several concerns existed: (1) these animals are an endangered species, and (2) they are very valuable as well as expensive experimental animals to maintain. Cotton-top tamarin colitis occurs spontaneously and is debilitating to affected animals. However, any increased mortality associated with colonic biopsies could cause a reevaluation of the risk-benefit aspect of using the procedure experimentally. Clinically, we had an occasional animal that appeared not to recover from the effects of the anesthesia and/or procedure and died within a few days. However, at necropsy, very rarely was there any

TABLE 1
Effect of Repeated Colonic Biopsies on Mortality in Four Age-Matched Cohorts of Cotton-Top Tamarins

Cohort	No.	Age range (as of 6/10/85) (years)	Mean age (as of 6/10/85) (years)	Mortality (%)	Colon biopsies			
					Mean	Range	Median	Mode
I	38	(2.7–7.9)	5.5	44.7	14.6	(1–23)[a]	16	17
II Total	58	(2.7–6.5)	4.4	63.8	1.1	(0–7)	1	1
A[b]	27	(2.7–6.5)	4.0	62.9	1.4	(0–6)	2	1
B[c]	31	(2.8–6.4)	4.6	64.5	1.0	(0–7)	1	1
III	10	(3.6–7.3)	5.6	70.0	0.6	(0–1)	1	1
		(as of 6/10/80)	(as of 6/10/80)					
IV	18	(3.6–7.3)	5.0	72.2	0.2	(0–2)	0	0

[a] One CTT died after 1 biopsy; a second after 2.
[b] CTTs not used as breeders.
[c] CTTs used as breeders.

indication that deaths occurring within a few days postbiopsy were biopsy related (only 1 to 2); in most cases, causes of death incuded pneumonia, acute colitis, etc., but there was no evidence of peritonitis. During colonoscopy, we had suspected perforation on five occasions (out of >2000 procedures); these animals were treated aggressively with antibiotic therapy, and by peritoneal lavage (when indicated), with a high survival rate (4/5 or 80%). Thus, we had preliminary information that there were no obvious deleterious effects, but we still needed assurance that the procedure was both safe and practical for this species.

We selected three cohorts (II, III, and IV) of cotton-tops that were biopsied minimally (mean number of biopsies ~1.0) to compare with 38 animals (cohort I) that we examined and biopsied repeatedly (mean ~15). Cohort II (N = 58) was comprised almost equally of breeding animals and nonbreeders; these two subsets of cohort II would hopefully answer two questions: during the same time period (1985 to 1990), (1) was there a difference in mortality between those living in the spacious breeding facility and the individual housing? and (2) was there a difference between the oft-biopsied CTTs (cohort I) and the rarely biopsied CTTs (cohort II)?

There was no difference in mortality between tamarins housed in the spacious MARCOR breeder facility in family groups (two to 3 × 3 × 5 ft cages for each family) and nonbreeders housed in individual caging during the 5-year period. Despite the small number of animals, this observation suggests that (1) the individual cages provide adequate space for the animals' well-being and (2) there is adequate socializing for CTTs in individually housed rooms without direct physical contact. Both of these environments appear to be adequate socially when cumulative mortality is the end-point of concern.

Cumulative 5-year mortality was determined for each of the groups with very low numbers of biopsies. The 58 CTTs in cohort II had 63.8% mortality. Cohort III was a small group (N = 10 beginning in 1985), but they were born in another colony and were transferred to MARCOR in 1982. The mortality at the end of the same 5-year observation period (1985 to 1990) was only slightly higher (70.0 vs. 63.8%) than the larger control cohort II. To determine if there was any difference in cumulative mortality between a previous 5-year period (1980 to 1985) and the current time period (1985 to 1990) in which cohorts I, II, and III were examined, we examined 18 age-matched CTTs that were alive in 1980. Mortality for cohort IV was 72.2% through 1985. Thus, cumulative mortality was nearly identical in three cohorts of CTTs with the frequency of mucosal biopsies averaging ~1 over a 5-year period (range of 63.8 to 72.2%). Mortality of those frequently biopsied animals (cohort I: a mean of 14.6 biopsies over a 5-year period) had a lower cumulative mortality (44.7%). Figure 1 shows the CTT deaths by 1-year periods in cohorts I and II; differences were accounted for by increased deaths in cohort II in years four and five of the period (1985 to 1990).

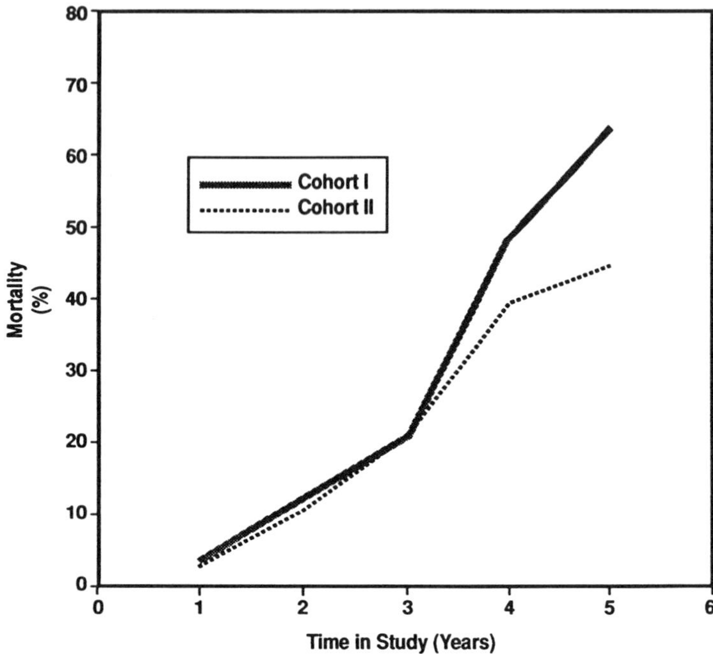

FIGURE 1. Percentage of cotton-top tamarin deaths by 1-year periods in two cohorts: I, mean number of 14.6 colonic biopsies; II, mean of 1.1 (1985 to 1990).

Thus, mortality was not increased in cotton-top tamarins that were biopsied repeatedly when their cumulative mortality was compared with cumulative mortality of either concurrent living age-matched animals or age-matched CTTs from a previous 5-year period. These data show that there was no deleterious effect as measured in increased numbers of deaths. The reason(s) for the reduced mortality in the repeatedly biopsied cohort (control mean ~70 vs. 44.7%) remains for speculation.

We can conclude from these data that the colonoscopy and mucosal biopsy technique as practiced in these studies can be safely performed without danger of increased mortality. These observations are reassuring in that this research offers hope to better understand the pathogenesis of CTT idiopathic ulcerative colitis with obvious application(s) toward successful therapeutics in CTT and man.

V. SUMMARY

From the data presented herein the question, "does repeated colonic mucosal biopsy cause increased mortality in cotton-top tamarins?" can be answered as "no". In fact the three rarely biopsied cohorts, including one that had both breeder-housed and individually caged MARCOR CTTs, had higher mortality during the same 5-year period than did the frequently biopsied cohort I (~70 vs. 44.7%). Cumulative mortality was very consistent over two 5-year periods, 1980 to 1985 and 1985 to 1990; this observation indicates that from 1980 to 1990 age-related causes of death were apparently very similar. Thus, we conclude that the colonoscopy and mucosal biopsy technique as practiced in these studies can be safely performed without danger of increased mortality. This information is extremely important, since cotton-top tamarins are endangered and, as nonhuman primates, they are also relatively expensive to maintain in captivity. These observations are reassuring in that this research offers hope to better understand the pathogenesis of CTT idiopathic ulcerative colitis with obvious application(s) toward successful therapeutics in CTT and man.

ACKNOWLEDGMENTS

This research was conducted in Oak Ridge Associated Universities' AAALAC-accredited Marmoset Research Center at Oak Ridge (MARCOR) and was approved and monitored by ORAU's Animal Care Standards Committee.

Research was supported, in part, by National Cancer Institute Contract NO1 CP21004 and the ORAU Corporation.

The authors acknowledge the excellent manuscript review by S. Tardif and R. Damian and manuscript preparation by Sandy Womble.

REFERENCES

1. **Clapp, N. K., Lushbaugh, C. C., Humason, G. L., Gangaware, B. L., and Henke, M. A.,** Natural history and pathology of colon cancer in *Saguinus oedipus oedipus, Digest. Dis. Sci.*, 30, 107S, 1985.
2. **Clapp, N. K., Henke, M. A., Hansard, R. M., Carson, R. L., Adams, L. E., and Nardi, R. V.,** Natural history, time course, and pathogenesis of idiopathic ulcerative colitis in cotton-top tamarins *(Saguinus oedipus)*, This volume, chapter 4.
3. **Clapp, N. K., Lushbaugh, C. C., Humason, G. L., Gangaware, B. L., and Henke, M. A.,** The marmoset as a model of ulcerative colitis and colon cancer, in *Colorectal Cancer and Its Precursors*, Ingalls, J. F. and Mastromarino, A., Eds., Allen R. Liss, New York, 1985, 247.
4. **Clapp, N. K. and Henke, M. A.,** Spontaneous colonic carcinoma observations in the Oak Ridge Associated Universities' 26-year-old cotton-top tamarin *(Saguinus oedipus)* colony, This volume, Chapter 11.
5. **Clapp, N. K., McArthur, A. H., Carson, R. L., Henke, M. A., and Peck, O. W.,** Endoscopy of the colon in tamarins and marmosets, *Lab. Anim. Sci.*, 35, 536, 1985.
6. **Clapp, N. K., Henke, M. A., Hansard, R. M., Adams, L. E., and Nardi, R. V.,** Does idiopathic ulcerative colitis in cotton-top tamarins (CTT) resemble the human disease?, *Gastroenterology,* submitted.
7. **Clapp, N. K., Henke, M. A., Hansard, R. M., Carson, R. L., and Nardi, R. V.,** Do repeated colonic biopsies increase mortality in colitic cotton-top tamarins (CTT)?, *Gastroenterology,* submitted.

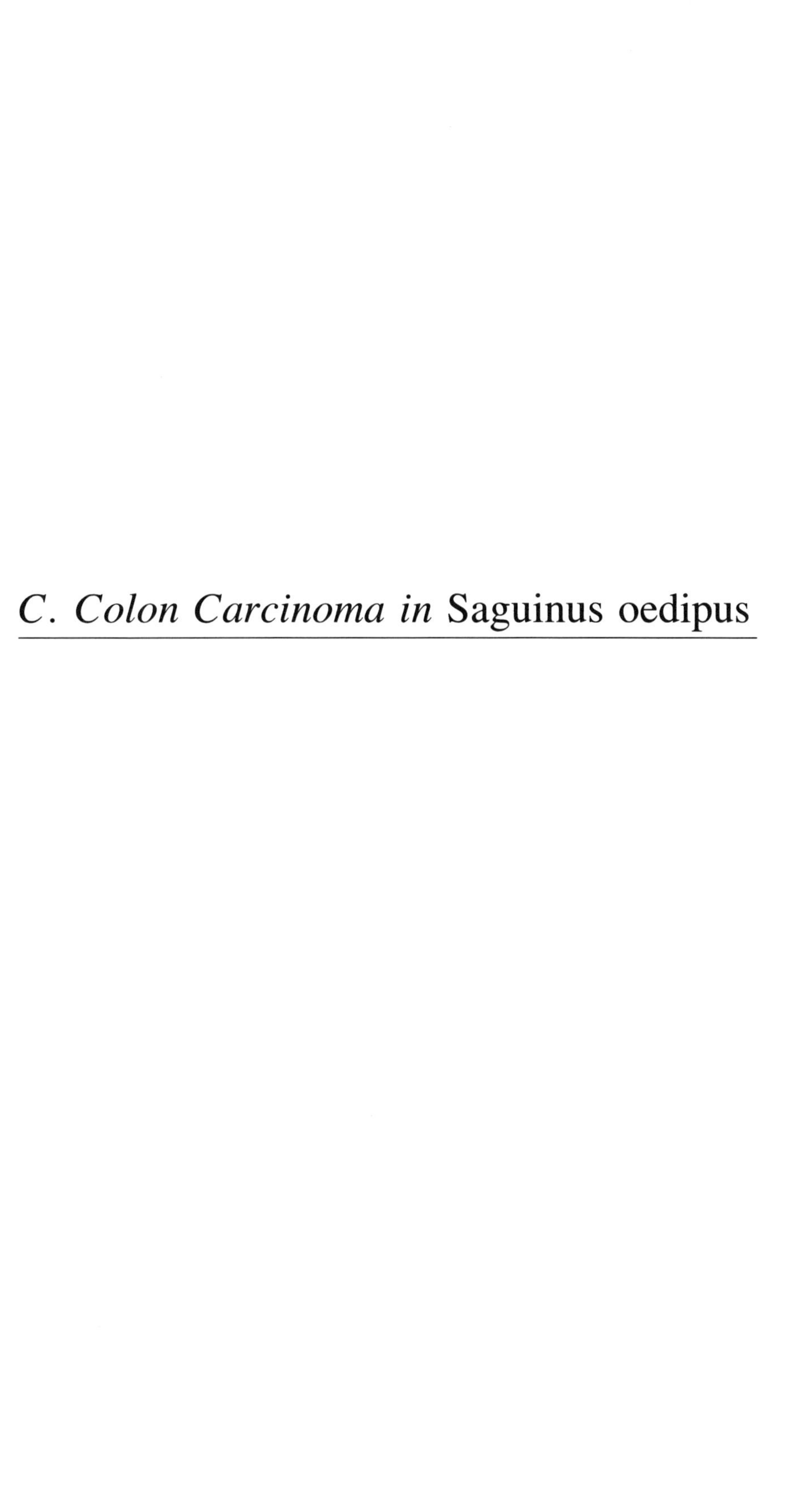

C. Colon Carcinoma in Saguinus oedipus

Chapter 11

SPONTANEOUS COLONIC CARCINOMA OBSERVATIONS IN THE OAK RIDGE ASSOCIATED UNIVERSITIES' 26-YEAR-OLD COTTON-TOP TAMARIN *(Saguinus oedipus)* COLONY

Neal K. Clapp and Marsha A. Henke

TABLE OF CONTENTS

0-8493-5363-7/93/$0.00 + $.50

I. INTRODUCTION

Cancer continues to threaten the human population throughout the world. Extensive biomedical research efforts have been conducted through government and private institutional financing, and results have been rewarding in specific cancerous processes. However, progress has been slow in a number of relatively high-incidence malignancies. Etiologies have been identified in a number of cancers, either at the "initiation" or "promotion" level of the cancer process. Still, we find that lung cancer remains as a prominent killer of men (a long-standing observation), and now increasingly of women, as the effect of increased smoking habits surfaces in increased lung cancer deaths.

Similarly, the colon cancer dilemma remains, in part, due to the difficulty in early diagnosis. Treatment of the cancer likewise has not progressed to desired levels, although combined modalities now offer some hope for improved cure rates. Strong emphasis has been placed on understanding polyp production and the transformation from a benign to malignant condition, both *in vivo* and *in vitro*. However, good colon cancer models are still lacking despite many excellent efforts to understand induced polyp-producing systems in rodents (e.g., as azoxymethane [AOM], 1,2-dimethylhydrazine [DMH], and *N*-methyl *N'*-nitro-*N*-nitrosoguanidine [MNNG]).[1] Contributions by dietary components such as fat and fiber have been also studied experimentally in rodents since they have been incriminated and/or suggested to alter the colon cancer process.[2]

The cotton-top tamarin (CTT), *Saguinus oedipus,* a small South American monkey that weighs up to 650 g, offers a truly unique opportunity for researchers to study a spontaneous colon cancer that develops in extremely high incidences. The cancer develops, most often, from a flat epithelium rather than from an adenoma/carcinoma sequence,[3,4] as is reported to occur in 80 to 90% of human colon cancer patients. The CTT pathogenesis may more closely follow the cancer family syndromes described by Lynch et al.[5,6] and the ulcerative colitis/carcinoma sequence in humans (both of which develop from a flat epithelium), than the adenoma/carcinoma process. However, the first polyp-bearing CTTs have been reported recently,[7] which suggests that CTT colon cancer pathogenesis may proceed by either the colitis/carcinoma or the adenoma/carcinoma route of transformation and may differ from humans only in taking the colitis/carcinoma route preferentially.

This report describes the occurrence of spontaneous colonic carcinoma and its demographic makeup in a long-standing (26-year-old) CTT colony; this colony includes large numbers of imported CTTs as well as colony-born progeny that also succumbed to this affliction. At this time, the occurrence of CTT colon cancer in the feral state remains uncertain, but the inflammatory condition that has been incriminated as a "promoter" in captive-held colonies[8] was also seen in animals endoscopically examined in the wild.[9] Therefore, it would seem reasonable to presume that the colon cancer process occurs in the wild as well. This suggestion is further supported by the fact that colon cancers have been reported in some 13 captive colonies. These cancers developed under diverse environmental conditions, including different caretakers, diets, husbandry, and water, and even on different continents.[10]

Since the CTT model for spontaneous colonic carcinoma had obvious merit, this report provides basic information about the colon carcinoma that will enable researchers to study the CTT process in light of the almost identical disease in humans. While interspecies extrapolation is always of great concern, the similarities between the disease in CTTs and humans continue to surface and seem to justify increased research efforts to better understand the CTT disease and to make first approximations toward the human condition. Ultimately, therapeutics against colon disease may be applied, tested, and evaluated in CTTs over a time span of a few years, whereas similar results in humans would require many years to obtain.

II. METHODS

A. ANIMAL NUMBERS

Cotton-top tamarins were imported into the Oak Ridge Associated Universities (ORAU) colony beginning in 1965 in small numbers and continued until 1976 when the CTT was declared endangered; they were placed upon the endangered species list and ORAU's importation of CTTs ceased. A total of 364 CTTs were imported from various suppliers. In 1982, ORAU was awarded a contract from the National Cancer Institute (NCI) to raise CTTs for cancer research, and 55 NCI-owned CTTs that had been housed at Rush Presbyterian-St. Luke's Medical Center in Chicago were transferred to ORAU's colony. In this chapter they will be included in the ORAU animals. Prior to their arrival at ORAU, no colonic carcinomas had been reported in the Rush colony, but one CTT with colon cancer died 4 months after its arrival. A few other CTTs (25) were received on breeder loan from other closed colonies, in particular the University of Wisconsin Department of Psychology.

Because of the imposed restrictions upon importation of CTTs from the wild, breeding of captive animals became essential if adequate numbers would be available for biomedical research efforts. The susceptibility of the CTT to Epstein-Barr virus infection, plus the newly discovered susceptibility of CTTs to spontaneous development of colonic carcinoma, expanded the use of and demands for this relatively new experimental species. Consequently, a newly designed breeding facility was built at ORAU for the express purpose of determining the limiting factors to successful breeding and then propagating CTTs in captivity for research purposes. Colony-born CTTs are an integral part of the data in this chapter.

From the total of 444 CTTs that were brought into the ORAU colony from other sources plus subsequent colony-born animals, data will be reported on 476 deaths of CTTs of both sexes that lived >1 year in the colony from 1965 to 1991. Excluded animals were predominantly neonatal deaths and imported animals that died as a result of shipment and relocation stresses; these CTTs were not considered to be at risk for colon cancer. Colony-born CTTs that survived early neonatal mortality are at risk as young adults; the youngest colony-born CTT diagnosed with colon cancer died at 15 months of age. A total of 249 imports and 227 colony-born CTTs comprise the data-set for this report.

B. NECROPSY PROCEDURE

Complete necropsies were performed on all CTTs immediately after death or euthanasia if they became moribund. All tissues (approximately 25 per animal) were preserved by 10% buffered-formalin fixation and/or freezing. Intestinal tissues were divided into duodenum, jejunum, and ileum (small intestine) and cecum and ascending, transverse, and descending colon (large intestine). The segments were opened longitudinally while pinned on the necropsy board; one half was rolled from the proximal to the distal end of the segment and fixed in formalin and the other half was quick frozen. Histological sections (5 μm) were prepared and tissues were routinely stained with periodic-acid Schiff's (PAS) reagent; this stain was of great benefit in identifying colon cancer metastases that were mucin-producing.

C. HISTOLOGY OF COLON CANCERS

The histological picture of CTT colonic carcinoma has been described in detail previously.[3,4] Primary colon cancers routinely developed from a flat epithelium in contrast with observations in humans where ~85% of the tumors are reported to develop from transformations in polyps.[11,12] CTT malignancies more closely follow the pathogenesis seen in the cancer family syndromes[5,6] and the hereditary nonpolyposis syndromes.[11] A recent report describes the first polyps seen in CTTs; after several visualizations and biopsies, one polyp was presumed to have become malignant.[7]

Primaries were most often anaplastic undifferentiated carcinomas with limited mucin production; however, malignant cells that were invasive or metastatic to other tissues were very high in mucin production. Most metastases were also undifferentiated, but, on rare occasions, metastatic cells formed aborted crypt-like structures. These were often from primaries with similar steps toward differentiation. Primary tumors were found in association with either active acute or chronic colitis,[8] but colon cancer was always found in association with colonic mucosa that showed evidence of either present or prior episodes of active colitis.

D. PARAMETERS EVALUATED

The effect of age, gender, and source of animals (imported vs. colony-born) will be discussed. The location of the malignancies within the colon and the predilection of metastatic sites will be shown and discussed.

Table 1

INCIDENCES OF COLON CANCER IN 476 COTTON-TOP TAMARINS *(Saguinus oedipus)* THAT DIED FROM 1965 THROUGH 1991 AFTER LIVING >1 YEAR IN ORAU COLONY

Category	No.	%
All cancer deaths	164	34.45%
All import cancer deaths	92	36.94% (92/249)
All colony-born cancer deaths	72	31.71% (72/227)

(through 12/31/91)

Table 2

EFFECTS OF AGE AND GENDER ON COLON CANCER IN IMPORTED AND COLONY BORN *S. oedipus*

	Age (Years)		Incidence (%)	
	Mean	Mode	Male	Female
Import	6.5	5	57	43
Colony-Born	11.1	8	53	47

(through 12/31/91)

III. RESULTS

In Table 1 are shown the number of cancer deaths in 476 import and colony-born CTTs that lived >1 year in the ORAU colony from 1965 to 1991. There were a total of 164 cotton-tops with colon cancers in 476 dead CTTs, a 34.4% incidence; a single CTT that died with colon cancer $3^1/_2$ months after importation was excluded from the data in Table 1 by the colony age restriction. Imported animal deaths with colon cancer were 36.9% (92/249) while colony-born deaths were 31.7% (72/227). Table 2 shows the cancer incidence and mean and mode age of occurrence in males and females within the import and colony-born CTTs. Males were slightly higher in incidence than females (57 vs. 43%, imports; and 53 vs. 47%, colony-born). The mean time of occurrence was 6.5 years of colony residence time for imports and 11.1 years (actual age) for colony-born CTTs with a mode of 5 and 8 years, respectively.

Figure 1 is a histogram of 93 colon cancer deaths by colony age (actual age is unknown) for imported CTTs and Figure 2 is a similar graph for 72

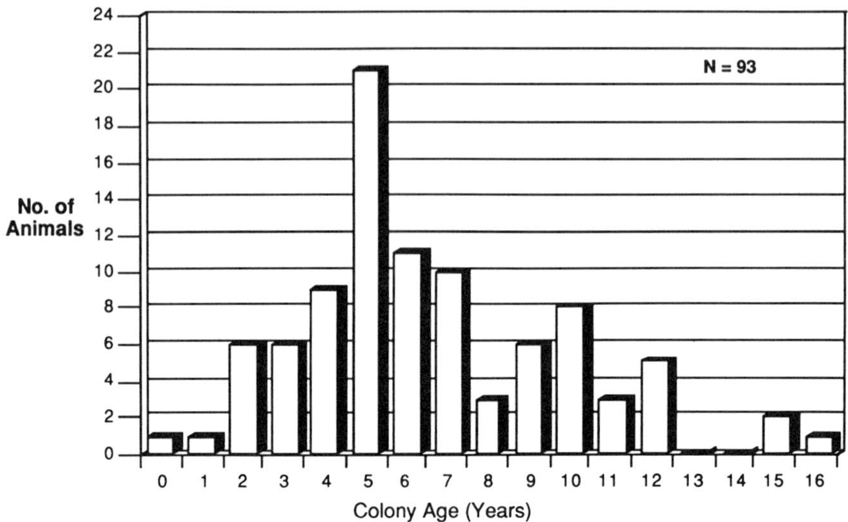

FIGURE 1. Histogram of 93 colon cancer deaths in imported cotton-top tamarins (*S. oedipus*) by colony age (1965 to 1991).

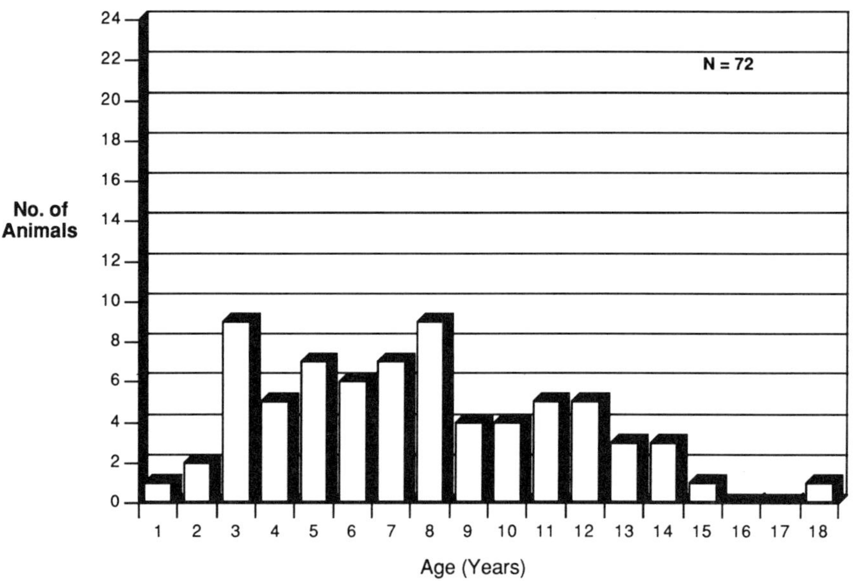

FIGURE 2. Histogram of 70 colon cancer deaths in colony-born cotton-top tamarins (*S. oedipus*) by age (1965 to 1991).

Table 3
FREQUENCY OF CARCINOMAS IN *S. oedipus* DEATHS BY AGE GROUPS. FROM 1981 THROUGH 1991

Year of Death	Colony Age (No. Cancers/No. Deaths)					
	(1-3 years)	(4-7 years)	(8-11 years)	(>12 years)		
1981	0/1	16/19	2/3	0/0		
1982	0/0	8/13	1/4	1/2		
1983	1/8	6/9	1/7	1/1		
1984	1/2	5/8	5/15	0/2		
1985	0/5	3/5	2/9	2/8		
1986	1/2	2/7	6/11	0/8		
1987	0/7	3/7	3/11	4/6		
1988	0/6	1/6	7/17	8/16		
1989	3/13	4/20	1/14	1/9		
1990	0/5	4/12	4/6	1/3		
1991	1/6	·2/5	3/6	4/10		
Totals	7/55	54/111	35/102	22/65	=	118/333
%	12.7	48.6	34.3	33.8	=	35.4%

(through 12/31/91)

colony-born CTTs (actual ages) through 1991. Both very young animals (15 months of age) (Figure 2) and relatively old animals (15 and 16 years) developed colonic cancer. From these data one could conclude that the preponderance of cancer deaths occurred in young adults. Nevertheless, some older animals in the 12- to 16-year range (human equivalent of ~60 to 80 years) were also susceptible.

Prior to 1981 different pathologists were responsible for necropsies and some differences naturally existed in sampling techniques and necropsy procedures. From 1981 to the present consistent tissue sampling procedures were used. CTT deaths with colon cancer from 1981 to the present are shown (Table 3) as a fraction of the number dying in 3-year age groups. For this table, colony ages for imports and actual ages for colony-born animals are used. Prior to 1981, no CTT over 6 years of age had died with colon cancer. Although the number of animals surviving to older ages is relatively small, we found that, in 1991, 4/10 CTTs dying at >12 years of age had colon cancer (Table 3). In the 10-year period from 1981 to 1991, the percentages of cancer positives/number of deaths for 4 to 7, 8 to 11, and >12 years of age were 48.6, 34.3, and 33.8%, respectively, with an overall percentage of

Table 4

LOCATION OF PRIMARY ADENOCARCINOMAS OF THE LARGE BOWEL *(S. oedipus)*

	All Cancer Animals
Number of Cancer Positive Animals	165
Colon Segment	
Cecum	78
Ascending Colon	71
Transverse	57
Descending Colon	90
Rectum	19
Segment Not Identified	4
Multiple Segments With Primaries	93

(through 12/31/91)

35.4% (118/333). This further supports the notion that the colon cancer occurred in slightly higher incidence in the 4- to 7-year group. Data in the table suggest that animals are living longer (dying later), which is due to two factors. First, the biological age of imported animals is unknown. An entry date for imported CTTs provides only a ''colony age'' (actual time in the colony); the largest number of import deaths was in the 4- to 7-year colony-age range. Secondly, colony-born CTTs have an ''older'' colony age than imports because of known actual ages; in addition, animals are generally living longer becuse of improved husbandry and general clinical care and knowledge. Some of our collaborators (Cheverud and co-workers) are currently studying ways to retrospectively approximate ages from skeletal collections through identifying the numbers of annulations in teeth. This information would provide more accurate estimtes of the imported animals' actual ages and would significantly improve the interpretation of age effects from these data.

Table 4 shows the distribution of primary adenocarcinomas by location (segments) within the large bowel. The number of animals is the total number of colon cancer-positive CTTs (165). The number for each colon segment is the total numbers of each segment that had identified primary tumors. Most of the cancer-positive segments had multiple primaries. For purposes of comparison with human data, the cecum, ascending, and transverse colon were considered ''right-side'' and the descending colon and rectum were ''left-side colon''; amounts of colonic tissue were approximately equal between

Table 5
SITES OF METASTASES OF 165 COLONIC ADENOCARCINOMAS
***(S. oedipus)* (1965-1991)**

Site	%
LN-Regional	75.1
Lung	13.9
Pancreas	12.1
Adrenal	3.6
Ovary	3.6
Uterus	1.2
Prostate	1.2
Liver	1.2
No Metastases Found	24.2

(through 12/31/91)

right and left sides. Right-sided cancer segments comprised 206/315 (65%) and left-sided were 109/315 (35%). The colon cancer distribution in right- and left-sided colon were comparable to those found in cancer family syndromes, hereditary nonpolyposis colorectal cancers, and ulcerative colitis/carcinoma patients.[5,6,13] They contrast with distribution of polyps and sporadic colon cancer incidences in humans, which are predominantly (80 to 85%) left-sided in location.[10] Use of the term "multiple segments" indicates where primary tumors were found in more than one colonic segment in an animal (93/165 = 56.3%).

CTT colonic carcinomas metastasized very early. In reviewing archival necropsy specimens collected prior to 1981, metastases were sometimes found in regional lymph nodes with PAS stain while no primary tumor was recognized in the original sections. Additional histological sections of the colon segments would then reveal the location of the colonic primary(s). With improved survival due to changes in sanitation and improved overall colony health and clinical care, cancers were larger, with more readily recognized metastatic foci (Table 5). The primary site of metastatic disease was the regional lymph nodes (75.1%) which varied in location depending upon the particular lymph nodes that drained the malignant segment(s). The highest incidence of distant metastasis was found in the lung (13.9%) with the abdominal organs being lesser affected sites that became involved when cancerous cells invaded through the colonic serosa. An obvious difference in metastastic predilection between CTTs and humans is the relative lack of liver metastases; while several conjectures have been offered, no satisfactory explanation has yet emerged.

IV. DISCUSSION

A. IMPORT VS. COLONY-BORN

The first colon cancers were reported in imported CTTs by Lushbaugh et al., in 1978.[14] Early on, the phenomenon was considered by some as strictly on ORAU colony problem. However, the 1981 report of 15 colonic cancers at the New England Regional Primate Research Center colony[15] confirmed a species susceptibility that was broader than a simple environmental contaminant problem in a single colony.

Whereas most of the early (1970s) cancers were found in imported CTTs,[3,4,15] the similar susceptibility of colony-born animals was soon confirmed, as was the lack of susceptibility of two other coexisting species at ORAU, the saddle-back tamarin and the common marmoset.[3] The cancer was also found in a number of other colonies, including the University of Bristol colony in Europe.[14] From the data in Table 1, colony-born animals have almost identical colon cancer prevalences as do imported animals (31.7 vs. 36.9%). Nearly all imported CTTs are now dead, since all importation ceased in 1976. The previously reported overall colon cancer incidence of 35%[3] that had been seen in the ORAU colony remained quite steady after some 26 total years of colony existence. One imported CTT died with colonic carcinoma 3½ months after arrival at ORAU, which strongly suggests, but certainly does not prove, that the malignancy developed prior to the animal leaving the wild. The question, "does colon cancer occur in feral animals?" is one of the interesting, but as yet unanswered, questions regarding the susceptibility of the species.

B. GENDER

Both sexes of CTTs are susceptible to development of colon cancer (Table 2), although males have slightly higher incidences, especially in imports (57 vs. 43%). The combined mean age at death for both sexes of imports (6.5 years) was less than that of colony-born (11.1 years and increasing). Data for imports are nearly complete with only seven still alive (as of January 1992). The observed modes also reflect the difference between colony age (age of entry into the colony) and the actual biological age, which was precisely known for colony-born animals. With an approximate maximum life span of 20 or so years for CTTs, one can considered that the age of greatest risk is the early to mid-adulthood; 5- to 8-year-old CTTs would reasonably compare agewise with 25 to 40-year-old humans. These ages are similar to the high-risk ages of human ulcerative colitis patients, but are younger than the majority of sporadic (not genetically related) colon cancer occurrences, which are primarily in later ages (>50 years of age) in the human population.[11,12]

C. AGE

The fact that older animals are now developing colonic cancer reflects the aging of the colony and the fact that import animals are "aged" beginning not at birth but at the time (and age) that they have entered the colony. As a result, the age for most cancers has changed during three somewhat arbitrary ~5-year "periods" of colony operation. First, prior to 1981, no colon cancer had been found in CTTs older than 6 years; these were mostly imported animals. At that time, a hypothesis was considered that CTT colon cancer might closely parallel those colon tumors of human genetically related incidences, e.g., familial polyposis coli, as the deaths were found only in young adults. This hypothesis became less attractive as a second period of thinking was entered beginning in 1981, and continuing through ~1985, in which colon cancer was also found in some older animals (>8 years of age). Most deaths and most colon cancers still occurred in the 4- to 7-year age period (Table 3); however, by 1985, all imports were >9 years of age and colony-born CTTs were "aging" and reaching what we now recognize as the higher-risk ages of 5 to 10 years. During this period, a second hypothesis was considered which stated that CTT colon cancers may occur in a biphasic pattern with early and late peaks. This distribution would closely parallel the human age distribution in which early colon cancers are genetically related but the largest number of sporadic colon cancers are late occurring; the numbers increased rapidly with aging of the population. During the next period, beginning in 1985 and continuing through 1991, most deaths were found in the 8- to 11- and >12-year age groups; ~35% of the deaths were still colon cancer related. As shown in the bar graphs of Figures 1 and 2, CTTs of all ages are susceptible to colon cancer; the current distribution across age closely resembles a normal statistical distribution with the only difference being that the most common observation (mode) in colony-born (age known) CTTs is actually ~3 years older than the import mode of 5 years.

D. DISTRIBUTION IN THE LARGE BOWEL

The long-standing dogmas in human colorectal cancer are that most, if not all, cancers develop from or in polyps and a majority of the cancers occur in the left side of the colon.[11,12] The location of adenomatous polyps appears to increase as one proceeds from the cecum through the descending colon and rectum. However, two new concepts have entered the picture: (1) the development of colonic tumors from a flat epithelium in ulcerative colitis and hereditary nonpolyposis colon cancer patients,[13] rather than going through a polyp stage, and (2) the increase in numbers of patients that have colonic malignancies of the right side.[5,6] Distribution of malignant primaries in the CTT colon follows the human colitis/carcinoma process very closely; only rarely do cancers develop from an adenomatous polyp. While the chemically induced rodent models of polyp induction, e.g., by the cycad derivatives, mimic the spontaneous and, to some degree, the genetically related familial polyposis coli syndrome, the cotton-top tamarin very closely parallels the nonpolypoid route of colon carcinogenesis. Based upon the obvious similarities between the CTT and at least some aspects of the human disease, the CTT model offers unique opportunities to study pathogenesis, therapeutics, and preventive actions in a more closely controlled experimental situation than would be possible in a human population.

E. METASTATIC POTENTIAL

The spontaneous CTT adenocarcinoma has a high metastic potential but has some most interesting differences from the human. The most obvious difference is that there is no apparent predilection for metastasis to the liver, a very serious, often fatal, complication of the human disease. In 1984, a number of prominent pathologists and colon cancer experts examined tissues from CTT colon cancers. One suggestion that was offered to explain the lack of liver metastases in CTTs was the apparent absence of angioinvasion by the CTT cancers. However, lymphatics and lymph nodes were commonly invaded by most CTT cancers, and these metastases would be expected to spread directly to the liver and eventually to the lung. Another interesting observation was that the malignancies spread to the lymphatics and lymph nodes very early but then proceed to distant sites later in the disease process. A possible explanation is that the CTT tumors may have strong antigenic potential that elicits sufficient host response to confine the tumor within the lymphatic system until later stages of the disease when immune surveillance is overwhelmed and distant metastasis occurs.

F. PRIMARY NEOPLASMS OF ORGANS OTHER THAN COLON

The incidences of primary neoplasms other than colon in 315 *Saguinus oedipus* and 101 *Callithrix jacchus* (common marmoset) that survived >1 year in the ORAU colony are listed in Table 6. Surprisingly, in CTTs only the remaining gastrointestinal tract (stomach and small intestine) joined the colon as sites for development of malignancies (a total of six carcinomas); primary tumors of these sites were still rare (incidences <2%). Other most frequent sites of CTT neoplasms (benign adenomas) were the thyroid (14.3%), adrenal cortex (3.2%), and uterus (1.9%). Similarly, common marmosets had few neoplasms, only three small intestine adenocarcinomas and 7.9% thyroid adenomas. The susceptibility of both callitrichid species to leukemias was very low; only a single reticulum cell sarcoma was diagnosed in CTTs and none were found in *Callithrix jacchus*. Both callitrichid species examined in this study were quite refractory to neoplasm induction of all organs except the colon; this lack of susceptibility to malignancies of other organs contrasts with most experimental species (especially rodents) which usually develop neoplasms of some organs in high incidences if survival is of sufficient time.[17]

Table 6

INCIDENCES OF PRIMARY NEOPLASMS, OTHER THAN COLON, IN *S. oedipus* AND *C. jacchus* SURVIVING > 1 YEAR IN ORAU COLONY (1981-1991)

	Saguinus oedipus	MAD+	Callithrix jacchus	MAD+
TOTAL DEATHS	315	2939	101	2135
Site of Neoplasm*	Incidence			
	(%)	MAD	(%)	MAD
Thyroid (A)	14.3	4515	7.9	3549
Adrenal [(A=9), (H=1)]	3.2	4905	–	–
Uterus [(A=4), (F=2)]	1.9	4012	–	–
Pancreas (A)	1.6	4372	–	–
Ileum [(A=1), (C=4)]	1.6	3892	–	–
Duodenum [(A=3), (C=1)]	1.3	4192	1.0	2096
Kidney [(A=2), (H=1)]	0.9	5824	–	–
Liver (A)	0.6	4846	–	–
Bladder (H)	0.3	2195	–	–
Salivary Gland (A)	0.3	2300	–	–
Testes (A)	0.3	3160	–	–
Mandible (O)	0.3	3812	–	–
Stomach (C)	0.3	5585	–	–
Ovary (A)	0.3	5585	–	–
Jejunum (C)	–	–	2.0	2365
Leukemias				
Reticulum Cell Sarcoma	0.3			

* – Pathology Codes:
A – Adenoma
C – Carcinoma
H – Hemangioma
O – Osteogenic sarcoma
F – Fibroma
\+ – Mean age at death (days)

V. SUMMARY

In summary, spontaneous colonic carcinoma develops in approximately 35% of adult CTTs; the cancers usually develop from a flat epithelium, are nonpolypoid, and occur in association with an idiopathic ulcerative colitis. The cancer can develop in all ages but is preferentially age dependent, in particular in young adult CTTs (5 to 10 years of age). The cancer has been found about equally in each gender and in colony-born and imported animals; it was predominatly (65 vs. 35%) a right-sided colon disease and metastasized readily to regional lymph nodes, less often to the lungs and pancreas, but rarely to the liver. Both callitrichid species, cotton-top tamarins and common marmosets, are refractory to spontaneous malignant neoplasms of most organs other than the gastrointestinal system, and only benign adenomas were found in rather low incidences in the thyroid and adrenal glands. Spontaneous CTT colon cancers closely mimic those in humans that arise in ulcerative colitis and hereditary nonpolyposis colon carcinoma patients and could serve as a valuable model for mechanistic, therapeutic, and preventive action research in CTTs and humans.

ACKNOWLEDGMENTS

The authors acknowledge the scientific contribution of Clarence C. Lushbaugh and Gretchen Humason for pathology diagnosis in the early years of the colony's existence; S. Tardif and R. Hansard for their assistance in data assimilation, analysis, and processing; S. Tardif and R. Damian for excellent manuscript review; and S. Womble for manuscript preparation.

REFERENCES

1. **Shamsuddin, A. K. M.,** In vivo induction of colon cancer dose and animal species, in *Experimental Colon Carcinogenesis,* Autrup, H. and Williams, G., Eds., CRC Press, Boca Raton, FL, 1983, chap. 3.
2. **Reddy, B. S.,** Dietary fat and colon cancer, in *Experimental Colon Carcinogenesis,* Autrup, H. and Williams, G., Eds., CRC Press, Boca Raton, FL, 1983, chap. 15.
3. **Clapp, N. K., Lushbaugh, C. C., Humason, G. L., Gangaware, B. L., and Henke, M. A.,** Natural history and pathology of colon cancer in *Saguinus oedipus oedipus, Digest. Dis. Sci.,* 30, 107S, 1985.
4. **Lushbaugh, C. C., Humason, G., and Clapp, N. K.,** Histology of colon cancer in *Saguinus oedipus oedipus, Digest. Dis. Sci.,* 30, 119S, 1985.
5. **Lynch, P. M., Lynch, H. T., and Harris, R. E.,** Hereditary proximal colonic cancer, *Dis. Colon Rectum,* 20, 661, 1977.
6. **Lynch, H. T., Lynch, P. M., Albano, W. A., and Lynch, J. F.,** The cancer family syndrome: a status report, *Dis. Colon Rectum,* 24, 311, 1981.
7. **Clapp, N. K., Henke, M. A., Hansard, R. M., Adams, L. J., Carson, R. L., Hawkins, J. V., and Nardi, R.,** Colonic polyps associated with colitis in cotton-top tamarins *(Saguinus oedipus):* progression to colonic carcinoma?, *Digest. Dis. Sci.,* submitted.
8. **Clapp, N. K., Henke, M. A., Lushbaugh, C. C., Humason, G. L., and Gangaware, B. L.,** Effect of various biological factors on spontaneous marmoset and tamarin colitis: a retrospective histopathologic study, *Digest. Dis. Sci.,* 33, 1013, 1988.
9. **Wood, J. D., Peck, O. C., Sharma, H. M., Mekhjian, H. S., Stone, D. W., Stonerook, M., Weiss, H. S., Hernandez, J., Rodriquez, J. V., and Rodriquez, M. A.,** Captivity promotes colitis in the cotton-top tamarin *(Saguinus oedipus), Gastroenterology,* 98, 1408, 1990.
10. **Clapp, N. K.,** Prevalence of colonic carcinoma in cotton-top tamarin colonies throughout the world, This volume, Chapter 13.
11. **Muto, T., Bussey, H. J. R., and Morson, B. C.,** The evolution of cancer of the colon and rectum, *Cancer,* 36, 2251, 1975.
12. **Morson, B.,** The polyp cancer sequence in the large bowel, *Proc. R. Soc. Med.,* 67, 451, 1974.

13. **Lynch, H. T., Kimberling, W., Albano, W. A., Lynch, J. F., Biscone, K., Schuelke, G. S., Sandberg, A. A., Lipkin, M., Deschner, E. E., Mikol, Y. B., Elston, R. C., Bailey-Wilson, J. E., and Danes, B. S.,** Hereditary nonpolyposis colorectal cancer (Lynch syndromes I and II). I. Clinical description of research, *Cancer (Philadelphia),* 56, 934, 1985.
14. **Lushbaugh, C. C., Humason, G. L., Swartzendruber, D. C., Richter, C. B., and Gengozian, N.,** Proceedings of the Conference, Oak Ridge, Tennessee 1977, *Primates Med.,* 10, 119, 1978.
15. **Chalifoux, L. V. and Bronson, R. T.,** Colonic adenocarcinoma associated with chronic colitis in cotton-top marmosets, *Sanguinus oedipus, Gastroenterology,* 80, 942, 1981.
16. **Kirkwood, J. K., Pearson, G. R., and Epstein, M. A.,** Adenocarcinoma of the large bowel and colitis in captive cotton-top tamarins *Saguinus o. oedipus, J. Comp. Pathol.,* 96, 507, 1986.
17. **Clapp, N. K.,** personal observations.

Chapter 12

GENETIC EPIDEMIOLOGY OF COLON CANCER

Gloria M. Petersen and Marie-Paule Roth

TABLE OF CONTENTS

0-8493-5363-7/93/$0.00 + $.50

I. INTRODUCTION

The cotton-top tamarin provides a unique opportunity for research into the genetic factors that predispose to colon cancer and their interaction with environmental agents. While a number of laboratory studies are important for identifying specific factors, a tremendous amount also can be learned from the genetic epidemiologic approach. In humans, the information provided by genetic and family studies of colorectal cancer have proved useful to demonstrate the existence of genetic predisposition. In this chapter, we will review such studies and show that relatives of an index case (propositus or proband) with common colorectal cancer are themselves at an increased risk for cancer, when compared to controls. Analogously, studies like this can shed light on the genetic predisposition to colon cancer in cotton-top tamarins, and help identify more productive lines of investigation that can optimize the use of this animal model in research.

II. GENETIC SUSCEPTIBILITY TO COLON CANCER IN HUMANS

A number of factors, both genetic and nongenetic, have been implicated in the development of colorectal cancer. Genetic susceptibility has been deduced from familial aggregation and the existence of inherited syndromes. Although colorectal cancer occurs in Gardner's syndrome, familial adenomatous polyposis, or cancer family syndrome, and in conditions with a genetic predisposition, such as ulcerative colitis, these diseases account for a small fraction of the total cases of colorectal cancer in humans. Several studies have attempted to estimate this fraction. For example, in one Finnish province during a 10-year period, 26/468 (5.5%) of all colorectal carcinoma patients had the diagnosis of cancer family syndrome.[1] Among their 584 family members, 150 (25.7%) had some form of malignancy, 86 (14.7%) being colorectal carcinomas. In this study, the frequencies of familial adenomatous polyposis and ulcerative colitis were 0.2 and 0.6%, respectively, so that approximately 4 to 6% of all colorectal carcinoma seemed to be due to specific genetic syndromes. Kee and Collins[2] evaluated 205 colon cancer cases (excluding familial polyposis) under age 55 in Northern Ireland between 1976 and 1978. They obtained an estimate of 1 to 2% being cancer family syndrome cases.

Hereditary colon cancers have been reported to be associated with earlier age of onset and proximal colon site.[3] However, Cannon-Albright et al.[4] tested these associations in 1800 colon cancer patients using a Utah population database. They estimated kinship coefficients in familial clusters of patients with early age of onset and proximal colon site and compared them to the distal or late-onset colon cancer families. If these features were hereditary, one would expect lower kinship coefficients in the latter group. They found that mean kinship coefficients were the same in both groups of patients, suggesting that early-onset and proximal colon site may not be hallmarks of familial cases, Kee and Collins[2] also have reported that proximal tumor excess was not a characteristic of colon cancer families. Thus, patients from colon cancer families may not have particular clinical characteristics, yet have a genetic predisposition. Family history may be the most important clue.

Only the rare genetic syndromes that have clearly recognized modes of inheritance may yield single inherited markers that are useful for accurate risk assessment. Most recently, the gene for familial adenomatous polyposis on the long arm of chromosome 5 has been identified[5,6] in humans. Although the Kidd blood group was reported to be linked to colon cancer syndrome,[7] a study in Finland could exclude linkage with the putative colon cancer gene, DCC.[8] The fact remains that the majority of colorectal cancer cases arise in families with no readily apparent specific inheritance patterns. A number of these families exhibit some familial aggregation, suggesting that hereditary factors may be important, but require interaction with environment factors. A number of retrospective studies have attempted to estimate the extent to which genetic factors infuence the incidence of common cancer of the large intestine. These are summarized in Table 1, and are detailed below. These studies rely primarily on analysis of family history of colorectal cancer.

Woolf's study of colon cancer pedigrees from Utah showed a higher number of deaths from colon carcinoma in the first-degree relatives of 242 patients who had died from colorectal cancer not associated with multiple polyposis, compared to control subjects.[9] Propositi were obtained from death certificates and family histories were determined from the records of the Mormon Genealogical Society. Causes of death for the relatives (145 fathers, 142 mothers, 209 brothers, 167 sisters) were also determined from death certificates. The control group consisted of sex-matched individuals who had died in the same country, the same year, and at approximately the same age as each of the deceased relatives of the propositi. Twenty-six first-degree relatives of the propositi (3.9%) had colorectal carcinoma compared to eight (1.2%) controls ($p < .01$). The number of deaths due to colorectal cancer was increased over the controls in all four classes of relatives.

Macklin studied the family histories of 145 patients who had surgery for carcinoma of the large intestine in Ohio.[10] He found a similar increase in death rates from the condition in both first-degree (118 fathers, 108 mothers, 82 brothers, 84 sisters) and second-degree relatives (139 grandfathers, 136 grandmothers, 369 uncles, 333 aunts) when compared with the general population of corresponding sex, age, and time-of-death distribution in Ohio. Thirty-one first-degree relatives (7.9%) and 47 second-degree relatives (4.8%) had colorectal cancer, compared to an expected 4.9 and 1.8%. There was also an excess of large bowel cancer in every category of the deceased relatives. In both of these retrospective studies, individuals were selected only when there was substantial evidence on the death certificate that carcinoma of the large intestine was present, as reported by the attending physician. Certificates were not included if there was any indication that multiple polyposis had been present, but case records were not examined and therefore

TABLE 1
Summary of Human Studies Documenting Increased Risk to Relatives of Patients with Colorectal Cancer (CRC) and Polyps

Location (Ref.)	No. of CRC propositi	First-degree relatives with CRC (%)	Patients with positive family history (%)	Controls with CRC (%)	Controls with positive family history (%)
Utah (9)[a]	242	26/663 (3.9%)	—	8/663 (1.2%)	—
Ohio (10)[a]	145	31/392 1st degree (7.9%) 47/977 2nd degree (4.8%)	—	19.4/392 (4.9%) 17.5/977 (1.8%)	—
London (11)[a]	209	41/352 (11.6%)	—	11.66/352 (3.3%)	—
Nebraska (12)[b]	50	15/470 (3.2%)	8/50 (16%)	3/460 (0.6%)	—
Scotland (13)[b]	50	8/349	8/50 (16%)	1/386 (0.3%)	1/50 (2%)
Melbourne (14)[b]	702	—	125/702 (18%)	—	—
Italy (15)[b]	100	—	11/100 (11%)	—	6/100 (6%)
Denmark (16)[b]	1,524 (<60 years)	186/2,650 (7%)	179/1,524 (11.7%)	—	—
France (18)[b,c]	170 CRC 170 Polyps	—	32/170 (18.8%) 25/270 (14.7%)	—	6/170 (3.4%)
Italy (19)[b,c]	139 CRC 151 Polyps	71/2,202 (3.2%)	—	16/2,203 (0.7%)	—
Italy (20)[b,c]	414 CRC 283 Polyps	—	47/414 (11.3%) 41/283 (14.5%)	—	44/855 (5.1%)
Utah (24)[d]	5 CRC 11 Polyps	67 Polyps/23 (20.7%)	—	25 Polyps/213 (11.7%)	—
Israel (25,26)[d]	—	38/471 asymptomatic 1st degree relatives (8.1%)	—	17/457 (3.7%)	—

[a] Death certificate data only.
[b] Data on all relatives, deceased and alive.
[c] Data included index cases with adenomatous polyps.
[d] Data on screened asymptomatic relatives included.

neither of these studies can claim to have successfully excluded patients with diseases such as polyposis coli.

Mortality figures have also been examined more recently by Lovett in London.[11] Death certificates were obtained for parents (161 fathers, 155 mothers) and siblings (57 brothers, 57 sisters) of 209 colorectal cancer patients. In all the groups of first-degree relatives there was a three- to fourfold increase in the death rate from intestinal cancer over that which would be expected in a comparable group of deaths in the general population (11.6 vs. 3.3%). This study also suggested that when a patient had multiple benign or malignant tumors in the large bowel, previous primary carcinoma or adenoma in the large bowel, or early age of onset of colorectal cancer, then he or she was more likely to have a positive family history of colorectal cancer.

However, mortality figures may not accurately estimate the incidence of colorectal cancer among first-degree relatives, because affected relatives may still be alive at the time of the study, or may have died from another cause. These problems were addressed by later studies. Lynch et al. studied 50 patients with histologically verified adenocarcinoma of the colon who were matched to patients of the same age and sex, admitted at approximately the same time with a diagnosis other than cancer, in Omaha, Nebraska.[12] Genealogy was documented as completely as possible through interviews of the patients and at least one of their first-degree relatives, and the information was verified through physician or hospital records. They found 15 first-degree relatives who suffered from the disease, vs. 3 in the control group. These 15 relatives, however, were distributed among 8 families; thus, 8/50, or 16%, of the index cases had a positive family history of colorectal cancer.

Duncan and Kyle studied 50 consecutive patients with adenocarcinoma of the colon or rectum in Scotland, excluding syndromic colon cancers.[13] Family histories on 349 first-degree relatives (parents, siblings, and children) were obtained. Comparable controls matched for sex and age, admitted for treatment of various nonmalignant conditions were identified. Family histories of 386 first-degree relatives were obtained. Eight of 50 patients in the cancer group (16%) and only one in the control group (2%) had a first-degree relative with colorectal cancer ($p < .05$). These investigators also examined clinical characteristics of their patients with positive family histories. They found that their mean age was similar to that of the whole group. In the patients with adenomatous polyps, 2 out of 12 (16%) had a positive family history of colorectal cancer, exactly the same percentage as the whole sample. There also was no right-sided predominance in the cancer group.

The Melbourne Colorectal Cancer Study, a population-based study, includes 702 colorectal cancer patients (excluding ulcerative colitis and familial polyposis).[14] In 125 cases (18%) at least one first-degree relative had a history of colorectal cancer. No statistically significant associations were found between those with a family history of colorectal cancer and age at detection, sex, country of birth, religion, number of cancers (single, synchronous, or metachronous), previously removed benign colorectal polyps, and adenomatous polyps found in the resection specimen. The family history rate of colorectal cancer for colon cancer cases was significantly higher than for rectal cancer cases ($p = .05$), and there was a gradient of decreasing rate from colon to rectum. The family history rate of colorectal cancer in parents of those who were less than 50 years old was twice that of those 50 or older. This difference approached statistical significance and appears to be congruent with the view that earlier age of onset is a chracteristic of those with a positive family history of colorectal cancer. This study also found that those who migrated from low-risk countries had rates more similar to their new country, consistent with findings of other migrant studies, and which suggests a role for environmental risk factors.

The incidence of colorectal cancer in Italy in first-degree relatives was evaluated in a study performed on 100 consecutive patients on whom surgery for colorectal cancer was performed, excluding familial polyposis.[15] One hundred patients matched for age and sex, in whom double-contrast enema and colonoscopy failed to show cancer, served as a control group. Colorectal cancer in at least one first-degree relative was found in 11% of the surgically treated patients and 6% of the control group. This difference failed to reach statistical significance, probably due to the small numbers involved. Adenomatous polyps found in patients operated for colorectal carcinomas (32%) were significantly more frequent than in the control group (18%) ($p < .05$), and remained so in the subgroups with negative family history. Small sample sizes did not allow detection of differences in incidence of polyps among those cases and controls with positive family history.

Sondergaard et al.[16] studied the incidence of colon cancer among 2650 parents of 1524 patients whose colon cancer occurred under age 60. They observed a significantly increased risk of colon cancer in both mothers and fathers. Compared to the general population, the standardized incidence ratios were 1.62 and 1.87, respectively. These authors also found no strong association between age at onset and site of the tumor in parents and patients.

All of the retrospective epidemiologic studies have shown that relatives of colorectal cancer patients have an elevated risk of developing this malignancy. The general impression is that the risk of large bowel neoplasia to an asymptomatic first-degree adult relative of a colorectal cancer patient is increased by two- to fourfold. Hereditary factors seem also to play an important etiological role in the increased incidence of occasional discrete adenomatous polyps in some kindreds.[17] Therefore, more recent proband studies have considered adenomatous polyps in examining the familiality of common colorectal cancer.

To evaluate the prevalence of colorectal cancer in France among first-degree relatives of patients with either common colorectal cancer or adenomatous polyps, Maire et al.[18] studied four groups: (1) 170 consecutive patients with histologically proved rectal ($N = 64$) or colonic ($N = 106$) adenocarcinoma, excluding cases of familial polyposis and cancer family syndrome;

(2) 170 control subjects matched for sex and age, in whom colonoscopy and barium enema were performed to exclude colorectal cancer or adenoma(s); (3) 170 consecutive patients with common rectal or colonic adenoma(s) and no evidence of polyposis coli and colorectal cancer; (4) 100 patients with cancer of various origins, excluding colorectal cancer and primary tumors known to be epidemiologically related to colorectal cancer as a check on recall biases. Results of family studies were expressed as "proved", when the pathological report was received, or "probable" colorectal cancer. Eighteen (10.6% of the 170 patients with colorectal cancer had at least one first-degree relative with past or present proved colorectal cancer and 14 (8.2%) with probable colorectal cancer. The corresponding figures included 11 proved (6.5%) and 14 probable (8.2%) in the group with polyps, 3 proved (1.7%) and 3 probable (1.7%) in the control group. The relative risk of colorectal cancer in close relatives was 6.3 and 4.7 ($p < .01$) in the colorectal cancer and adenoma groups, respectively. The present data indicate that colorectal cancer is more frequent in close relatives of patients not only with colorectal cancer, but also with colorectal adenoma(s), compared with relatives of controls.

Ponz de Leon et al. used a tumor registry in Italy to determine whether close relatives of patients with colorectal cancer or polyps are more likely to develop large bowel cancer than members of the general population.[19] For each patient, a careful clinical history was taken, as well as a genealogy of first-degree realtives. Controls matched on age and sex, and hospitalized for diseases other than neoplastic or colonic, were selected. A total of 139 cases of cancer and 157 of polyps were registered in one year; there were 2202 first-degree relatives in the disease group (1325 alive) and 2203 in the controls (1328 alive). Among the relatives of patients with tumors, 71 cases of colorectal cancer were found as compared to 16 in the controls ($p < .001$). Large bowel cancer occurs four times more often in relatives of patients with colorectal cancer or polyps than in controls. When considered separately, an increased frequency of cases of colorectal cancer among first-degree relatives was found both in the cancer and in the polyp group.

Bonelli et al.[20] studied family histories of 283 patients with adenomatous polyps, 414 patients with colon cancer, 399 polyp-free subjects, and 456 hospital controls. Both the polyp and colon cancer groups had positive family histories of 11.3 and 14.5%, respectively, while the controls had an overall rate of 5.1%.

The hypothesis that there is also a genetic basis for isolated colorectal adenomas, the precursors of colon cancer,[21] remained untested until recently because both polyps and cancer occur late in life, and only a small fraction of polyps cause clinical symptoms. Screening for polyps with flexible sigmoidoscopy is a way to overcome these difficulties and clarify the underlying genetic factors. Burt et al. examined the inheritance of susceptibility to colonic polyps and cancer in a large Utah pedigree (over 5000 members spanning six generations) with 15 cases of common colorectal cancer, but no recognizable inheritance pattern when cancer cases alone were considered.[22] Inheritance was clarified, however, by systematic screening for colonic polyps in pedigree members and spouse controls. All available first-degree relatives of subjects with colorectal cancer or adenomatous polyps who were over 25 years old were selected for study, and spouses of family members studied were used as controls to ensure similarity of demographic and lifestyle characteristics. One or more adenomatous polyps were found in 21% of family members (41 of 191) but only in 9% of controls (12 of 132) ($p < .005$). Pedigree analysis suggested that the observed excess of discrete adenomatous polyps and colorectal cancer was the result of an inherited dominant gene for susceptibility, rather than an inherited recessive gene for susceptibility or a chance occurrence. These findings point to the importance of more extensive surveillance for adenomatous polyps and colorectal cancer in susceptible families. Hyperplastic polyps are common non-neoplastic growths that are often indistinguishable from adenomatous polyps on gross examination. Hyperplastic polyps were found in 46 of 191 family members (24%) and in 38 of 132 controls (29%), a difference that is not statistically significant and which obviates bias in the screening process. There was also no significant difference in the prevalence of hyperplastic polyps among individuals with adenomas (28%) compared to those without adenomas (27%), and hyperplastic polyps did not cosegregate with adenomas in either randomly ascertained individuals (controls) or in individuals with an inherited susceptibility to adenomatous polyp formation.[23]

Prospective studies that screen first-degree relatives for polyps or colorectal cancer have also been initiated. Cannon-Albright et al.[24] extended the study of Burt et al.[22] by ascertaining 4 additional cancer cluster pedigrees and 11 pedigrees through a proband with adenoma (6 were spouse pedigrees, in which spouses found to have adenomas were considered as probands). Flexible proctosigmoidoscopy was used to identify polyps. Sixty-seven adenomas were found in 323 family members (20.7%), and 25 in 213 spouse controls (11.7%) ($p < .01$). Rozen et al. studied 471 asymptomatic adults in Israel who were first-degree relatives of patients having large bowel "neoplasia" (adenomatous polyps and/or cancer), but without polyposis syndromes.[25,26] These first-degree relatives were screened by fecal occult blood examinations and flexible sigmoidoscopy, followed by colonoscopy when indicated. Adenomatous polyps or cancer were found in 8.1% of the study group as compared with 3.7% in a control group of 457 volunteers not having the same family history of neoplasia and undergoing similar screening tests. Of the study group, the age-adjusted rate for colorectal adenomas and cancer increased threefold ($p < .001$) for subjects older than 40 years, and an even higher fivefold relative risk was found for large bowel cancer alone ($p = .01$). Analysis by the number of affected first-degree relatives showed that the screenees have a significant linear trend of increasing risk of colorectal neoplasia with increasing number of affected relatives. If only one relative was affected with large bowel neoplasia the risk was threefold ($p < .01$), whereas with more than one affected relative, the risk increased to fivefold ($p < .01$). When considering cancer only, the screenees with only one affected relative again had a threefold increased risk for colorectal cancer but this did not reach statistical significance. However, the screenees with more than one relative were 9 times more at risk for cancer ($p < .01$).

These results confirm the usefulness of the genetic epidemiologic approach to study colon cancer. From a pragmatic view, obtaining a family history is important for identifying a group at risk for these lesions. This group could benefit from regular cancer and adenomatous polyp screening, particularly when older than 40 years. Identification of a constitutional genetic marker could facilitate selective screening for colorectal cancer in identifying the genetically predisposed persons.[27] One could then attempt to determine who among the genetically predisposed persons remain unaffected, who are affected with polyps, and who are affected with colon cancer. One could also attempt to clarify whether the absence of polyps or cancer expression in some persons could be attributed to modifying genes, a late age at onset of the lesions, or environmental modulation of a genetic predisposition.

III. GENETIC SUSCEPTIBILITY TO COLON CANCER IN TAMARINS

As has been well described elsewhere in this volume, the cotton-top tamarin appears to have an increased risk of developing colon cancer when compared to other related species. The exact nature of this susceptibility is not clearly indentified. While some workers have suggested that infectious agents may be the proximal cause of colitis in marmosets and tamarins, other evidence suggests that cotton-top tamarins are uniquely susceptible to colon cancer, with genetic factors being more important than envrionmental factors in the development of disease.[28,29] The most suggestive line of evidence is the report of Clapp and co-workers that no colon cancer was detected in other tamarin species (*Saguinus fusicollis illigeri* and *Callithrix jacchus*), although housed in the same facility with presumably the same exposure to environmental agents.[29]

Similar to human colon cancer studies, the genetic epidemiologic approach in cotton-top tamarins has yielded interesting observations. DuFrain reported some evidence that suggested a familial component in the susceptibility to colon cancer in tamarins.[30] Of ten cases of colony-born tamarins with colon cancer, three had an affected parent, and there were two sib-pairs in the remaining seven. The sib-pairs had similar ages of onset, and the relative pairs in general appeared to have similar sites of primary tumors. In addition, there was the suggestion that the histopathology of the tumors themselves were similar to that found in inherited human adenocarcinomas. This apparent clustering was suggestive, but whether a distinct group at higher risk for colon cancer compared to cotton-top tamarins remained unresolved.

Using a different study design, Petersen et al. extended this observation by studying a six-year cohort of 176 colony-born cotton-top tamarins.[31,32] Of the colony-born tamarins in this cohort, 14% developed colon cancer. However, careful examination of the data showed that offspring of parents who had died of colon cancer were not at increased risk of developing cancer compared to offspring with unaffected parents. In addition, it was found that the coefficient of relationship between two pairs of tamarins with colon cancer was not increased over that of any two animals randomly sampled from the cohort. This finding has been confirmed by Cheverud, who used a larger sample of the colony and estimated a 17% heritability of colon cancer.[42] This suggests that there is not an increased familial clustering of colon cancer; in fact, all cotton-top tamarins are at an equally high risk of developing colon cancer compared to other related species. The risk for colon cancer in the tamarin is pan-specific and likely genetically mediated. Whether this risk is etiologically heterogeneous, as in humans, is equivocal. Two possible means of this pathogenesis have been suggested. Clapp et al.[33] have observed colonic polyps in cotton-top tamarins, suggesting a polyp-to-cancer pathway. Another potential avenue of genetic predisposition may be through colitis, from data indicating that colitis and colon cancer are associated in the tamarin.[34,35] The evidence that ulcerative colitis in humans has a genetic component is documented, as well as its being a risk factor for colon cancer.[36-39] While the data thus far suggest a genetic etiology for colon cancer in the cotton-top tamarins, more studies are needed to clarify pathogenesis and identify more specific markers or genetic predispositions. Some promising lines of research are afforded by human studies, showing that genetic factors do affect colonic tumor development.[40,41]

IV. SUMMARY

In summary, genetic epidemiology has provided important methodological approaches to understanding genetic factors that predispose to colorectal cancer in humans and the cotton-top tamarin. In humans, it is quite clear that colorectal cancer encompasses a number of disorders with different etiological bases. While there are several inherited syndromes that involve colon cancer, there appears to be some genetic predisposition even to common colon cancer. We have reviewed the studies that have demonstrated that first-degree relatives of a patient with common colon cancer are at increased risk for developing cancer. Application of similar methods to the cotton-top tamarin may yield productive avenues of research using this animal model to in turn understand human disease.

ACKNOWLEDGMENTS

Supported in part by National Institutes of Health grants NH4789, CA44688, the Cancer Research Foundation of America, and the Clayton Fund.

REFERENCES

1. **Mecklin, J. P.,** Frequency of hereditary colorectal carcinoma, *Gastroenterology,* 93, 1021, 1987.
2. **Kee, F. and Collins, B. J.,** How prevalent is cancer family syndrome?, *Gut,* 32, 509, 1991.
3. **Lynch, H. T., Lynch, P. M., Albano, W. A., and Lynch, J. F.,** The cancer family syndrome: a status report, *Dis. Colon Rectum,* 24, 311, 1981.
4. **Cannon-Albright, L. A., Thomas, T. C., Bishop, D. T., Skolnick, M. H., and Burt, R. W.,** Characteristics of familial colon cancer in a large population data base, *Cancer,* 64, 1971, 1985.
5. **Kinzler, K. W., Nilbert, M. C., Su, L. K. et al.,** Identification of FAP locus genes from chromosome 5q21, *Science,* 253, 661, 1991.
6. **Groden, J., Thliveris, A., Samowitz, W. et al.,** Identification and characterization of the familial adenomatous polyposis coli gene, *Cell,* 66, 589, 1991.
7. **Boman, B. M., Lynch, H. T., Kimberling, W. J., and Wildrick, D. M.,** Reassignment of a cancer family syndrome gene to chromosome 18, *Cancer Genet. Cytogenet.,* 34, 153, 1988.
8. **Peltomaki, P., Sistonen, P., Meklin, J. P. et al.,** Evidence supporting exclusion of the DCC gene and a portion of chromosome 18q as the locus for susceptibility to hereditary nonpolyposis colorectal carcinoma in five kindreds, *Cancer Res.,* 51, 4135, 1991.
9. **Woolf, C. M.,** A genetic study of carcinoma of the large intestine, *Am. J. Hum. Genet.,* 10, 42, 1958.
10. **Macklin, M. T.,** Inheritance of cancer of the stomach and large intestine in man, *J. Natl. Cancer Inst.,* 24, 551, 1960.
11. **Lovett, E.,** Family studies in cancer of the colon and rectum, *Br. J. Surg.,* 63, 13, 1976.
12. **Lynch, H. T., Guirgis, H., Swartz, M., Lynch, J., Krush, A. J., and Kaplan, A. R.,** Genetics and colon cancer, *Arch. Surg.,* 106, 669, 1973.
13. **Duncan, J. L. and Kyle, J.,** Family incidence of carcinoma of the colon and rectum in north-east Scotland, *Gut,* 23, 169, 1982.
14. **Kune, G. A., Kune, S., and Watson, L. F.,** The Melbourne colorectal cancer study. Characterization of patients with a family history of colorectal cancer, *Dis. Colon Rectrum,* 30, 600, 1987.
15. **Aste, H., Saccomano, S., Bonelli, L., and Pugliese, V.,** Adenomatous polyps and familial incidence of colorectal cancer, *Eur. J. Cancer Clin. Oncol.,* 20, 1401, 1984.
16. **Sondergaard, J. O., Bulow, S., and Lynge, E.,** Cancer incidence among parents of patients with colorectal cancer, *Int. J. Cancer,* 47, 202, 1991.
17. **Woolf, C. M., Richards, R. C., and Gardner, E. J.,** Occasional discrete polyps of the colon and rectum showing an inherited tendency in a kindred, *Cancer,* 8, 403, 1955.
18. **Maire, P., Moricheau-Beauchant, M., Drucker, J., Barboteau, M. A., Barbier, J., and Matuchansky, C.,** Prevalence familiale du cancer du colon et du rectum: resultats d'une enquete "cas-temoins" de 3 ans, *Gastroenterol. Clin. Biol.,* 8, 22, 1984.
19. **Ponz De Leon, M., Ascari, A., Antonioli, A., Manenti, F., Melotti, G., Pezcoller, C., Piccagli, I., Grisendi, A., Mazzeo, D., and Miselli, A.,** Frequency of colorectal cancer among the first-degree relatives of patients with cancer or polyps of the large bowel, *Gut,* 26, A1153, 1985.
20. **Bonelli, L., Martines, H., Conio, M., Bruzzi, P., and Aste, H.,** Family history of colorectal cancer as a risk factor for benign and malignant tumors of the large bowel. A case-control study, *Int. J. Cancer,* 41, 513, 1988.
21. **Stryker, S. J., Wolff, B. G., Culp, C. E., Libbe, S. D., Ilstrup, D. M., and MacCarty, R. L.,** Natural history of untreated colonic polyps, *Gastroenterology,* 93, 1009, 1987.
22. **Burt, R. W., Bishop, D. T., Cannon, L. A., Dowdle, M. A., Lee, R. G., and Skolnick, M. H.,** Dominant inheritance of adenomatous colonic polyps and colorectal cancer, *N. Engl. J. Med.,* 312, 1540, 1985.

23. **Black, J., Skolnick, M. H., and Burt, R. W.,** Lack of association between hyperplastic and adenomatous polyps of the colon, *Gastroenterology,* 92, 1319, 1987.
24. **Cannon-Albright, L. A., Skolnick, M. H., Bishop, D. T., Lee, R. G., and Burt, R. W.,** Common inheritance of susceptibility to colonic adenomatous polyps and associated colorectal cancers, *N. Engl. J. Med.,* 319, 533, 1988.
25. **Rozen, P., Fireman, Z., Terdiman, R., Hellerstein, S. M., Rattan, J., and Gilat, T.,** Selective screening for colorectal tumors in the Tel-Aviv area: relevance of epidemiology and family history, *Cancer,* 47, 827, 1981.
26. **Rozen, P., Fireman, Z., Figer, A., Legum, C., Ron, E., and Lynch, H.,** Family history of colorectal cancer as a marker of potential malignancy within a screening program, *Cancer,* 60, 248, 1987.
27. **Henochowicz, S., Macrae, F. A., Lukeis, R. E., Garson, O. M., and Whitehead, R. H.,** Dominant inheritance of adenomatous colonic polyps and colorectal cancer, *N. Engl. J. Med.,* 313, 1160, 1985.
28. **Lushbaugh, C. C., Humason, G. L., Swartzendruber, D. C., Richter, C. B., and Gengozian, N.,** Spontaneous colonic adenocarcinoma in marmosets, *Primates Med.,* 10, 119, 1978.
29. **Clapp, N. K., Lushbaugh, C. C., Humason, G. L., Gangaware, B. L., and Henke, M. A.,** Natural history and pathology of colon cancer in Saguinus oedipus oedipus, *Digest. Dis. Sci.,* 30, 107S, 1985.
39. **DuFrain, R. J.,** Is cancer of the colon familial in cotton-top tamarins?, *Cancer Genet. Cytogenet.,* 14, 83, 1985.
31. **Petersen, G. M., Clapp, N. K., and Tardif, S. D.,** Cotton top tamarins are genetically susceptible to colon cancer, *Gastroenterology,* 92, 1575, 1987.
32. **Petersen, G. M., Clapp, N. K., and Tardif, S. D.,** Genetic susceptibility to colon cancer in cotton-top tamarins, *Clin. Res.,* 35, 185A, 1987.
33. **Clapp, N. K., Henke, M. A., Hansard, R. M., Adams, S. L., Carson, R. C., Hawkins, J. V., and Nardi, R.,** Colonic polyps associated with colitis in cotton-top tamarins (*Saguinus oedipus*): progression to colonic carcinoma?, *Gastroenterology,* 100, A355, 1991.
34. **Richter, C. B., Lushbaugh, C. C., and Swartzendruber, D. C.,** Cancer of the colon in cotton-topped tamarins, *Comparative Pathology of Zoo Animals,* Montali, R. J. and Migaki, G., Eds., Smithsonian Institution Press, Washington, D.C., 1980, 567.
35. **Chalifoux, L. V. and Bronson, R. T.,** Colonic adenocarcinoma associated with chronic colitis in cotton top marmosets (Saguinus oedipus), *Gastroenterology,* 80, 942, 1981.
36. **McConnell, R. B.,** Ulcerative colitis — genetic features, *Scand. J. Gastroenterol.,* 18(Suppl. 88), 14, 1983.
37. **Sherlock, P., Bell, B. M., Steinberg, H., and Almy, T. P.,** Familial occurrence of regional enteritis and ulcerative colitis, *Gastroenterology,* 45, 413, 1963.
38. **Singer, H. D., Anderson, J. G. D., Frischer, H., and Kirsner, J. B.,** Familial aspects of inflammatory bowel disease, *Gastroenterology,* 61, 423, 1971.
39. **Kirsner, J. B.,** Inflammatory bowel disease — clinical, etiological, and genetic aspects, in *Genetics and Heterogeneity of Common Gastrointestinal Disorders,* Rotter, J. I., Samloff, I. M., and Rimoin, D. L., Eds., Academic Press, New York, 1980, 261.
40. **Vogelstein, B., Fearon, E. R., Hamilton, S. R., Kern, S. E., Presinger, C., Leppert, M., Nakamura, Y., White, R., Smits, A. M. M., and Bos, J. L.,** Genetic alterations during colorectal tumor development, *N. Engl. J. Med.,* 319, 525, 1988.
41. **Fearon, E. R. and Vogelstein, B.,** A genetic model for colorectal tumorigenesis, *Cell,* 61, 759, 1990.
42. **Cheverud, J. M., Tardif, S., Henke, M. A., and Clapp, N. K.,** Genetic epidemiology of colon cancer in the cotton-top tamarin *(Saguinus oedipus).* Submitted.

Chapter 13

PREVALENCE OF COLONIC CARCINOMA IN COTTON-TOP TAMARIN COLONIES THROUGHOUT THE WORLD

Neal K. Clapp

TABLE OF CONTENTS

0-8493-5363-7/93/$0.00 + $.50

I. INTRODUCTION

The use of animal models is extremely important to the study of human diseases; in fact, progress in biomedical research is often delayed or even inhibited because a suitable animal model is not available or has not been recognized and/or well understood. Ideally, the animal model would exactly mimic all aspects of the human disease, but such is rarely the case. In fact, the investigator usually selects the particular model that best duplicates his research interest(s). Further, essential elements of an animal model include that it must be reproducible in results from laboratory to laboratory and it should be reasonably available to reach investigators.

In the early 1970s, the first report of spontaneous large bowel neoplasms in a relatively new colony of cotton-top tamarins (CTT) (*Saguinus oedipus*) (first imported ~1966) identified a spontaneous animal malignancy with extremely important human ramifications.[1] Understanding this unique tamarin affliction could well contribute to the improvement of tamarin health and well-being as well as offer hope for successful treatment and recovery of people afflicted with this very serious human disease. In the 1970s, this primate species was relatively new in research laboratories; little was known of its physiology and pathobiology. Consequently, the discovery of a non-human primate with spontaneous colonic carcinoma was received with mixed reviews; cautious optimism arose from those who recognized the potential value for such a research tool, but scepticism also surfaced among others who had some unanswered questions regarding the etiology, frequency, and true spontaneity of occurrence.

As the disease was reported in the literature results were discussed, a dilemma developed tht existed for several (~10) years; the malignancy had been diagnosed only in the cotton-top tamarin colony housed at the Oak Ridge Associated Universities (ORAU), Oak Ridge, TN. The ORAU callitrichid colony had been started in 1961 by Dr. Nazareth Gengozian but only a few cotton-tops had been imported before 1966. Other colonies had been started at even a later date, and most of them were smaller in numbers. At that time, similar observations of colonic carcinoma had not been made in other colonies. Questions were even raised at scientific meetings as to why the neoplasm had not been diagnosed in other colonies; no simple answer surfaced. The cause of this malignancy was not identified.

Most large bowel cancer investigators in both humans and experimental animals believe that environmental factors contribute significantly to the etiology of colonic carcinoma. Thus, the ORAU tamarin/marmoset diet and environment were closely scrutinized for any possible carcinogenic contaminants. The drinking water was also considered as possibly bearing some mutagen/carcinogen (or foreign, physical, or chemical agent) that could be the etiologic agent of this "spontaneous" disease. Every aspect of the husbandry and general health of the marmoset colony was examined for the causal "agent(s)". None were identified.

II. HISTORICAL PERSPECTIVES

What were the complicating factors to this intriguing scientific question? Admittedly, the ORAU colony was somewhat larger than the other colonies in the U.S. in that it housed some 400 to 500 animals of several different species of callitrichids, and it was the oldest established cotton-top tamarin colony. However, an unusual quirk in demographics was that, since 1961, the largest number of callitrichids in the ORAU colony had been saddle-back tamarins (*Saguinus fuscicollis*) and not cotton-top tamarins. Significant numbers of cotton-tops were imported first in the early 1970s. Most zoo populations contained relatively small numbers (10 to 20) of CTTs. In addition to ORAU's colony, only the colonies at the New England Regional Primate Research Center (NERPRC), Southborough, MA, Rush Presbyterian-St. Luke's Medical Center in Chicago, IL, and Texas A & M University, College Station, TX were very large (~50 to 100 or larger).

In 1968, the first large bowel malignancy was diagnosed at ORAU in a *Callimico goeldii;* the first colon carcinoma in a cotton-top tamarin was diagnosed in 1970.[1] Subsequently, some 12 colonic neoplasms were described and reported by Lushbaugh et al. in 1978.[1] As the prevalence of cotton-top colon carcinomas increased in the 1970s and early 1980s, a second ORAU report identified a then-current total of 14 colonic malignancies in 109 CTT necropsies;[2] no colonic neoplasms were found in the other species, *Saguinus fuscicollis,* saddle-back tamarin, or *Callithrix jacchus,* the common marmoset.

Also, in 1980 a confirmatory study described 15 colonic tumors in cotton-top tamarins from the New England Regional Primate Research Center; these carcinomas were identical histologically with those found at ORAU.[3] This report further suggested that a species susceptibility to colon cancer existed and that the malignancy was probably related to the intercurrent occurrence of colitis. In 1986, two similar colonic malignancies were reported in the CTT colony at the University of Bristol, England.[4]

To explore the status of the cotton-top tamarin as an experimental model for human colonic diseases, an international workshop was hosted by ORAU in April, 1984.[5] The theme for the presentations and discussions was "Is the Marmoset an Experimental Model for the Study of Gastrointestinal Disease?"; marmoset was often used generically to include all callitrichids. At that time, one report summarized the observations of colonic carcinoma in four independently established colonies in the U.S. and the U.K.[6] These colonies were, in addition to ORAU's, a National Cancer Institute (NCI)-owned colony that had been located at St. Luke's Medical Center in Chicago but which was transferred to Oak Ridge under an NCI contract, the New England Regional Primate Research Colony operated by Harvard University, and the Unitersity of Bristol, England, colony which was operated by Dr. M. A. Epstein and Dr. James Kirkwood. Thus, "spontaneous" colonic carcinoma was found in four independently established cotton-top tamarin colonies that operated under different housing conditions, diets, and husbandry practices and even on two different continents.[6]

As time passed and these results became better known, the basic tenet was finally accepted that some peculiarity existed in the cotton-top tamarin species that predisposed it to a high prevalence of colonic carcinomas. These figures were far in excess of the high-risk figures for susceptible human populations (~35 vs. 0.03% in humans). With this knowledge, more people examined CTTs, both living and dead, for this condition. Not surprisingly, colonic carcinoma was diagnosed in other colonies and was reported in the literature and through personal communications, e.g., at the University of Wisconsin Psychology Department, the Regent's Park Royal Zoo in London, England, Washington, D.C. Zoo, and the Seattle, Washington Zoo. The susceptibility of CTTS had now been observed in zoo populations and in facilities with somewhat different environmental conditions than were found in the larger research colonies. In particular, the University of Wisconsin Department of Psychology (Dr. Charles Snowdon) staff and students have more personal contact with the animals which could conceivably reduce some of the presumed stress-related conditions associated with individual housing.

III. CURRENT STATUS OF COTTON-TOP TAMARIN COLONIES WITH DIAGNOSED COLONIC CARCINOMA

As knowledge of colonic carcinoma diagnosis became more widespread, attention was directed toward recognition of this disease. Presumably, more complete necropsies were performed with appropriate histologic examination, the histological material was more diligently examined, and colonic carcinoma diagnosis has now been confirmed in 13 colonies that, to the best of our knowledge, were begun independently. Granted, some very small animal interchange has occurred between colonies,[12] but, by and large, the CTT colonies have remained independent in their operation and production.

Recently, a "current-status" telephone survey was conducted and the information was tabulated in Table 1; the pesonnel providing the colony information are recognized for their cooperation in the acknowledgment section of this chapter. A total of >245 colon carcinoma cases was reported in this survey. Institutions reported data from colonies at six zoos, three universities, and four predominantly research colonies.

That 35% of adult CTTs die with colon cancer in ORAU's colony may, to some degree, reflect the age of the colony population rather than a greater colony susceptibility;[6,7] prevalences in other colonies may adjust upward with longer life of the colony. Several reports have suggested that the CTT has a unique and, as yet, unidentified susceptibility to colonic carcinoma; the recognition of colon cancer under such diverse housing and environmental conditions as described herein further supports this inference.

TABLE 1
Thirteen Independently Founded *Saguinus oedipus* Colonies in which Colonic Carcinomas Have Been Diagnosed (Through 12/91)

		Location	Mean colony size[a]	No. of cases
Research colony				
1.	MARCOR — ORAU-owned	Oak Ridge, TN	225	149
2.	MARCOR — NCI-owned/St. Luke's	Oak Ridge, TN	12	16
3.	New England Regional Primate Center	Southborough, MA	328	58
4.	University of Bristol	Bristol, England	168	>25
5.	University of Wisconsin	Madison, WI	64	7
6.	The Ohio State University	Columbus, OH[b]	30	10
7.	German Primate Center	Gottingen, Germany[c]	88	5
Zoo colony				
8.	Buffalo Zoological Gardens	Buffalo, NY	21	2
9.	Woodland Park Zoo	Seattle, WA	~10	2
10.	Zoological Society of London, Regent's Park	London, England	29	1
11.	Los Angeles Zoo	Los Angeles, CA	31	3
12.	San Diego Zoo	San Diego, CA	1	2
13.	National Zoo	Washington, D.C.	0	1

[a] Data obtained from *International Cotton-Top Tamarin Studbook,* 3rd ed., 1990.[12]
[b] Colony formerly at Texas A&M, College Station, TX, Dr. Frank Stein.
[c] Also reported one *S. fuscicollis* with colonic carcinoma.[13]

IV. DISCUSSION

During the years since the first diagnosis of spontaneous colonic carcinoma in cotton-top tamarins, several pieces of the puzzle have fallen in place.

First, the phenomenon is not a local contaminant problem in Oak Ridge, Tennessee, as was thought by some, but rather a universal species problem. The condition has been confirmed in at least 13 different colonies with essentially independent origin.

Several possible causes can be discounted or, at the very least, do not account for the worldwide species susceptibility:

1. A common infectious agent, e.g., virus, bacterium, protozoan, etc.
2. Dietary factors, since diets vary widely between colonies
3. Caging, either as individuals or as family groups
4. Certain high-risk families, since the risk is high in all CTTs

The probability seems very low that a single extrinsic infectious agent could etiologically be the sole cause of either CTT idiopathic colitis or spontaneous colon cancer. It is remotely conceivable that each cotton-top tamarin in the world could be carrying the same virus in its genetic make-up that might account for the susceptibility to one or both diseases. However, the fact that the histology of not only the colitis but also the colonic cancer appears to be quite similar from colony to colony as well as from animal to animal within a colony suggests that the susceptibility is a species problem rather than a sporadic-occurring event.

As suggested by Morin,[8] tamarins and marmosets receive almost as many dietary formulations as there are colonies. Several reports from different colonies indicate that the nutrient composition is quite comparable although the ingredients of the diet may vary considerably. Supplementation is also widely varied which makes the diet an unlikely source of any universal "contamination".

Similarly, housing varies from individual caging of approximately 18 × 20 × 20 in. to large cages in which a family unit may reach 8 to 10 animals. Likewise, variations exist in breeding facilities from double or slightly larger single cages to large (3 × 3 × 5 ft) double apartments for a single family.[9] These differences suggest that neither breeding cages with family groups nor individual housing predisposes CTTs to colonic disease over the other forms of housing.

The notion that the colon cancer has a familial contribution is a logical assumption based upon human data. An interesting study of the differences in susceptibility to colon cancer between first-degree cancer family relatives and those not so associated showed that the risk was not familial but was panspecies in nature.[10] The abundant data point to some hereditary factor that is not presently identified, but some postulations include a possible inability to repair DNA damage, increased response to proliferative stimuli such as inflammatory bowel disease, viral infection, etc.

Since most CTT colonies also have intercurrent colitis, this colonic disease may well be strongly implicated, if not absolutely incriminated, as the (or a) "promoting" agent in the multistage hypothesis of colonic cancer.[7,11] These inferences should not be construed to totally eliminate any possible contribution of environmental (including dietary) factors from any of the aforementioned hypotheses. A number of unanswered questions remain.

V. SUMMARY

While the mechanisms to explain CTT susceptibility to colonic carcinoma remain as yet unidentified, the data collected from 13 independently established colonies strongly infer a panspecies susceptibility. Whereas some environmental factors are similar between colonies, diversity in diets, type of housing, sanitation, caging size and structure, etc. strongly suggest that the cotton-top tamarin will develop colon cancer regardless of the environment.

These observations should not be construed to eliminate all contributions to colon carcinogenesis by environmental factors but rather suggest that the predisposing "initiation" event may be some genetically related change that is not identified at this time. Exacerbations of colitis could then serve as a "promoting" event. Some specific research efforts are underway that will address the causality of the susceptibility as well as the contribution of some potentially involved environmental factors.

ACKNOWLEDGMENTS

This research was conducted in ORAU's AAALAC-accredited Marmoset Research Center at Oak Ridge (MARCOR) and was approved and monitored by ORAU's Animal Care Standards Committee.

Research was supported, in part, by the ORAU Corporation.

The authors acknowledge the excellent manuscript review by J. Crook and R. Damian and manuscript preparation by Sandy Womble.

Organizations and staff contributing colonic carcinoma and total colony information to this chapter:

- New England Regional Primate Research Center — Dr. Norval King, Laura Chalifoux
- University of Bristol, Comparative Pathology Laboratory — Prof. I. A. Silver, Drs. Bryan Warren and Paul Watkins
- University of Wisconsin, Department of Psychology — Dr. Charles Snowdon and Rebecca S. Roush
- Ohio State University, Department of Physiology, College of Medicine — Dr. Jackie Wood, Dr. Doug Stone

- Buffalo Zoological Gardens — Dr. Jerry Aquilina, Dr. Allen Prowten
- Seattle Zoo — Dr. Robert Russell, University of Washington (currently at University of Maryland)
- Zoological Society of London, Regent's Park — Dr. James Kirkwood
- Los Angeles Zoo — Pathology Department
- Zoological Society of Sand Diego — Pathology Department
- German Primate Center — Prof. H. J. Kuhn, Dr. M. Brack
- National Zoo — Dr. Richard Montali

REFERENCES

1. **Lushbaugh, C. C., Humason, G. L., Swartzendruber, D. C., Richter, C. B., and Gengozian, N.,** Spontaneous colonic adenocarcinoma in marmosets, *Med. Primatol.,* 10, 119, 1978.
2. **Richter, C. B., Lushbaugh, C. C., and Swartzendruber, D. C.,** Cancer of the colon in cotton-top tamarins, in *Proc. Symp. Comparative Pathology of Zoo Animals 1978,* Montali, R. J. and Migaki, G., Eds., Smithsonian Institution Press, Washington, D.C., 1980, 567.
3. **Chalifoux, L. V. and Bronson, R. T.,** Colonic adenocarcinoma associated with chronic colitis in cotton-top marmosets, *Saguinus oedipus, Gastroenterology,* 80, 942, 1981.
4. **Kirkwood, J. K., Pearson, G. R., and Epstein, M. A.,** Adenocarcinoma of the large bowel and colitis in captive cotton-top tamarins, *Saguinus o. oedipus, J. Comp. Pathol.,* 96, 507, 1986.
5. **Clapp, N. K. and Vener, K. H.,** Co-Chairmen, Is the marmoset an experimental model for the study of gastrointestinal disease?, *Digest. Dis. Sci.,* 30, 1985.
6. **Clapp, N. K., Lushbaugh, C. C., Humason, G. L., Gangaware, B. L., and Henke, M. A.,** Natural history and pathology of colon cancer in *Saguinus oedipus oedipus, Digest. Dis. Sci.,* 30, 107S, 1985.
7. **Clapp, N. K. and Henke, M. A.,** Spontaneous colonic carcinoma observations in the Oak Ridge Associated Universities' 26-year-old cotton-top tamarin *Saguinus oedipus* colony, This volume, Chapter 11.
8. **Morin, M. L.,** Colony management problems encountered in using marmosets and tamarins in biomedical research, *Digest. Dis. Sci.,* 30, 14S, 1985.
9. **Clapp, N. K. and Tardif, S. D.,** Marmoset husbandry and nutrition, *Digest. Dis. Sci.,* 30, 17S, 1985.
10. **Petersen, G. M. and Roth, M.-P.,** Genetic epidemiology of colon cancer, This volume, Chapter 12.
11. **Clapp, N. K., Henke, M. A., McArthur, A. H., and Carson, R.,** Colonic epithelial changes associated with acute colitis and the development of colon carcinoma in tamarins, in *Int. Symp. Future Research Approaches in IBD: Mechanisms of Chronic Infection and Inflammation,* McDermott, R. P., Ed., Elsevier, Amsterdam, 1988, 713.
12. **Tardif, S. D. and Colley, R.,** *International Cotton-Top Tamarin Studbook,* 3rd ed., Oak Ridge Associated Universities, Oak Ridge, TN, 1990.
13. **Brack, M.,** Intestinal carcinomas in two tamarins *(Saguinus fuscicollis, Saguinus oedipus)* of the German Primate Centre, *Lab. Anim.,* 22, 144, 1988.

Chapter 14

EARLY COLONIC CARCINOMA DEVELOPMENT IN COTTON-TOP TAMARINS: EVIDENCE OF PROMOTION BY COLITIC EPISODES

Neal K. Clapp and Marsha A. Henke

TABLE OF CONTENTS

0-8493-5363-7/93/$0.00 + $.50

I. INTRODUCTION

Colorectal carcinoma is a devastating disease of the affluent Western world: the U.S., Canada, Western Europe, Australia, and New Zealand. Despite extensive research and experimentation, this disease remains one of the most important causes of cancer-related deaths. The study of mechanisms and hereditary and environmental contribution(s) in development of colon cancer in humans and experimental models is only part of intensive on-going research.

Although many questions remain unanswered, much recent progress has been made. An early milestone was the discovery that certain colonic adenomas (polyps) in human patients could, in fact, develop into colonic carcioma.[1,2] The obvious experimental route was to study the causes and pathogenesis of polyp production; thus, one could ultimately modify colon cancer incidences by controlling polyps.

Discovery of some hereditary contributions to colonic polyps and carcinomas, e.g., familial polyposis coli and Gardner's syndrome,[3] plus the cancer family and hereditary nonpolyposis colorectal carcioma syndromes,[4,5] made the proposed disease pathogenesis somewhat more complex. Current reports indicate that even the so-called sporadic colon cancer occurrences cause increased risk in first- and second-degree relatives.[6] Exciting discoveries resulting from *in vitro* studies have even suggested important sequences that may exist in the chromosome changes during both polyp and cancer development.[7-9]

Idiopathic ulcerative colitic (UC) patients often develop multicentric primary foci of colonic carcinoma[10] as do those members of the cancer family syndromes.[4,5] While some hereditary or familial influence may well be involved in UC susceptibility, the ulcerative colitis/carcinoma sequence could be considered mechanistically as a "promotion" by colitis of colonic epithelial cells at multiple sites, with the resulting expression of multiple malignant foci. This contrasts with observations in familial polyposis coli patients who have hundreds or even thousands of polyps and still develop only a single or, at most, a very few primary colonic cancers. The difference observed in the numbers of primary tumor foci between these two high-risk human subsets may be explained by the following: ulcerative colitis patients receive, by the nature of their disease process, a repeated or "pulsed" inflammatory insult to the colon which clearly increases the risk for developing colon cancer.

The cotton-top tamarin (CTT) (*Saguinus oedipus*) develops high incidences of spontaneous colonic carcioma (35% of adult deaths in captivity).[11,12] The development of this condition closely parallels the human ulcerative colitis/carcinoma pathogenesis. The CTT process routinely develops from a flat epithelium without polyp formation. Only recently, after over 2000 colonoscopic examinations, have any polyps been identified in CTTs.[13] One adenomatous polyp was followed for several months and was believed to have become malignant. This CTT primate model offers the opportunity to study this aggressive malignancy in relation to the human counterpart.

Despite extensive research efforts, many important pieces of the colonic cancer puzzle remain unanswered; some putative or "expected" intermediate stages of the process have not as yet been identified or recognized. Most CTTs that die with advanced colonic carcinomas have late-stage multiple primarites,[11,12] with metastases. However, two individual cotton-top tamarins have been observed with multiple primary tumors that appeared histologically of different ages (or stages) of development in separate colonic segments. This chapter presents a histological picture of early colonic carcinoma development with suggestive evidence of colon cancer expression in cotton-top tamarins which could have resulted from a series of active colitic episodes.

II. METHODS

Animals: two imported middle-aged cotton-top tamarins, (1740) a 6-year, 10-month-old female and (4595) a 12-year, 4-month-old male, died with colon carcinoma. One of the last cotton-top tamarins received, CTT FO-1740, was imported into the Oak Ridge Associated Universities' (ORAU) colony in November 1976. Clinically, she had intermittent diarrhea for several months and was hemoccult positive. In July 1983, a large abdominal mass was palpated in the transverse colon; the tumor was confirmed by barium air contrast radiography. At necropsy, a 2-cm mass was found in the transverse colon, the cecum was thickened, and a cecal tumor was suspected.

CTT MO-4595 was imported to Litton's in November 1973, transferred to Kensington, MD, and then to Rush Presbyterian-St. Luke's Medical Center in Chicago in 1980. Finally, he was transferred from Rush to ORAU in 1982. Tamarin 4595 had loose stools for 4 months in 1982 and again in 1984. In October 1985, a small abdominal mass was palpated, but barium air contrast radiography results were inconclusive for a colon tumor. At necropsy, the colon was distended with feces, but there was no gross evidence of a colon tumor; the suspected mass was not found.

Necropsy procedure: a complete necropsy was performed on each CTT and histological sections were obtained from ~25 different organs. Routinely, colons were opened longitudinally; half of each colon segment was quick-frozen and half of the colon was rolled (as a "jelly roll") from proximal to distal with the mucosa inside, fixed in buffered formalin, and prepared (5-μm sections) for pathological observation. Routine histological staining with periodic acid Schiff's reagent was used to identify mucin in colon cancers and their metastases.

III. RESULTS

Case No. 1 (Animal FO-1740): A gross photograph (Figure 1) of a 6-year-old female cotton-top tamarin shows a large 2-cm napkin-ring colon

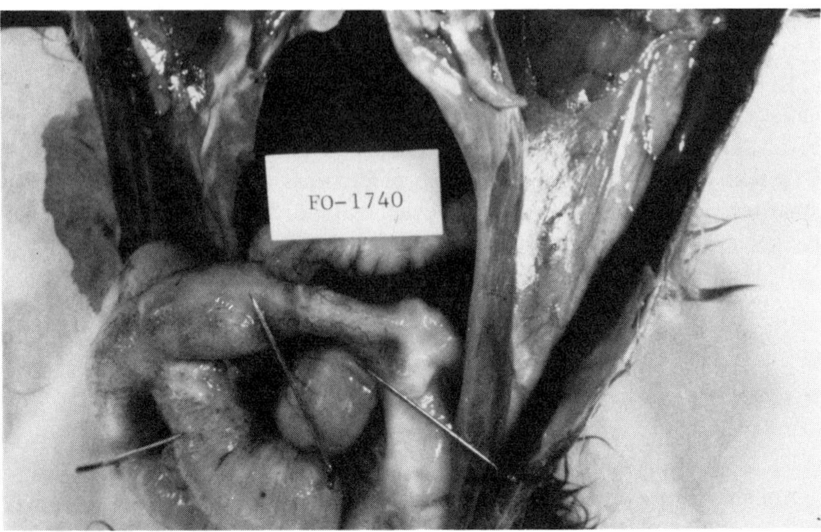

FIGURE 1. Gross photograph of a 2-cm napkin-ring colonic tumor of the transverse colon in cotton-top tamarin 1740.

tumor of the transverse colon; the cecum and ceco-colic junction were markedly thickened. Histologically, the large primary tumor in the transverse colon was a mucin-producing undifferentiated adenocarcinoma that displayed attempts to form abortive crypts (Figure 2); the histological picture was identical with previous descriptions.[4,11,12] Cancer cells exhibiting increased mucin production had invaded the muscle layers, and metastases were seen in the lymphatics that drained the colon.

The histological changes in the cecum were quite different from those seen in the transverse colon. Figure 3 is a montage of a part of the cecal mucosa which showed, in a single 5-μm histological section, multiple primary tumor foci that were identified; each was less than, or equal to, the thickness of the colonic mucosa. The 22 foci in the cecal mucosa were composed of anaplastic undifferentiated epithelial cells as previously described for primary CTT colon tumors;[11,12,14] uniquely, however, these multiple foci were almost identical in size, were spread throughout the cecum, and were essentially confined within the mucosa. None of the tumors appeared to extend beyond the muscularis mucosa (Figure 4).

However, in the ascending colon, a different picture was seen. Neither a large tumor mass like that found in the transverse colon nor the multiple intramucosal tumor foci as described in the cecum were seen. Within a large number of individual crypts, the epithelial cells of the basal two thirds of the crypts were flattened (low cuboidal) and mucin-depleted (Figure 5). As described by Yardley,[15] anaplastic undifferentiated malignant cancer cells, often mucin-producing, ''budded off'' into the crypt lumen, producing a very early

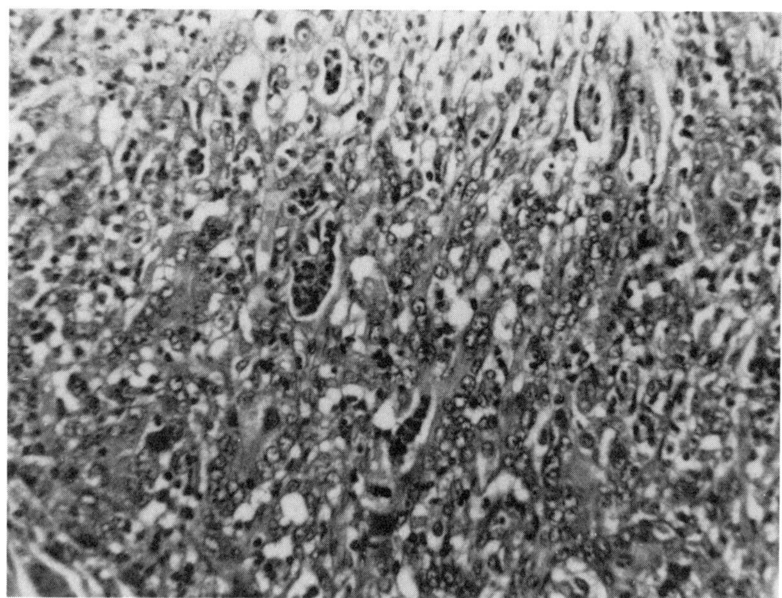

FIGURE 2. Photomicrograph of a primary highly undifferentiated adenocarcinoma with attempts to form abortive crypts. Crypt abscesses are also evident. Very little mucin is seen in the cancer cells. PAS 250×.

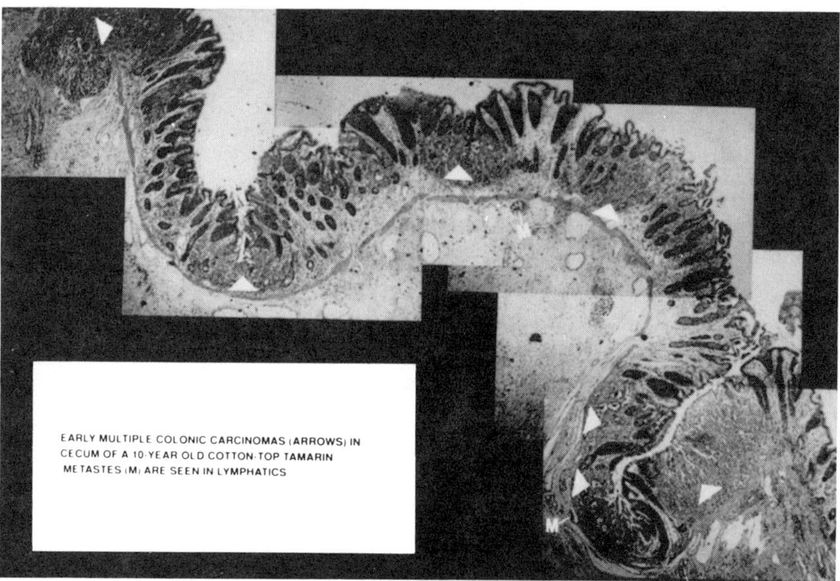

FIGURE 3. Montage of multiple primary carcinomas (arrows) of the cecum (CTT FO-1740). Tumors are confined within the mucosa. PAS 60×.

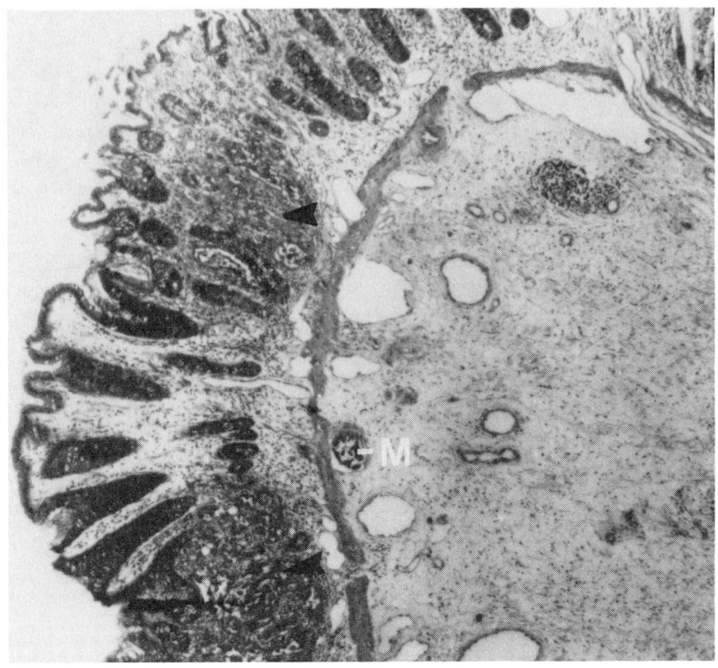

FIGURE 4. Photomicrograph of CTT in Figure 3, showing two primary carcinomas (arrows) in the cecal mucosa that are approximately the same size. Animal has chronic colitis with minimal infiltration of mononuclear cells. Mucosa has numerous architectural malformations that have resulted from repair following a previous episode of active colitis. A metastatic focus (M) is seen in one submucosal lymphatic. PAS 100×.

"intracrypt" stage of colon cancer (Figure 6). This proliferation of crypt epithelium occurred at the base of many crypts (Figure 7). The third of the crypt nearest the gut lumen very often appeared relatively normal with near-normal cellular basilar orientation and nearly normal amounts of mucin production (Figure 5).

On occasion, 3 to 4 adjacent crypts had these proliferative changes (Figure 7). In some instances, cancer cells were confined within crypts, but, in other areas of the ascending colon, small-to-large foci of cancer cells had invaded the lamina propria with apparent destruction of the colonic epithelium (Figure 7). On a single 5-μm section, at least 100 crypts in the ascending colonic segment were found to be in nearly identical stages of tumor development.

A summary of the findings in this unique cotton-top tamarin follows. There were what appeared to be three histologically distinct phases, or stages, of colon cancer development in three separate colonic segments. These stages ranged from a very early multicentric intracrypt proliferation, possibly "dysplastic to preneoplastic", in the ascending colon, through multiple primaries that had coalesced to somewhat larger sizes that attained the thickness of the

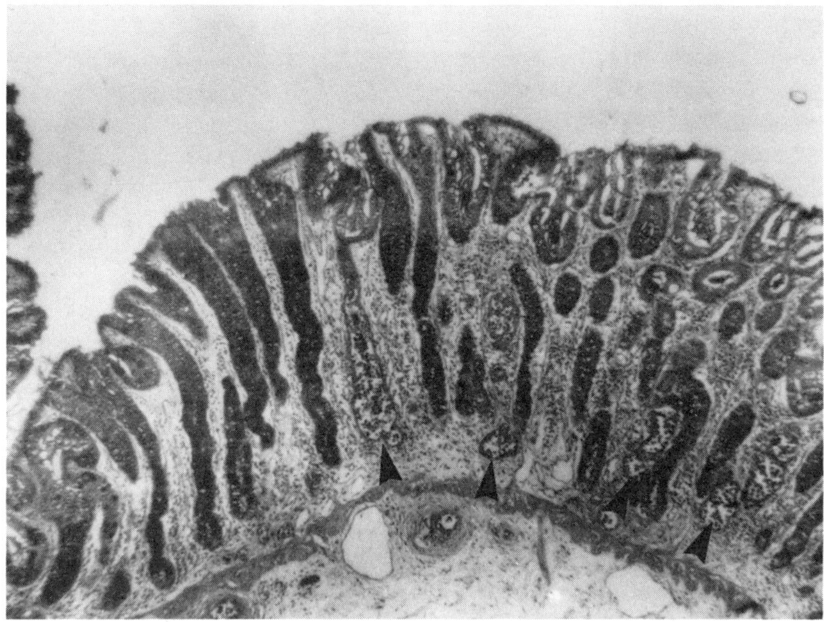

FIGURE 5. Photomicrograph of the ascending colon of the same CTT in Figure 3. Cancer cells are budding from the crypt epithelium into the crypt lumen (arrows), especially at the base of the crypts. Some crypts are tortuous and branching is evident, which is the result of remodeling following active colitic episode. PAS 60×.

cecal mucosa; finally, a large, grossly visible neoplastic mass was found in the transverse colon.

Case No. 2 (Animal MO-4595): The second cotton-top tamarin showed no gross evidence of a colonic tumor at necropsy. Histologically, the cecum, ascending colon, and descending colon exhibited a mild chronic (inactive) colitis but no evidence of malignancy.

A small portion of the transverse colon contained numerous accumulations of malignant cells that were somewhat intermediate between the "intracrypt" size and the "mucosal" size of primaries found in the ascending colon and cecum, respectively, in CTT 1740. The epithelium of a number of the crypts was destroyed by the progressive growth of the cancer cells and some primary foci encompassed the width of several crypts. The area that contained these small primaries comprised approximately 10% of the transverse colon segment, a much smaller portion of the total segment than was found in the 1740 tamarin. It would appear that, although the stage of the colon cancer development was comparable to CTT-1740, the total mucosa that progressed from nonrecognizable "initiation only" to early cancer is significantly less. This observation implies that only a very small area was affected by the promoting agent and/or process, i.e., it was simply a focal activity.

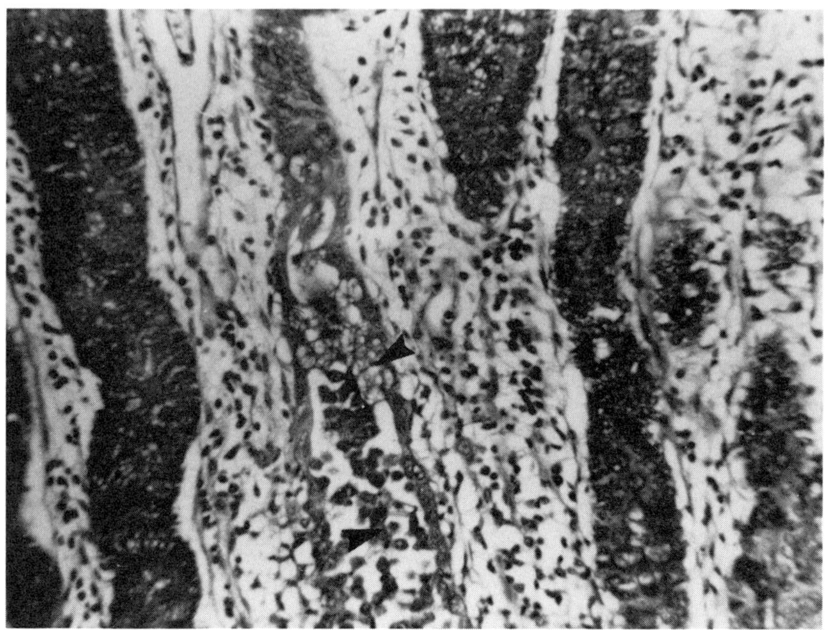

FIGURE 6. Enlargement of photomicrograph of CTT in Figure 5. Crypt epithelium that contains cancer cells (arrows) is flattened with loss of mucin. PAS 150×.

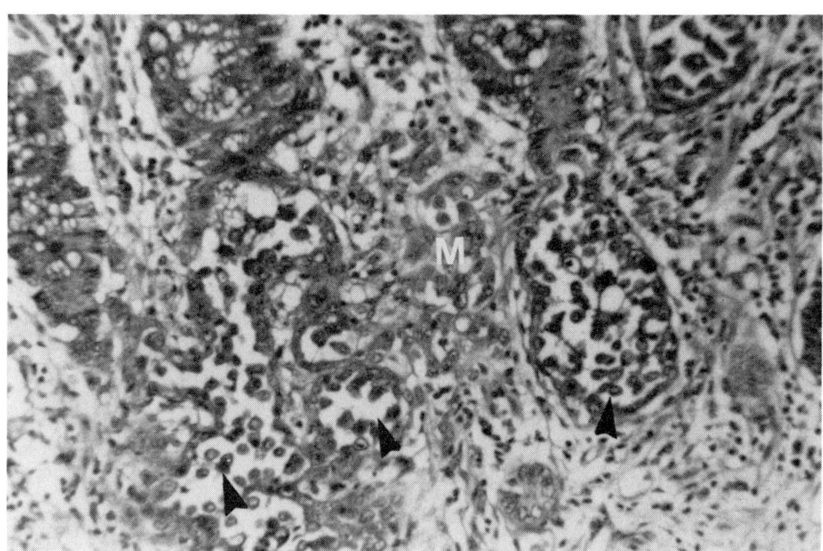

FIGURE 7. Photomicrograph of an adjacent area of the ascending colon in CTT in Figure 5. At least 3 crypts (arrows) are evident and all have budding cancer cells within the crypt lumen. Malignant cancer cells have broken through the epithelium and invaded the lamina propria (M). PAS 400×.

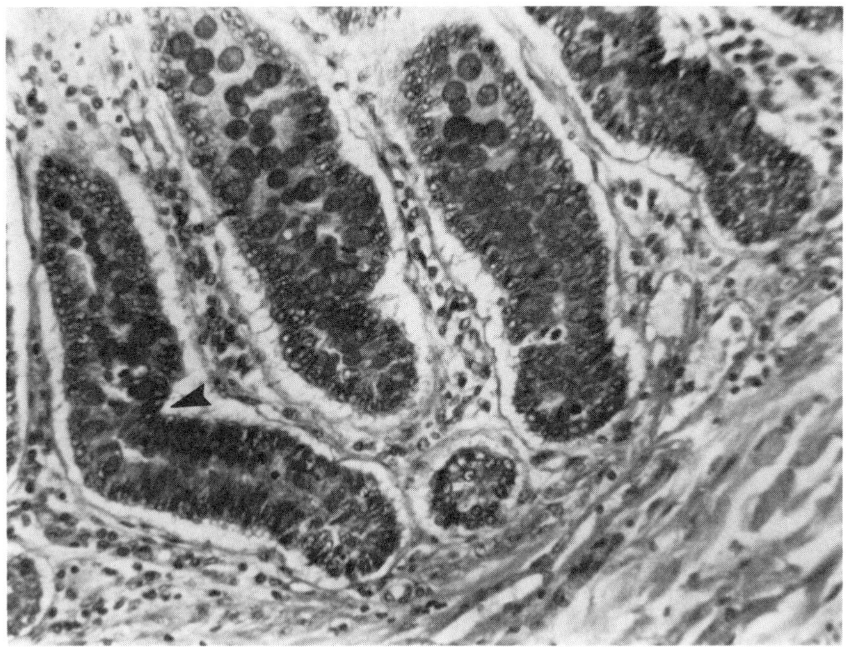

FIGURE 8. Photomicrograph of remodeled crypt epithelium showing a boot-shape remodeling (arrow). PAS 400×.

IV. DISCUSSION

A majority of the CTT colonic carcinomas had relatively large tumor masses at necropsy that are histologically similar when compared with the intracrypt and intramucosal stages of carcinoma seen in these two CTTs. Most often,[11,12] the tumors have been multiple and have been relatively extensive in each colonic segment with metastatic foci present in the regional lymph nodes and possibly other body organs. Finding these two animals with early stages of cancer development has shed light upon the early transition from benign to malignant state while offering an opportunity to assemble some ideas that might give insight into the process of early cancer development.

Both tamarins had chronic colitis but no evidence of active colitis at necropsy. Architectural mucosal remodeling, representing changes associated with repair following prior acute colitic episodes, was evident and included boot-like crypt formations (Figure 8), branching crypts (Figures 9, 10), and tortuous crypts (Figure 5). However, only mild to moderate infiltration of mononuclear inflammatory cells was seen (Figure 5).

Most ''spontaneous'' cancers occur as single primary tumors that are presumed to result from a single initiated cell that becomes autonomous and

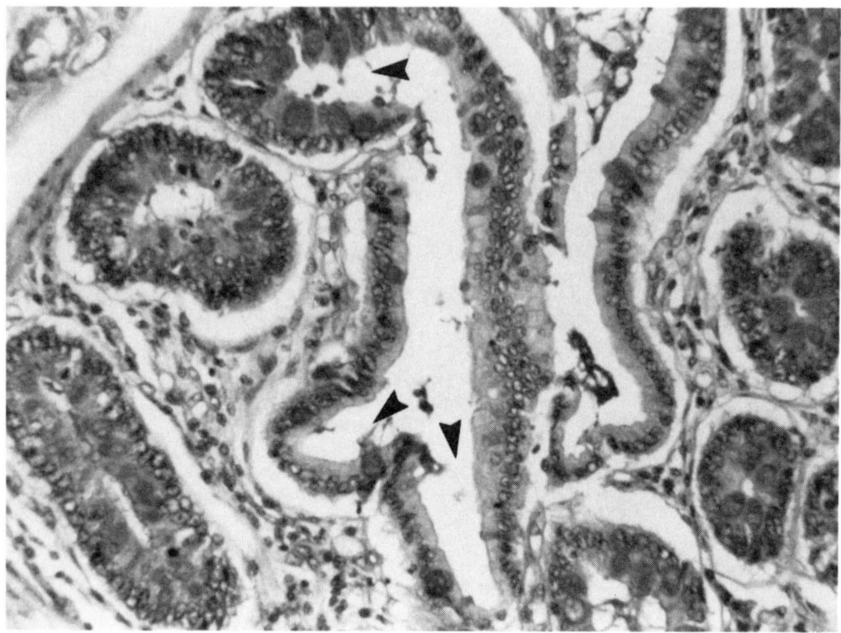

FIGURE 9. Photomicrograph of remodeled crypt epithelium showing branching crypts (arrows). PAS 400 ×.

rejects ''normal'' tissue growth restraints (e.g., immunological surveillance, contact inhibition, etc.). Occasionally, multiple ''primaries'' may be observed in a human or an animal colon, but the inference often made is that only one is ''primary'' and the other tumor nodules are most probably metastases. In chemically induced tumor systems, such as 1,2-dimethylhydrazine (DMH) or azoxymethane (AOM), the presence of multiple primary foci suggests that the chemical treatment causes intracellular changes (probably initiation and promotion after treatment with complete carcinogens) and primary tumors develop simultaneously at multiple sites.

The observation in these two tamarins of possibly three subsets (which appear to be of different ''age'' [or stage] after the insult) of ''spontaneous'' cancer development within a single animal is intriguing. Is more than one etiologic process represented or are the three subsets or stages resulting from the same process occurring at different times? The authors propose that the latter best describes the histological pictures that were observed. For example, an early colitic episode may have resulted in the large ''older'' tumor mass in the transverse colon; the multiple tumor foci in the cecum of animal CTT 1740 could have been ''promoted'' to cancer expression by a second episode of colitis (or typhlitis), even though at death the inflammatory grade was mild

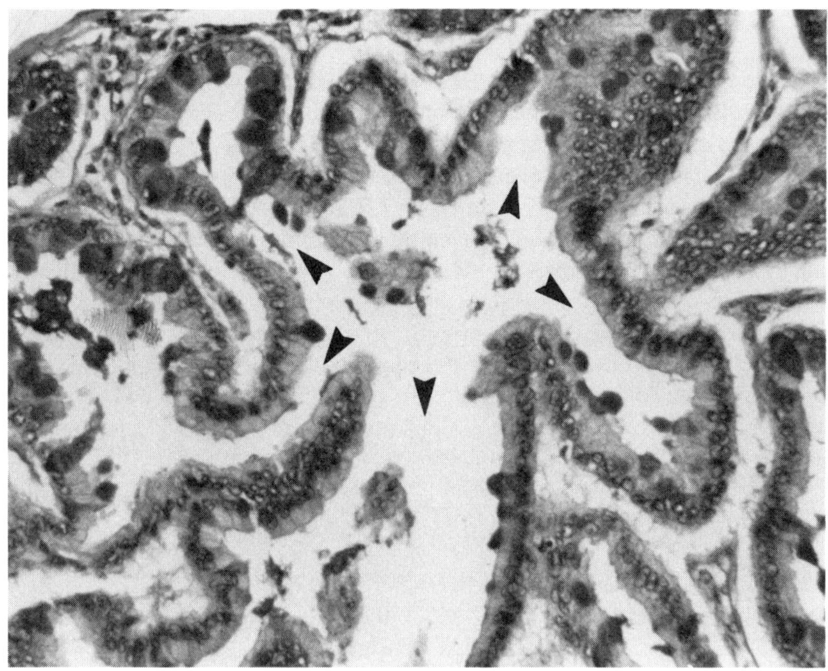

FIGURE 10. Photomicrograph of remodeled crypt epithelium showing extensive branching of crypts (arrows). PAS 400×.

chronic. A third later-occurring exacerbation of colitis (in the ascending colon) could cause the intracrypt changes which appear closer chronologically and developmentally (the malignancy was still confined to single crypts) to the most recent episode of "promoting" event(s). Clinically, these inflammatory events could have been either asymptomatic or mildly symptomatic and might not have been detected. Currently, we simply have been unable to identify the causative events or the exact time of their occurrence. However, the histological observations seem to be explained best as the result of three colitic events separated in time but which caused tumor expression in three different locations.

It would seem reasonable to assume that the events either could be identical with the same causal agent, e.g., virus, stress, dietary changes, etc., or could be different but with the same result (neoplastic expression). The experience in human ulcerative colitis patients who often develop multicentric colonic cancer primaries throughout the colon suggests that a remarkably similar situation may occur in the coexisting tamarin colonic diseases, ulcerative colitis and colonic carcinoma.

V. SUMMARY

Whereas several events that lead from benign mucosal changes to colonic carcinoma have been identified and/or postulated, the exact processes and the variations that might occur are not all known. The cotton-top tamarin offers an opportunity to study the events that occur in the colitis/carcinoma sequence in CTTs with application to man. Two CTTs died with colonic carcinoma and had what appeared to be at least three histologically different stages of cancer development in one animal. It was postulated that the three distinct stages in three colonic segments could have resulted from exacerbations of colitis at different times. The histologic evidence could help to better understand the contribution of colitis (promotion) to the expression of colonic carcinoma. The cotton-top tamarin offers an animal model that can be studied to understand this important process and possibly offer practical solutions that might eventually reduce human colon cancer incidences.

ACKNOWLEDGMENTS

This research was conducted in ORAU's AAALAC-accredited Marmoset Research Center at Oak Ridge (MARCOR) and was approved and monitored by ORAU's Animal Care Standards Committee.

Research was supported, in part, by the ORAU Corporation.

The authors acknowledge the excellent manuscript review by J. Crook, S. Tardif, and R. Damian and manuscript preparation by Sandy Womble.

REFERENCES

1. **Muto, T., Bussey, H. J. R., and Morson, B. C.,** The evolution of cancer of the colon and rectum, *Cancer,* 36, 2251, 1975.
2. **Morson, B.,** The polyp cancer sequence in the large bowel, *Proc. R. Soc. Med.,* 67, 451, 1974.
3. **Gardner, E. J.,** Familial polyposis coli and Gardner syndrome — is there a difference?, in *Progress in Clinical and Biological Research,* Vol. 115, *Prevention of Hereditary Large Bowel Cancer,* Ingall, J. R. F. and Mastromarino, A. J., Eds., Alan R. Liss, New York, 1983, 39.
4. **Lynch, H. T., Kimberling, W., Albano, W. A., Lynch, J. F., Biscone, K., Schuelke, G. S., Sandberg, A. A., Lipkin, M., Deschner, E. E., Mikol, Y. B., Elston, R. C., Bailey-Wilson, J. E., and Danes, B. S.,** Hereditary nonpolyposis colorectal cancer (Lynch syndromes I and II). I. Clinical description of research, *Cancer (Philadelphia),* 56, 934, 1985.
5. **Lynch, H. T., Lynch, P. M., Albano, W. A., and Lynch, J. F.,** The cancer family syndrome: a status report, *Dis. Colon Rectum,* 24, 311, 1981.
6. **Petersen, G. M. and Roth, M.-P.,.** Genetic epidemiology of colon cancer, This volume, Chapter 12.

7. **Vogelstein, B., Fearon, E. R., Hamilton, S. R., Kern, S. E., Preisinger, A. C., Leppert, M., Nakamura, Y., White, R., Smits, A. M. M., and Bos, J. L.,** Genetic alterations during colorectal tumor development, *N. Engl. J. Med.*, 319, 525, 1988.
8. **Paraskeva, C. and Williams, A. C.,** Are different events involved in the development of sporadic versus hereditary tumours? the possible importance of the microenvironment in hereditary cancer, *Br. J. Cancer,* 61, 828, 1990.
9. **Paraskeva, C., Corfield, A. P., Harper, S., Hague, A., Audcent, K., and Williams, A. C.,** Colorectal carcinogenesis: sequential steps in the *in vitro* immortalization and transformation of human colonic epithelial cells (review), *Anticancer Res.*, 10, 1189, 1990.
10. **Lynch, H. T., Lynch, P. M., Lynch, J. F., and Danes, B. S.,** What is hereditary colon cancer?, in *Progress in Clinical and Biological Research,* Vol. 115, *Prevention of Hereditary Large Bowel Cancer,* Ingall, J. R. F. and Mastromarino, A. J., Eds., Alan R. Liss, New York, 1983, 3.
11. **Clapp, N. K., Lushbaugh, C. C., Humason, G. L., Gangaware, B. L., and Henke, M. A.,** Natural history and pathology of colon cancer in *Saguinus oedipus oedipus, Digest. Dis. Sci.*, 30, 107S, 1985.
12. **Clapp, N. K. and Henke, M. A.,** Spontaneous colonic carcinoma observations in the Oak Ridge Associated Universities' 26-year-old cotton-top tamarin *(Saguinus oedipus)* colony, This volume, Chapter 11.
13. **Clapp, N. K., Henke, M. A., Hansard, R. M., Adams, L. J., Carson, R. L., Hawkins, J. V., and Nardi, R.,** Colonic polyps associated with colitis in cotton-top tamarins *(Saguinus oedipus):* progression to colonic carcinoma?, *Digest. Dis. Sci.*, submitted.
14. **Lushbaugh, C. C., Humason, G., and Clapp, N. K.,** Histology of colon cancer in *Saguinus oedipus oedipus, Digest. Dis. Sci.*, 30, 119S, 1985.
15. **Yardley, J. H.,** Comments on comparative pathology of colonic neoplasia in cotton-top marmoset *(Saguinus oedipus oedipus), Digest. Dis. Sci.*, 30, 126S, 1985.

Chapter 15

DEATH RATES WITH AGE FROM ALL CAUSES AND FROM COLONIC CARCINOMA IN WILD-CAUGHT AND COLONY-BORN COTTON-TOP TAMARINS

Neal K. Clapp and John B. Storer

TABLE OF CONTENTS

0-8493-5363-7/93/$0.00 + $.50

I. INTRODUCTION

It is well established that cotton-top tamarins (CTT) (*Saguinus oedipus*), maintained in captivity, spontaneously develop adenocarcinomas of the colon.[1-9] Thus, this animal species may provide an excellent model for experimental studies having relevance to the problem of colon carcinomas in man. When designing such studies it would be helpful to know the expected death rate by age from colon cancer and from all causes. To date it has not been possible to provide these estimates, for two reasons. First, many of the animals in research colonies were originally imported from the wild and their actual ages were unknown. Second, colony-born animals of known age have not been maintained long enough nor in sufficient numbers to provide good estimates.

In the present study we have utilized data from 539 cotton-top tamarins imported to or born in the Oak Ridge Associated Universities' (ORAU) Marmoset Research Center at Oak Ridge (MARCOR) research colony. We have indirectly inferred the age of the animals at the time of importation, and, by pooling all the data, we have obtained estimated death rates from all causes and from colon cancer as a function of age. We have also calculated the median age at death from all causes.

II. METHODS

This analysis has been performed on data from 539 cotton-top tamarins that either died in the ORAU colony between January 1, 1977 and April 15, 1988, or were alive in the colony on April 15, 1988 (Table 1). Death rates by age interval were calculated from: number dead in the interval/number of animal-days at risk in the interval. In tabulating days at risk, only the days at risk for animals in the colony between the above dates were included, i.e., if an animal was born before January 1, 1977, the days at risk prior to this date were not included. Similarly, if the animal was imported or transferred from another facility, only the days at risk were counted while the animal was in the ORAU facility.

The ages of animals born in captivity (''colony-born'') are, of course, their true ages. For imported animals we have used the term ''colony-age'', which is dated from the time of their receipt at the MARCOR facility. The true age of these animals is unknown, but is the sum of their age at the time of receipt plus their colony-age. We excluded data on any animals that died at less than 300 days of age whether true age or colony age. In this way we avoided distorting the data because of any high neonatal and/or juvenile death rates or high mortality associated with the stress of capture and acclimatization to captivity.

Table 1
ORIGIN AND SEX OF ANIMALS USED IN ANALYSIS

Origin	Sex	Total Number	Dead (all causes) No. (%)	Dead (Ca colon) No. (%)	Alive* (No.)
Imported	F	87	75 (87%)	31 (41%)	12
Imported	M	121	106 (88%)	43 (40%)	15
Colony-born	F	162	54 (33%)	14 (28%)	108
Colony-born	M	169	60 (35%)	15 (25%)	109
Totals		539	295 (55%)	104 (35%)	244

*Alive April 15, 1988

The death rates by age interval were found to increase exponentially with age and could be described by the equation

$$R_t = R_o e^{kt}$$

where R_t = death rate at age t, R_o = intercept constant, and k = rate constant.

This relationship also holds throughout much of the life span in human populations and in populations of domestic and experimental mammals. Weighted, least-square regression lines were calculated using the number dead in each interval as the appropriate weighting factor. Goodness-of-fit was evaluated from the residual sum of squares using standard chi-square tables.

Even though only 55% (295/539) of the animals had died, it was possible to estimate cumulative survival or cumulative mortality curves from the data used to calculate the death rates. These estimates were based on the following considerations. The death rate was assumed to be constant across each age interval, and the midpoint of each interval was used in the calculations of death rate with age. This means that half the animals dying in each interval were assumed to die before the midpoint and half were assumed to die after the midpoint. To estimate the number alive at the midpoint, it is necessary only to divide the days lived in the interval by the width of the interval. By adding one half the number dead (all causes) in the interval to the number alive at the midpoint we obtain the number entering the interval. Dividing the number dead by the number entering gives the fractional number dead. Successive multiplication of the fractions surviving gives the cumulative survival and one minus these values gives cumulative mortality. When this

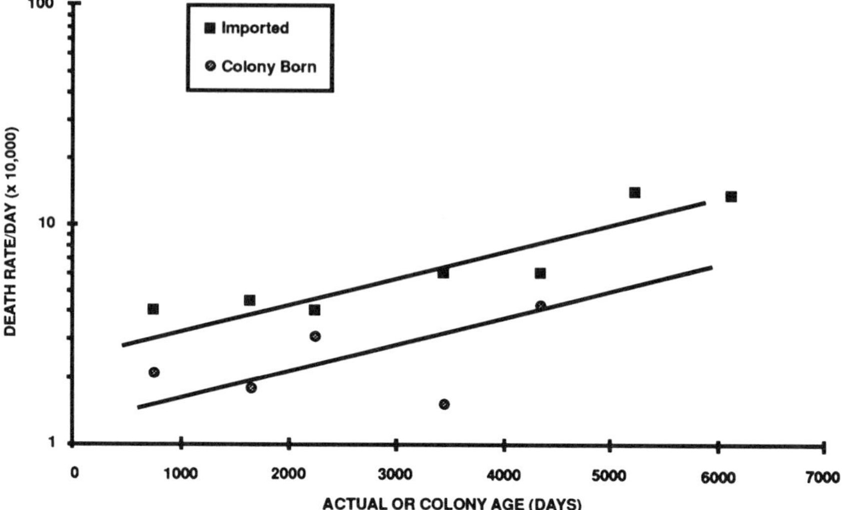

FIGURE 1. Death rate/day (all causes) with age in imports (■——■) and colony-born (●——●) tamarins; sexes combined. The death rate is in terms of dead per day at risk ($\times 10^4$). Ages for wild-caught animals are "colony ages".

approach is applied to deaths from colon cancer, the resulting cumulative mortality is automatically corrected for competing causes of death (see Kaplan-Meier modification in Reference 10).

III. RESULTS AND DISCUSSION

A. DEATH RATES (ALL CAUSES)

Death rates with age were initially calculated separately for male and female animals. The numbers of animals were small, however, and there was considerable scatter in the points. Since there were no major or consistent differences in death rates by sex, the data were pooled for further analysis. Age intervals of 300 and 600 days were tried, but there were too few deaths in some intervals to give adequate death rate estimates; therefore, 900-d intervals were used.

The death rates from all causes as a function of true age for colony-born animals and of colony-age for imported animals are shown in Figure 1. The equations for the regression lines were

$$\text{colony-born } R_t = .000160\, e^{.000216t} \qquad p > .30$$

$$\text{imported } R_t = .000286\, e^{.000217t} \qquad p > .10$$

It is obvious from the regression coefficients as well as visual inspection that the slopes of these two lines do not differ significantly and that the line

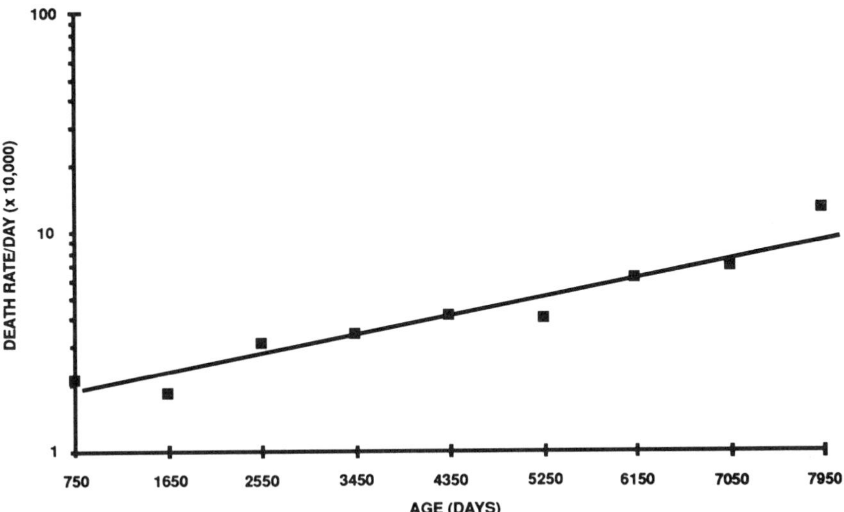

FIGURE 2. Death rate/day (all causes) with age in tamarins. All data pooled. For the imported animals, inferred ages used were "colony age" plus 2685 d.

for the imported animals is simply displaced to the left on the age scale. Since the regression coefficients are not significantly different, we calculated a common slope of 0.0002165 and recalculated the intercepts for the two lines. The extent of the lateral displacement of the line for imported animals was then calculated from:

$$\text{displacement} + (\text{days}) = \frac{\ln R_o\ (\text{imports}) - \ln R_o\ (\text{colony-born})}{k}$$

The displacement so calculated amounted to 2685 d (7.3 years). In other words, if we add 2685 d to the colony age of the imported animals, the lines will superimpose.

Accordingly, we added 2685 d to the colony-age of each imported animal, resorted the data by age interval, and pooled it with the data for colony-born animals. Death rates from all causes as a function of known (colony-born) or inferred (imported) age for all animals are shown in Figure 2. The equation for the relationship is

$$R_t = .000164\ e^{.000211t} \qquad p > .70$$

The rate constant for this equation is lower than we would have expected for experimental animals with the longevity of tamarins. The doubling time for the death rate (.693/.000211) is 3284 d or 9 years. This doubling time is longer than that for human populations (about 7 years) and far in excess of that for mice (about 100 d). The flat slope suggests that, while many of the problems associated with the maintenance of tamarins in captivity have been solved, there remains a large component of early (young adult but not neonate) mortality that presumably may be further reduced. A significant contribution to this observation is that, not only have the CTTs not been inbred at MARCOR, but also they have been intentionally outbred in that known related animals are not allowed to mate. This outbreeding policy may contribute to greater variability in the population as a whole and, hence, increased resistance to different disease entities at varying ages. However, immunogenetic evidence indicates that callitrichids are unusual in that they naturally possess a high level of homogeneity at the major histocompatibility complex.[11] Histopathologic findings in these young adult animals need to be examined intensively to see if the reasons for this early component of mortality can be identified; to date, no unusual disease entities have been identified.

The median survival time (MST) for the animals can be estimated from:

$$MST = l/k \ln \frac{.693k}{R_o} + 1$$

The median survival time for the pooled data (Figure 2) is 3022 d or 8.3 years.

B. DEATH RATES (COLON CARCINOMA VS. ALL CAUSES)

The relationship between age and the death rate from carcinoma of the colon was then examined. The pooled data for all animals are plotted in Figure 3. It is apparent that the death rate from this disease increases (albeit erratically) with age and reaches a plateau. It is not clear whether there is a true decrease at the oldest age since this point is based on only four cancer cases. No simple regression relationship described the death rate with age in colon cancer cases, and no attempt was made to fit a complicated model. One possibility is that the cancer incidence is bimodal with early and late-appearing peaks. The analysis is complicated by the fact that the adjustment of implied actual ages of imports plus pooling the data causes the first three data points to be based solely on cancer cases in colony-born animals and the last five points to be heavily weighted by cancers in the imports. In any case, the question of the exact relationship of colon cancer to age can probably not be resolved until such time as a large number of colony-born animals of known age have lived out their life spans.

Since many cancer investigators are more familiar with cumulative survival or mortality curves with age than with death rates, such curves are provided. Figure 4 shows the cumulative percent survival (death from all causes) with increasing actual or inferred age (data pooled). The surprising aspect to this curve is the lack of the chracteristic shoulder (at early ages) on

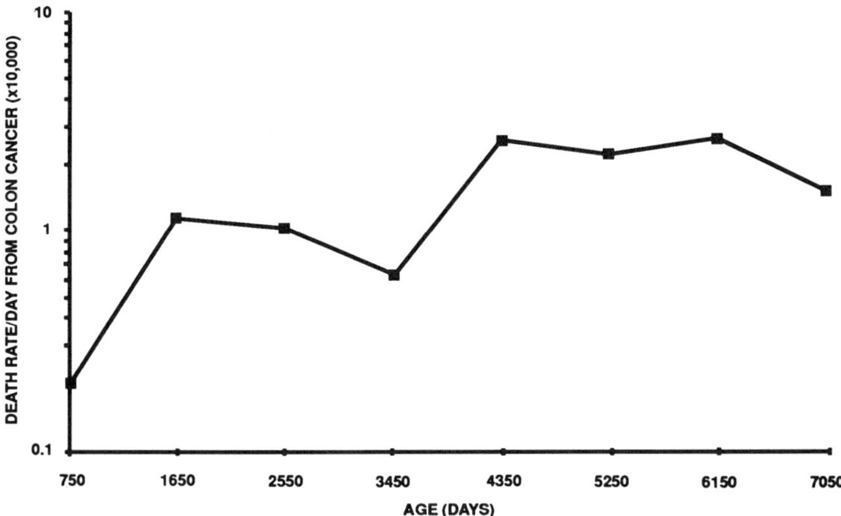

FIGURE 3. Death rate/day from colon carcinoma with age in tamarins. All data pooled. Death rate increases with age and plateaus. No simple regression relationship described death rate with age for colon carcinoma.

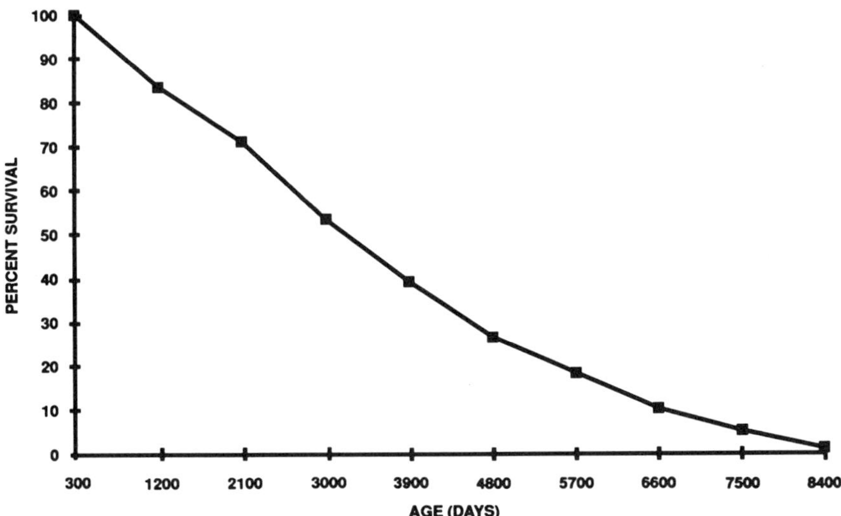

FIGURE 4. Estimated cumulative percent survival with age in tamarins (all causes). All data pooled. Ages are actual (colony-born) or inferred (imports).

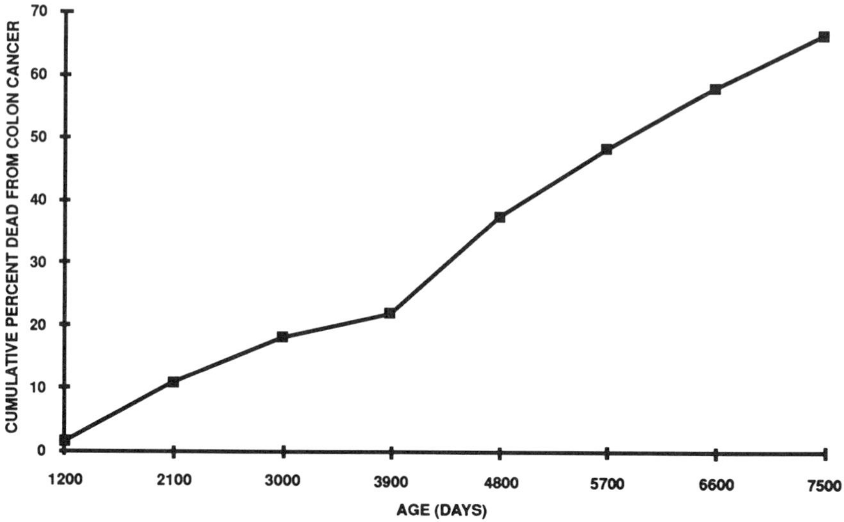

FIGURE 5. Estimated cumulative percent mortality from colon cancer with age in tamarins. All data pooled. Ages are actual (colony-born) or inferred (imports).

the left side of the curve. This finding reinforces our earlier conclusion that there is a large component of early mortality that has not been eliminated despite continuing improvements in colony management practices.[12] In Figure 5 we show the corrected (for competing risks) cumulative incidence of colon cancer with age. The very high attained incidence at late ages is indicative of the high susceptibility of this species to carcinoma of the colon. From these two tables, it should be possible for investigators to make a rough estimate of the expected mortality and incidence of colon cancer in animals of various ages and thus enable them to judge required sample sizes for specific experiments.

IV. SUMMARY

The cotton-top tamarin (*Saguinus oedipus*) provides an excellent model for experimental studies relevant to colonic carcinomas in man. However, determining death rates for colon cancer vs. all causes in a captive population is complicated by the unknown actual ages of imported animals and by the inadequate numbers of colony-born CTTs currently available to provide good estimates. Data were obtained from 539 cotton-top tamarins that lived over 300 days in the colony and that either died in the MARCOR facility between January 1, 1977 and April 15, 1988, or were alive in the colony on April 15, 1988. Death rates for imports and colony-born animals have identical slopes except for a displacement of 2685 d for imported animals (suggesting an average estimated age on arrival at MARCOR of ~7.3 years). The flat (nonsigmoid) slope suggests that a large component of young adult mortality exists that contributes to "early" deaths and that potentially may be further reduced in numbers. Death rates from colon cancer increase, albeit somewhat erratically, with age. Mortality curves are more or less linear with age, suggesting diverse causes of death across the life span of the animals. These data will allow investigators to estimate expected mortality and incidence of colonic carcinoma in various ages and thus more accurately determine required sample sizes for specific experiments.

ACKNOWLEDGMENTS

This research was conducted in ORAU's AAALAC-accredited Marmoset Research Center at Oak Ridge (MARCOR) and was approved and monitored by ORAU's Animal Care Standards Committee. Research was supported, in part, by the ORAU Corporation.

The authors acknowledge the excellent manuscript review by J. Crook, S. Tardif, R. Damian, M. Henke, and C. Jaquish, and manuscript preparation by S. Womble.

REFERENCES

1. **Lushbaugh, C. C., Humason, G. L., Swartzendruber, D. C., Richter, C. B., and Gengozian, N.,** Spontaneous colonic adenocarcinoma in marmosets, in *Primates in Medicine,* Vol. 10, Gengozian, N. and Deinhardt, F., Eds., S. Karger, Basel, 1978, 119.
2. **Richter, C. B., Lushbaugh, C. C., and Swartzendruber, D. C.,** Cancer of the colon in cotton-top tamarins, in *Comparative Pathology of Zoo Animals,* Montali, R. J. and Migaki, G., Eds., Smithsonian Institution Press, Washington, D.C., 1980, 567.
3. **Chalifoux, L. V. and Bronson, R. T.,** Colonic adenocarcinoma associated with chronic colitis in cotton-top marmoset *Saguinus oedipus, Gastroenterology,* 80, 942, 1981.
4. **Clapp, N. K., Littlefield, L. G., and Lushbaugh, C. C.,** Colon carcinoma in subhuman primates, *Gastroenterology,* 83, 519, 1982.
5. **Clapp, N. K., Lushbaugh, C. C., Humason, G. L., Gangaware, B. L., and Henke, M. A.,** Natural history and pathology of colon cancer in *Saguinus oedipus oedipus, Digest. Dis. Sci.,* 30, 107s, 1985.
6. **Clapp, N. K., Lushbaugh, C. C., Humason, G. L., Gangaware, B. L., and Henke, M. A.,** The marmoset as a model of ulcerative colitis and colon cancer, in *Colorectal Cancer and Its Precursors,* Ingalls, J. F. and Mastromarino, A., Eds., Allen R. Liss, New York, 1985, 247.
7. **Kirkwood, J. K., Pearson, G. R., and Epstein, M. A.,** Adenocarcinoma of the large bowel and colitis in captive cotton-top tamarins *Saguinus o. oedipus, J. Comp. Pathol.,* 96, 507, 1986.
8. **Clapp, N. K., Lushbaugh, C. C., Humason, G. L., Gangaware, B. L., and Henke, M. A.,** The cotton-top tamarin as an animal model of colorectal cancer metastasis, in *Biology and Treatment of Colon Cancer Metastasis,* Mastromarino, A., Ed., Martinus Nijhoff, Hingham, MA, 1986, 31.

9. **Clapp, N. K., Henke, M. A., McArthur, A. H., and Carson, R. L.,** Colonic epithelial changes associated with acute colitis and the development of colon carcinoma in tamarins, in *Int. Symp. Future Research Approaches in IBD: Mechanisms of Chronic Infection and Inflammation,* McDermott, R. P., Ed., Elsevier, Amsterdam, 1988, 713.
10. **Hoel, D. G. and Walburg, H. E., Jr.,** Statistical analysis of survival experiments, *J. Natl. Cancer Inst.*, 49, 361, 1972.
11. **Watkins, D. I. and Letvin, N. L.,** Immunobiology of the cotton-top tamarin, This volume, Chapter 21.
12. **Clapp, N. K. and Tardif, S. D.,** Marmoset husbandry and nutrition, *Digest. Dis. Sci.*, 30, 17S, 1985.

Chapter 16

TAMARIN COLON CANCER AND FLOW CYTOMETRY

Joseph E. Fuhr, Stuart Van Meter, Richard B. Andrews, and Neal K. Clapp

TABLE OF CONTENTS

0-8493-5363-7/93/$0.00 + $.50

I. INTRODUCTION

The cotton-top tamarin (CTT) is proposed as a potentially important animal model for the study of colon cancer, because the tamarin, like the human, develops ulcerative colitis which in time undergoes tissue changes and progresses with a high incidence to colonic cancer. The full application of the tamarin model to human disease is under continuing investigation.[1]

In humans, regular follow-ups are necessary to provide adequate surveillance of a disease progression which may develop over a decade or more. A definitive marker for a premalignant or early malignant change is a desired goal for research in the area of human colon cancer in the ulcerative colitis patient. While most pathologists may agree on the classification and interpretation of early and severe dysplasia, a grey area remains between.[2] Flow cytometry has been, and continues to be, studied as a potential technique to provide an objective assessment of premalignant or early malignant transformation in patients with ulcerative colitis.[3,4]

The results and conclusions incorporated in this chapter thus must be considered preliminary. The tamarin model must still be further understood and developed, and the prognostic value of flow cytometry even in human surveillance is still under investigation.[5] The results, however, provide additional data for comparison of tamarin colon cancer to human, and help to sharpen the focus for areas of further investigation.

II. GENERAL CONSIDERATIONS OF FLOW CYTOMETRY

Although virtually everyone is now familiar with the basic tenets of flow cytometry, it is important to remember that this technique is basically one of cytology. Cells, or in the case of deparaffinized tissue, fragments of cells, must be individually dispersed in order to permit individual analyses. Cells, or nuclei, must stream past an incident light source, generally a laser, in single file. By means of an associated computer, the manner is recorded in which each cell or nucleus reacts to the light, either by scatter (for size and complexity) or by excitation of a bound fluorochrome.

In studies of DNA content, as reported in this chapter, the tissue is recovered from a paraffin block, disaggregated, and stained with a fluorochrome which binds in a relatively stoichiometric fashion to double-stranded nucleic acid. Thus, the total amount of fluorescence associated with each nucleus should be proportional to the amount of DNA present within the single nucleus. Virtually all somatic cells of an individual contain the same amount of DNA (diploid) and should yield equivalent levels of fluorescence after staining with a DNA-specific dye, such as propidium iodide. As cells proceed through the cell cycle, there is an incremental gain in DNA content as the cell doubles its DNA prior to completing mitosis. Since flow cytometry can assess the amount of DNA per cell, it is capable of determining which cells were actively involved in the process of cell division, and in what part of the cell cycle the cell was. Flow cytometry thus can reveal what portion of the cells in a tissue were in cell cycle at the time the tissue was obtained. It, of course, cannot indicate how rapidly a cell was progressing through the cell cycle, only that the cell was in cycle. Nonetheless, by calculating the numbers of cells in S phase and in G_2/M phase, and dividing that number by the number of all cells (G_0, G_1, S, G_2/M) a value can be obtained which has been labeled as the proliferative index of a specific tissue. In addition, cancer cells are frequently characterized by an abnormal complement of DNA (DNA aneuploid).[6] The ability of flow cytometry to detect DNA aneuploid populations has been utilized to evaluate prognosis for a number of tumor types, as well as a potential objective marker for the diagnosis of cancer.

III. COTTON-TOP TAMARINS AND FLOW CYTOMETRY

Before studies could be initiated to assess the value of flow cytometry in monitoring dysplastic changes in the tamarin colon, it was necessary to confirm that colon cancer in the tamarin was characterized by the same incidence of DNA aneuploid cell populations as was encountered in humans. Because of the small size of the animal and the availability of archival tissues, the decision was further made to perform all analyses on deparaffinized tissues. In this manner, histological confirmation could be obtained that the tissue was malignant. In addition, a second 4-μm slice for H&E staining was made in order to establish that the malignant tissue penetrated through the thick section which was cut for flow cytometry DNA analysis.

A. TISSUE PREPARATION

Sections were selected for analysis based on histological evaluation of a 4-μm H&E section. From these selected blocks a 50-μm slice was prepared for analysis. A second thin slice confirmed the presence of the tumor throughout the section. The basic procedure of Hedley et al.,[7] as modified by Sickle-Santanello et al.,[8] was followed, with only slight variation. A 50-μm slice was obtained from each histological block for analysis. After excess paraffin was trimmed, the remaining specimen was wrapped in a piece of laboratory tissue (Kimwipe). The wrapped tissue was then locked within a plastic histology cassette used for embedding specimens. The cassette was immersed in a beaker with Histoclear with constant mixing. After 10 min, the Histoclear was decanted and the procedure repeated. After the second deparaffinizing stage, the tissue was hydrated by passage successively through solutions of 100% ethanol, 95% ethanol, 70% ethanol, and 50% ethanol for 10 min each. The tissue was finally fixed using two washes of distilled water.

The sample was then removed from the plastic cassette and from the tissue paper. The sample was minced and incubated with 1 ml of 0.5% pepsin in saline at a pH of 1.5 for 30 min at 37°C. The sample was then chilled on ice and an equal volume of cold 3% polyethylene glycol (PEG) in phosphate-buffered saline was added. The sample was filtered through a 65-μm nylon mesh and rinsed in a test tube by the addition of cold 3% PEG in phosphate-buffered saline. All pellets were collected by centrifugation at 2000 rpm for 10 min. Nuclear preparations were made by resuspending the cells in 0.6% non-idet P40, 0.1% albumin in saline. Ribonucleic acid was removed by treatment with 0.1% RNase for 10 min at room temperature. Propidium iodide was added (50 μg/ml) to stain DNA. After at least 30 min on ice, the sample was analyzed on a flow cytometer.[9]

B. FLOW CYTOMETRY INSTRUMENTATION

Nuclei were analyzed for DNA content on an Ortho 50H Cytofluorograf with a 2151 computer (Data General). Software and circuitry of the unit allow simultaneous analyses of the integrated fluorescence signal (area) and the amplitude of the signal (peak). In this manner, by trapezoidal gating the signal from doublets and debris can be reduced in the generated histogram. The machine was focused with standard beads each day to yield a coefficient of variation of 2.5 or better for right-angle fluorescence. DNA was analyzed at a flow rate of approximately 50 nuclei per second.

Proliferation rate for each tissue was determined manually. In practice, this was obtained by dividing the numbers of cells in S and G_2/M by all the cells in the gated histogram.

IV. PLOIDY PATTERNS AND HISTOLOGY FROM TAMARIN COLON CANCERS

Colon cancers from 10 tamarins were analyzed. The results summarized in Table 1 indicate that cancer was confirmed in each, and that the type varied from poorly differentiated to fairly well differentiated with mucin production. A DNA aneuploid population, however, was detected in only one section (Figure 1D). The remainder of the tissues were exclusively diploid. It should be noted that even the one DNA aneuploid pattern was more diffuse than that which has been recovered from deparaffinized human colon cancers studied by this laboratory. This may suggest that aneuploid nuclei from tamarin colon cancer cells are more friable than those from humans. A typical histogram from a deparaffinized human colon cancer containing DNA aneuploid population is shown in Figure 1C. It seems unlikely that the failure to detect abnormal DNA populations is due to general dissolution of nuclei during the processing stages because the signal from the diploid G_0/G_1 was relatively tight (Figures 1A and 1B) and comparable to that obtained from human tissues. In addition, it would be expected that if a selective loss of a DNA aneuploid population had occurred, then there should have been a significant increase in the amount of nuclear debris excluded from the processed histograms. This was also not the case as the amount of debris excluded from each histogram ranged from 15% to a high of 31%. These values are consistent with signals

TABLE 1
Marmoset Colon Cancers

Animal no.	Ploidy	Proliferation rate (%)	Histology
MO-4028	Diploid	9.4	Focal adeno ca. in mucosa with focal submucosal extensions (lymphatics)
MO-4423	Diploid	11.5	Adeno ca. poorly differentiated extending through muscular wall
MO-4292	Diploid	5.9	Adeno ca. poorly differentiated extending through muscular wall
MO-4720	Diploid	11.5	Adeno ca. poorly differentiated extending through bowel wall
FO-4586	Diploid	12.4	Adeno ca. poorly differentiated extensive
MO-4597	Diploid	9.8	Adeno ca. poorly differentiated with mucin production, extending through bowel wall
MO-4515	Diploid	7.1	Adeno ca. fairly well differentiated, intramucosal
	Diploid	6.8	Focal area of poorly differentiated adeno
FO-4825	Aneuploid	16.7	Adeno ca. mucin producing, poorly differentiated extending through bowel wall
MO-4053	Diploid	8.0	Adeno ca. mucin producing, poorly differentiated extending through bowel wall
MO-4945	Diploid	5.2	Adeno ca. poorly differentiated, focally extending through bowel wall

to be expected from a deparaffinized specimen in which two entire planes of nuclei have been sliced. The conclusion then seems reasonable that DNA aneuploid populations did not exist in the majority of tamarin colon cancers studied.

Proliferation rates obtained were also variable, as indicated in Table 1, with rates ranging from low (7% or less) to high (15% or greater). It should also be noted that each tissue sample contained normal tissue as well as cancer. In order to prevent dilution of proliferation rate ascribed to the malignant cells by inclusion of a majority of normal cells, slices were divided, and regions enriched for tumor cells were processed separately from regions relatively poor in malignant cells. Selections were based on evaluation of histology slides. With one exception, proliferation rates from malignant sections were only slightly elevated above the adjacent region. Examination of the histology slides indicated the tumor penetrated the thickness of the flow cytometry slice. Therefore, proliferation rate was not diluted because of the inclusion of significant numbers of normal nuclei.

V. DISCUSSION

A number of reports have been published which indicate a majority of human colon cancers are characterized by the presence of gross changes in DNA content per nucleus (DNA aneuploid).[6] In some studies, in fact, the

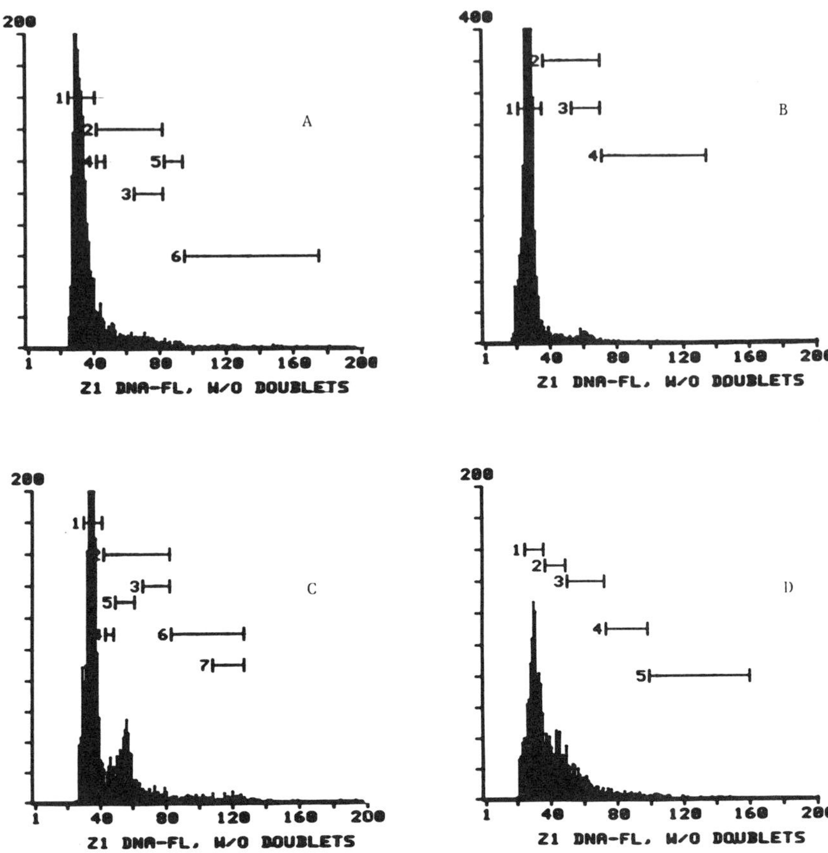

FIGURE 1. DNA histograms from paraffin-embedded colon tissue. (A) Histogram from marmoset colon cancer with approximately 12% proliferation rate; (B) histogram from marmoset colon cancer with approximately 7% proliferation rate; (C) histogram from human colon cancer showing typical DNA aneuploid population; (D) histogram from marmoset colon cancer showing diffuse DNA aneuploid population.

incidence of DNA aneuploidy in this condition has been reported to be as high as 85%.[10] It has been consistently shown that with worsening Duke's classification, the level of DNA aneuploidy increases. As would be expected, an inverse relationship has also been found between the presence of DNA aneuploid cells and survival.[11] This relationship, however, existed even when cancers were analyzed according to Duke's classification.[12]

Beyond staging or evaluating possible prognosis, flow cytometry-determined DNA content has been investigated as a screening test. The goal was that relatively objective ploidy (diploid vs. aneuploid) determination of colon biopsies could supplement the customary histological evaluation of tissue obtained during surveillance colonoscopy of the ulcerative colitis patient.[5] In this manner, additional information could be obtained to assist in the interpretation of tissues with varying levels of dysplasia. Development of this application is of course predicated on the presence of DNA aneuploidy at an early, even dysplastic, stage of colon carcinogenesis.

The failure to detect a high incidence of DNA aneuploidy in the current limited analysis of documented cotton-top tamarin colon cancers suggests a different cellular transformation pathway may exist in the tamarin than in the human. Although further studies will be necessary to confirm these early results, they do indicate that flow cytometry of colon biopsies from tamarins with ulcerative colitis may be more productive if additional parameters are included in the analysis. The successful recovery of tamarin colon nuclei from paraffin-embedded blocks is encouraging and indicates flow cytometry analyses can be performed.

A common hypothesis about colon carcinogenesis is that an early event involves an increase in the rate of cellular proliferation. The rates observed in the current series were clearly elevated in some animals. Additional restriction of the amount of noninvolved tissue in the analysis and establishment of a base proliferation rate for normal cotton-top tamarin colon tissue may result in a useful marker for premalignant changes in colon cells from tamarins. In addition, monoclonal antibodies are available against proliferation-specific proteins, such as PCNA, which can be used on nuclei recovered from paraffin. Screening for the presence and eventual loss of tumor suppressor antigens such as p53 can also be a productive area for future investigation.

VI. CONCLUSION

Colon cancer nuclei can be recovered from paraffin-embedded tissue in a quality and quantity suitable for flow cytometry analysis. In a preliminary study, DNA aneuploid populations were detected with low frequency even in histologically established invasive tamarin carcinomas. This frequency pattern appears to be different from that found in human colon cancers, but further evaluation may be helpful in understanding the causes and significance of DNA aneuploid populations in human colon cancers. Further investigations are needed in this colon cancer model to evaluate proliferation patterns and specific antigen expressions. These studies may well contribute to establishment of colon cancer in the cotton-top tamarin as a valuable model of human cancer, but with sufficient differences to lead to new insights into the pathogenesis and progression of colon cancer.

REFERENCES

1. **Clapp, N. K., Lushbaugh, C. C., Humason, G. L., Gamgaware, B. L., and Henke, M. A.,** The marmoset as a model of ulcerative colitis and colon cancer, in *Colorectal Cancer and its Precursors,* Ingalls, J. E. and Mastromario, A., Eds., Allen R. Liss, New York, 1985, 274.
2. **Ridell, R. H., Goldman, H., Ransohoff, D. F., Appelman, H. D., Fenoglio, C. M., Haggitt, R. C., Ahren, C., Correa, P., Hamilton, S. R., Morson, B. C., Sommers, S. C., and Yardley, J. H.,** Dysplasia in inflammatory bowel disease: standardized classification with provisional clinical applications, *Hum. Pathol.,* 14, 931, 1983.
3. **Lofberg, R., Brostrom, O., Karlen, P., Tribukait, B., and Ost, A.,** Colonoscopic surveillance in long standing total ulcerative colitis — a 15 year follow-up study, *Gastroenterology,* 99, 1021, 1990.
4. **McKinley, M. J., Budman, D. R., and Kahn, E.,** High grade dysplasia in Crohn's colitis characterized by flow cytometry, *J. Clin. Gastroenterol.,* 9, 452, 1987.
5. **Meling, G. L., Clausen, O. P. F., Bergan, A., Schjolberg, A., and Rognum, T. O.,** Flow cytometric DNA ploidy pattern in dysplastic mucosa, and in primary and metastatic carcinomas in patients with longstanding ulcerative colitis, *Br. J. Cancer,* 64, 339, 1991.
6. **Barologie, B., Drewinko, B., Schumann, J., Gohde, W., Dosik, G., Latreille, J., Johnson, D. A., and Freireich, E. J.,** Cellular DNA content as a marker of neoplasia in man, *Am. J. Med.,* 69, 105, 1980.
7. **Hedley, D. W., Friedlander, M. L., and Taylor, I. W.,** Application of DNA flow cytometry to paraffin-embedded archival material for the study of aneuploidy and its clinical significance, *Cytometry,* 6, 327, 1985.
8. **Sickle-Santanello, B., Farra, W. B., DeCenzo, J. F., Keyhani-Rofagha, S., Klein, J., Pearl, D., Laufman, H., and O'Toole, R. V.,** Technical and statistical improvements for flow cytometric DNA analysis of paraffin-embedded tissue, *Cytometry,* 9, 594, 1988.
9. **Fuhr, J. E., Frye, A., Kattine, A. A., and Van Meter, S.,** Flow cytometric determination of breast tumor heterogeneity, *Cancer,* 67, 1401, 1991.
10. **Harlow, S. P., Eriksen, B. L., Poggensee, L., Chmiel, J. S., Scarpelli, D. G., Murad, T., and Bauer, K. D.,** Prognostic implications of proliferative activity and DNA aneuploidy in Astler-Coller Dukes stage c colonic adenocarcinomas, *Cancer Res.,* 51, 2403, 1991.
11. **Wolley, R. C., Schrieiber, K., Koss, L. G., Karas, M., and Sherman, A.,** DNA distribution in human colon carcinomas and its relationship to clinical behavior, *J. Natl. Cancer Inst.,* 69, 15, 1982.
12. **Armitage, N. C., Robins, R. A., Evans, D. F., Turner, D. R., Baldwin, R. W., and Hardcastle, J. D.,** The influence of tumor cell DNA abnormalities on survival in colorectal cancer, *Br. J. Surg.,* 72, 828, 1985.

D. Physiologic Changes and Markers Associated with Colon Disease

Chapter 17

FECAL STEROIDS IN TAMARINS AND MARMOSETS

Bertram I. Cohen, Erwin H. Mosbach, Marsha A. Henke, and Neal K. Clapp

TABLE OF CONTENTS

0-8493-5363-7/93/$0.00 + $.50

I. INTRODUCTION

Cancer of the colon is among the most prevalent malignancies of many "westernized" populations of North America and Europe.[1] Despite concerted attempts to study this disease (such as the National Large Bowel Cancer Project, 1975 to 1986) and establish its cause and treatment, colon cancer continues to rank as the second most deadly form of cancer in the U.S.[2]

Over the past decade, hypotheses have been proposed suggesting that large bowel cancer is related to diet, geographic location, socioeconomic status, and/or heredity.[3-9] Many studies have focused on diet in general as well as individual dietary components in particular (fat, fiber, and/or protein) in order to elucidate the etiology of colon cancer.[4,9-14] However, the effect(s) of diet on cancer remains undetermined.

Animal models have been used to study whether certain dietary components accelerate or retard colon cancer.[15,16] Most studies in animals have used rats in which colon cancer can be induced by treatment with chemical carcinogens (1,2-dimethylhydrazine, DMH; *N*-methyl-*N'*-nitrosourea, NMU), often in conjunction with dietary modifications.[16-23] In rats, sterols and bile acids are found to be promoters of tumor development both in germfree and conventional animals.[10,24-33] An animal model in which tumors develop spontaneously (in the absence of chemical carcinogens) enables us to evaluate whether these steroids (or their metabolites) initiate and/or promote colon cancer. The cotton-top tamarin, *Saguinus oedipus,* offers such an opportunity to study spontaneously developing colon cancer in a subhuman primate. This chapter will examine the relationship between steroids and colon cancer in tamarins.

II. STEROLS AND BILE ACIDS

A. STRUCTURE AND FUNCTION

Bile acids, steroids which are abundantly found in feces, are formed in the liver of mammals from the 27-carbon-atom molecule cholesterol (**I,** Figure 1) by a complex series of biochemical reactions.[34] The two primary bile acids formed from cholesterol are chenodeoxycholic acid (**II,** Figure 1) and cholic acid (**III,** Figure 1). These compounds are amidated in the liver with glycine or taurine and secreted into the bile. Most of the bile salts entering the intestine are reabsorbed via active or passive transport mechanisms.[35,36] The bile salts then return to the liver via the portal vein and undergo reamidation and reexcretion into bile; the enterohepatic circulation is the mechanism whereby 97% of the bile salts are conserved.[36]

In the large bowel the primary bile acids come into contact with the fecal flora and undergo a series of structural modifications. The most prominent bile acids in the feces are formed by the bacterial 7α-dehydroxylation of the primary bile acids.[37,38] As a result of this reaction, cholic acid is converted to deoxycholic acid (**IV**, Figure 1) and chenodeoxycholic acid is transformed

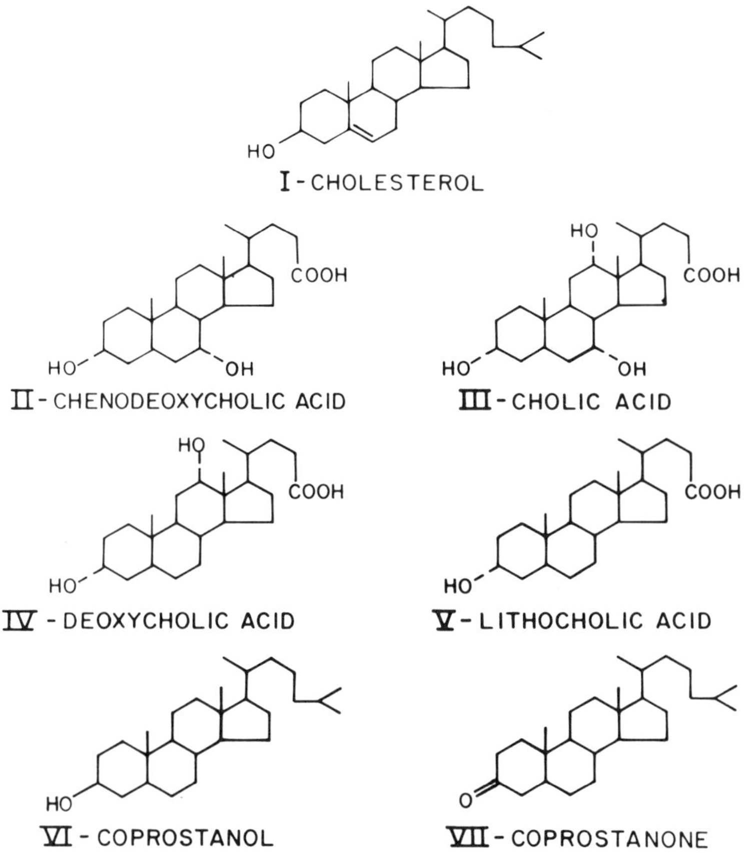

HO
I - CHOLESTEROL

HO OH
II - CHENODEOXYCHOLIC ACID

HO COOH HO OH
III - CHOLIC ACID

HO COOH HO
IV - DEOXYCHOLIC ACID

COOH HO
V - LITHOCHOLIC ACID

HO
VI - COPROSTANOL

O
VII - COPROSTANONE

FIGURE 1. Structures of steroids.

into lithocholic acid (**V,** Figure 1). In addition to dehydroxylation, the fecal flora can transform bile acids via dehydration, oxidation, and isomerization, producing perhaps as many as 20 to 30 different metabolites.[38] In man, bile acid excretion is found to average between 500 and 750 mg per day.[35,36] These amounts have been shown to increase in diseases of the large bowel, as well as in individuals given bile acids for gallstone dissolution.[39,40]

B. BILE ACIDS AND COLON CANCER

Bile acids are involved in the absorption of fat from the intestine. The realization that an increased intake of fat leads to an increase in intestinal bile acid concentration and that this is associated with an increased incidence of colon cancer led to the hypothesis that bile acids play a role in the etiology of this disease.[21,28] Metabolic epidemiological studies have shown that high-risk populations have increased concentrations of bile acids and cholesterol (or its metabolites) in the feces.[41-44] In addition, these populations have increased concentrations of intestinal anaerobic bacteria and an enhanced metabolic activity of these bacteria.[42] Thus, in individuals consuming high-fat diets (rich in meat), the bacterial metabolism of bile acids as well as neutral sterols was greater in individuals who consumed a low-meat, low-protein diet.[41] Patients with either colorectal cancer and/or adenomatous polyps have higher concentrations of fecal bile acids and cholesterol metabolites than control patients.[41] The daily excretion of secondary bile acids in stool was higher in patients with colon cancer. In addition, the bacterial transformation of cholesterol to coprostanol (**VI,** Figure 1) and coprostanone (**VII,** Figure 1) in the large bowel was high for the American population (80% of the fecal sterols are either coprostanol or coprostanone)[41-44] compared to other groups. These data, taken collectively, suggest a relationship between steroids in feces and colonic cancer.

In animals, studies showed that rats fed a high-fat diet and given a carcinogen (DMH) were more prone to large bowel cancer than rats fed a low-fat diet;[21,30] the levels of coprostanol as well as the bacterial modifications of the acidic steroids by the intestinal flora were enhanced by a high-fat diet. Bile acids administered in the diet or given intrarectally acted as tumor promoters in rats treated with carcinogens. Intrarectal instillation of lithocholic acid or taurodeoxycholic acid in rats treated with MNNG increased the incidence of colonic neoplasms.[31] Similarly, intrarectal instillation of sodium cholate and sodium chenodeoxycholate increased tumor production in germ-free rats treated with MNNG. Thus, bile acids and neutral sterols were implicated in the etiology of colon cancer induced chemically in experimental animals.

The relationship of fecal steroids to colorectal cancer has been ascribed to several aspects of sterol metabolism. These include the type and quantity of neutral sterols and bile acids entering the colon and/or the composition of the gut bacteria which might metabolize the fecal steroids to carcinogenic or procarcinogenic compounds. It would be advantageous to study these phenomena in a model where cancer develops without pretreatment with a chemical carcinogen/toxin. Consequently, we have studied such a model, namely, the cotton-top tamarin, to compare the amounts of fecal steroids in species with a high susceptibility and two species that are not susceptible to spontaneous colon cancer.

III. STEROLS AND BILE ACIDS IN TAMARINS AND MARMOSETS

A. METHODS OF ANALYSES

Fecal steroids were analyzed by the series of steps summarized in Table 1.[45-48] Fresh fecal samples (collected in Oak Ridge, TN) were freeze-dried for 48 h prior to chemical analyses and shipped to Beth Israel Medical Center, New York. An aliquot of the powdered fecal material was placed into a

TABLE 1
Steps Used in Fecal Analysis

Procedures in sequence[a]	Results
• Freeze dry and grind fresh fecal sample	Removal of water and preparation for extraction
• Soxhlet extraction with 95% ethanol-0.1% NH_4OH for 48 h	Complete removal of steroids from fecal sample
• Save portion of fecal extract for determination of compounds that may be destroyed by subsequent analysis	
• Mild alkaline hydrolysis of extract from step 2	Hydrolysis of sterol esters
• Hexane extraction	Removal of neutral and plant sterols
• TLC, GLC, and GLC-MS of neutral and plant sterols	Identification and quantitation of sterols
• Removal of organic solvents after hexane extraction	To prevent formation of artifacts in bile acid workup
• Vigorous alkaline hydrolysis	Deconjugation of bile acids
• Acidification	Protonation of fecal bile salts prior to organic solvent extraction
• $CHCl_3$-MeOH extraction; store at 0°C for 6–12 h	Hydrolysis of bile acid sulfates
• Extraction with chloroform and combination with Folch extract	Removal of all fecal bile acids
• Methylation of bile acids (methanol/5% HCl)	Derivatization required for quantitative analysis and identification
• TLC	Removal of hydroxy fatty acids
• GLC (TMS ether derivatives on 3% SE-30)	Further derivatization for quantitation of total fecal bile acids
• GLS-MS	Definitive identification of all fecal bile acid components

[a] TLC, Thin-layer chromatography; GLC, gas-liquid chromatography; GLC-MS, gas-liquid chromatography-mass spectrometry; TMS, trimethylsilylether.

cellulose extraction thimble; the thimble was then placed in a Soxhlet extractor. The sample was extracted with 95% ethanol and 0.1% ammonium hydroxide for 48 h to remove the steroids from the fecal residue. All subsequent reactions, centrifugations, and extractions were performed using the fecal extract.

The neutral sterols (cholesterol, coprostanol, coprostanone) were separated from the acidic steroids (bile acids) for quantification and identification. The total fecal extract was reduced to 20 ml in volume by evaporation under a stream of nitrogen. Ten milliliters of this extract were stored for future analyses. The remaining fraction was subjected to mild alkaline hydrolysis and the free natural sterols were removed by hexane extraction. Thin-layer chromatography on florisil was used to separate cholesterol, coprostanol, and coprostanone. The individual neutral sterols were quantitated by gas-liquid chromatography as their trimethylsilylether (TMS) derivatives using 5α-cholestane as an internal standard.[46] In certain cases, positive identification of the neutral sterols was made by gas-liquid chromatography-mass spectrometry.

The acidic steroids remained in the aqueous phase after extraction of the neutral sterols. Since the acidic compounds may be present as amidates, they were hydrolyzed under vigorous alkaline conditions. Next, the free bile acid fraction was protonated by acidification with HCl followed by extraction with chloroform-methanol (2:1, v:v, 50 ml, 1 time) and chloroform (50 ml, 2 times). The free bile acids were esterified with methanol; the methyl esters were purified by thin-layer chromatography and quantitated by gas-liquid chromatography using published procedures.[48]

B. STEROIDS IN TAMARINS AND MARMOSETS

This study represents the first attempt to identify and quantitate the fecal steroids in three species of tamarins and marmosets. Since the common marmoset (*Callithrix jacchus*) and saddle-back tamarin (*Saguinus illigeri*) develop ulcerative colitis but do not develop colon cancer spontaneously,[49-51] they were treated collectively as controls (Table 2). A third species, the cotton-top tamarin (*Saguinus oedipus*) (CTT) has a high susceptibility to develop colonic carcinoma (35% of adults die with this cancer).[49,50,52] Neutral and acidic steroids are reported in milligrams per gram dry feces (Table 2). The proportions of coprostanol and deoxycholic acid in each fraction are also reported.

The weight of the neutral sterol fraction averaged 1.13 mg/g feces in the controls; this amount more than doubles in the CTT species (2.65 mg/g) (Table 2). The proportion of coprostanol in the neutral sterol fraction is lower in the controls (8%) than in the CTTs (25%). Thus, the bacterial flora of the CTTs appears more active in converting cholesterol to coprostanol; the significance of this finding relative to the development of colon cancer and ulcerative colitis remains unknown. Several studies have shown that the major bacterial metabolites of cholesterol (such as coprostanol and coprostanone) are not carcinogens themselves but the possibility that these compounds may be metabolized to "activated molecules" which are carcinogens *in situ* warrants further study.[42] Reddy et al.[44] have demonstrated the presence of the cholesterol metabolite, cholestane-3β,5α,6β-triol in the feces of patients with colon cancer. The triol is presumably formed by the bacterial flora, but its involvement in colon cancer is unknown.

IV. DISCUSSION

The type and/or quantity of the fecal bile acids in the colon may play a role in the etiology of large bowel cancer. We examined the bile acid spectrum in the feces of tamarins and marmosets and determined bile acid concentration (mg/g) as well as the proportion of deoxycholic acid (% of total bile acid)

TABLE 2
Fecal Sterols in Marmosets

Animal no.[a]	Species	Status—1987/age (years)	Neutral sterols		Acidic steroids	
			mg/g dry feces	Coprostanol %	mg/g dry feces	Deoxycholic acid %
			Group 1			
3846	*jacchus*	Alive/10	0.50	0	0.91	61
3824	*jacchus*	Alive/10	1.34	0	1.91	11
4071	*jacchus*	Alive/8	0.30	0	0.54	23
4129	*illigeri*	Dead/4	1.64	0	1.44	40
3662	*illigeri*	Alive/11	1.89	40	1.49	40
			1.13 ± 0.35[b]	8 ± 9[b]	1.26 ± 0.27[b]	35 ± 10[b]
			Group 2			
4023	*oedipus*	Alive/9	2.54	0	1.09	28
4053	*oedipus*	Alive/10	2.10	0	0.87	26
1717	*oedipus*	Dead/5	2.17	2	0.85	25
3210	*oedipus*	Alive/10	4.41	3	1.13	53
1616	*oedipus*	Dead/6	2.26	4	0.66	33
4356	*oedipus*	Alive/7	1.15	23	0.40	12
1435	*oedipus*	Alive/13	1.47	25	0.38	4
4022	*oedipus*	Dead/6.5	0.78	37	0.83	22
1095	*oedipus*	Dead/13	3.66	58	1.66	45
1639	*oedipus*	Dead/5.7	3.93	60	0.46	12
0924	*oedipus*	Dead/14	5.76	64	0.67	10
			2.65 ± 0.52[b]	25 ± 8[b]	0.81 ± 0.12[b]	25 ± 5[b]

[a] Individual animal numbers at Oak Ridge.
[b] Average ± standard error of the mean.

(Table 2). The average total fecal bile acid concentration is higher in the control animals than in those developing cancer (CTTs) (1.26 vs. 0.81 mg/g) (Table 2). In addition, deoxycholic acid was more abundant in the controls as compared with the colon cancer-susceptible species (35 vs. 25%). This finding is unexpected and is not in accord with results obtained in other species, where increased cellular turnover and tumorigenesis in the colon is associated with increased fecal deoxycholic acid concentration.[40] Rats administered carcinogen and given deoxycholic acid had more tumors than those treated with carcinogen alone. Feeding cholic acid (which increases fecal concentrations of deoxycholic acid) to NMU-treated rats results in an increased incidence of colon tumors compared to animals treated with carcinogen alone.[19] Deoxycholic acid has been suggested as a possible compound which is capable of promoting colon tumor development.[10,19,27,31] There may also be a causal association between bacterial flora, fecal bile acids, and colon cancer. One important difference between the CTT model and the rat is that CTTs develop cancer *spontaneously* without using a chemical carcinogen. Thus, bile acids may play a different role in the initiation and/or promotion of cancer in the CTT (where the cancer develops spontaneously) than in the carcinogen-treated rat. It seems evident that the role of bile acids in the etiology of colonic disease requires further study.

V. CONCLUSIONS

The cotton-top tamarin model of colon cancer and ulcerative colitis offers a new avenue to study the role of bile acids in tumor development. Other animal models show that bile acids act as tumor promoters when the tumors are induced chemically; CTTs fail to show increased bile acid excretion or degradation even though they develop colon cancer spontaneously. The role of neutral sterols and their degradation products in tumor development is also unknown. Studies on the nature of the bacterial flora, intestinal cellular turnover, tumor number and size, and the effect of dietary manipulation (e.g., bile acid or sterol feeding) may allow us to determine whether steroids affect spontaneous tumor formation in this primate colon cancer model.

ACKNOWLEDGMENT

This work was supported in part by U.S. Public Health Services grant HL 24061 from the National Heart, Lung and Blood Institute and DK 43204 from the National Institute of Diabetes and Digestive and Kidney Diseases.

REFERENCES

1. **Correa, P. and Haenszel, W.,** The epidemiology of large-bowel cancer, *Adv. Cancer Res.,* 26, 1, 1978.
2. **Zaridze, D. G.,** Guest editorial: Environmental etiology of large bowel cancer, *J. Natl. Cancer Inst.,* 70, 389, 1983.
3. **Armstrong, B. and Doll, R.,** Environmental factors and cancer incidence and mortality in different countries, with special reference to dietary practices, *Int. J. Cancer,* 15, 617, 1975.
4. **Carroll, K. K. and Khor, H. T.,** Dietary fat in relation to tumorigenesis, *Prog. Biochem. Pharmacol.,* 10, 308, 1975.
5. **Cummings, J. H., Wiggins, H. S., Jenkins, D. J. A., Houston, H., Jivraj, T., Drasar, B. S., and Hill, M. J.,** Influence of diets high and low in animal fat on bowel habit, gastrointestinal transit time, fecal microflora, bile acid and fat excretion, *J. Clin. Invest.,* 61, 953, 1978.
6. **Dales, L. G., Friedman, G. D., Ury, H. K., and Thistle, J. L.,** A case-control study of relationships of diet and other traits to colorectal cancer in American Blacks, *Am. J. Epidemiol.,* 109, 132, 1979.
7. **Jain, M., Cook, G. M., Davis, F. G., Grace, M. G., Howe, G. R., and Miller, A. B.,** A case-control study of diet and colo-rectal cancer, *Int. J. Cancer,* 26, 755, 1080.
8. **Jensen, O. M., MacLennan, R., and Wahrendorf, J.,** Diet, bowel function, faecal charcteristics and large bowel cancer in Denmark and Finland, *Nutr. Cancer,* 4, 5, 1982.
9. **Phillips, R.,** Role of life-style and dietary habits in risk of cancer among Seventh-Day Adventists, *Cancer Res.,* 35, 3513, 1975.
10. **Cohen, B. I. and Mosbach, E. H.,** The role of bile acids in colon cancer, in *Basic and Clinical Aspects of Dietary Fiber,* Vahouny, G. and Kritchevsky, D., Eds., Plenum Press, New York, 1985, 487.
11. **McCay, P. B.,** Dietary fat and cancer — an overview, in *Diet, Nutrition and Cancer: from Basic Research to Policy Implications,* Alan R. Liss, New York, 1983, 7.
12. **Newmark, H. L., Wargovich, M. J., and Bruce, W. R.,** Colon cancer and dietary fat, phosphate, and calcium: a hypothesis, *J. Natl. Cancer Inst.,* 72, 1323, 1984.
13. **Reddy, B. S.,** Dietary fat and its relationship to large bowel cancer, *Cancer Res.,* 41, 3700, 1981.
14. **Visek, W. J., Clinton, S. K., and Truex, C. R.,** Nutrition and experimental carcinogenesis, *Cornell Vet.,* 68, 3, 1971.
15. **Reddy, B. S., Narisawa, T., Maronpot, R., Weisburger, J. H., and Wynder, E. L.,** Animal models for the study of dietary factors and cancer of the large bowel, *Cancer Res.,* 35, 3421, 1975.
16. **Boffa, L. C., Lupton, J. R., Mariani, M. R., Ceppi, M., Newmark, H. L., Scalmati, A., and Lipkin, M.,** Modulation of colonic epithelial cell proliferation, histone acetylation, and luminal short chain fatty acids by variation of dietary fiber (wheat bran) in rats, *Cancer Res.,* 52, 5906, 1992.
17. **Bird, R. P., Mercer, N. J. H., and Draper, H. H.,** Animal models for the study of nutrition and human disease: colon cancer, atherosclerosis and osteoporosis, *Adv. Nutr. Res.,* 7, 155, 1985.
18. **Bull, A. W., Soullier, B. K., Wilson, P. S., Hayden, M. T., and Nigro, N. D.,** Promotion of azoxymethane-induced intestinal cancer by high fat diets in rats, *Cancer Res.,* 39, 4956, 1979.
19. **Cohen, B. I., Raicht, R. F., Deschner, E. E., Takahashi, M., Sarwal, A. N., and Fazzini, E.,** Effect of cholic acid feeding on N-methyl-N-nitroso-urea-induced colon tumors and cell kinetics in rats, *J. Natl. Cancer Inst.,* 64, 573, 1980.

20. **LaMont, J. F. and O'Gorman, T. A.,** Experimental colon cancer, *Gastroenterology,* 75, 1157, 1978.
21. **Reddy, B. S.,** Dietary fat and colon cancer, in *Experimental Colon Carcinogenesis,* Autrup, H. and William, G. M., Eds., CRC Press, Boca Raton, FL, 1983, 225.
22. **Nigro, N. D., Bhadrachari, N., and Chomchai, C.,** A rat model for studying colonic cancer: effect of cholestyramine on induced tumors, *Dis. Colon Rectum,* 16, 438, 1973.
23. **Shamsuddin, A. K. M.,** In vivo induction of colon cancer, dose and animal species, in *Experimental Colon Carcinogenesis,* Autrup, H. and William, G. M., Eds., CRC Press, Boca Raton, FL, 1983, 51.
24. **Chomchai, C., Bhadrachari, N., and Nigro, N. D.,** The effect of bile on the induction of experimental intestinal tumors in rats, *Dis. Colon Rectum,* 17, 310, 1974.
25. **Cruse, J. P., Lewin, M. R., and Clark, C. G.,** The effects of cholic acid and bile salt binding agents on 1,2-dimethylhydrazine-induced colon carcinogenesis in the rat, *Carcinogenesis,* 2, 439, 1981.
26. **Cruse, J. P., Lewin, M. R., Ferulano, G. P., and Clark, C. G.,** Experimental evidence against the bile salt theory of colon carcinogenesis, *Eur. Sug. Res.,* 13, 117, 1981.
27. **Narisawa, T., Magadia, N. E., Weisburger, J. H., and Wynder, E. L.,** Promoting effect of bile acid on colon carcinogenesis after intrarectal instillation of MNNG in rat, *J. Natl. Cancer Inst.,* 53, 1093, 1974.
28. **Reddy, B. S.,** Diet and excretion of bile acids, *Cancer Res.,* 41, 3766, 1981.
29. **Reddy, B. S. and Watanabe, K.,** Effect of cholesterol metabolites and promoting effect of lithocholic acid in colon carcinogenesis in germfree and conventional F344 rats, *Cancer Res.,* 39, 1521, 1979.
30. **Reddy, B. S. and Ohmori, T.,** Effect of intestinal microflora and dietary fat on 3,2'-dimethyl-4-aminobiphenyl-induced colon carcinogenesis in F344 rats, *Cancer Res.,* 41, 1363, 1981.
31. **Reddy, B. S., Narisawa, T., Weisburger, J. H., and Wynder, E. L.,** Promoting effect of sodium deoxycholate on colonic adenocarcinomas in germfree rats, *J. Natl. Cancer Inst.,* 56, 441, 1976.
32. **Reddy, B. S., Watanabe, K., Weisburger, J. H., and Wynder, E. L.,** Promoting effect of bile acids in colon carcinogenesis in germfree and conventional F344 rats, *Cancer Res.,* 37, 3238, 1977.
33. **Sarwal, A. N., Cohen, B. I., Raicht, R. F., Takahashi, M., and Fazzini, E.,** Effects of dietary administration of chenodeoxycholic acid on N-methyl-N-nitrosourea-induced colon cancer in rats, *Biochim. Biophys. Acta,* 574, 423, 1979.
34. **Carey, M. C.,** The enterohepatic circulation, in *The Liver: Biology and Pathobiology,* Arias, I., Popper, H., Schachter, D., and Shafritz, D. A., Eds., Raven Press, New York, 1982, 429.
35. **Hofmann, A. F.,** The enterohepatic circulation of bile acids in man, *Clin. Gastroenterol.,* 6, 3, 1977.
36. **Hofmann, A. F.,** Chemistry and enterohepatic circulation of bile acids, *Hepatology,* 4, 4S, 1984.
37. **Gustafsson, B. E.,** The physiological importance of the colonic microflora, *Scand. J. Gastroenterol. Suppl.,* 77, 117, 1982.
38. **Macdonald, I. A., Bokkenheuser, V. D., Winter, J., McLernon, A. M., and Mosbach, E. H.,** Degradation of sterols in the human gut, *J. Lipid Res.,* 24, 675, 1983.
39. **Bell, G. D., Whitney, B., and Dowling, R. H.,** Gallstone dissolution in man using chenodeoxycholic acid, *Lancet,* 2, 1213, 1972.
40. **Danzinger, R. G., Hofmann, A. F., Schoenfield, L. J., and Thistle, J. L.,** Dissolution of cholesterol gallstones by chenodeoxycholic acid, *N. Engl. J. Med.,* 286, 1, 1972.
41. **Reddy, B. S. and Wynder, E. L.,** Metabolic epidemiology of colon cancer: fecal bile acids and neutral sterols in colon cancer patients and patients with adenomatous polyps, *Cancer,* 39, 2533, 1977.

42. **Reddy, B. S., Weisburger, J. H., and Wynder, E. L.,** Effects of high risk and low risk diets for colon carcinogenesis on fecal microflora and steroids in man, *J. Nutr.*, 105, 878, 1975.
43. **Reddy, B. S., Mastromarino, A., Gustafson, C., Lipkin, M., and Wynder, E. L.,** Fecal bile acids and neutral sterols in patients with familial polyposis, *Cancer,* 38, 1694, 1976.
44. **Reddy, B. S., Martin, C. W., and Wynder, E. L.,** Fecal bile acids and cholesterol metabolites of patients with ulcerative colitis, a high risk group for development of colon cancer, *Cancer Res.*, 37, 1697, 1977.
45. **Miettinen, T. A., Ahrens, E. H., Jr., and Grundy, S. M.,** Quantitative isolation and gas-liquid chromatographic analysis of total dietary and fecal neutral steroids, *J. Lipid Res.*, 6, 411, 1965.
46. **Cohen, B. I., Raicht, R. F., and Mosbach, E. H.,** The effect of dietary bile acids, cholesterol and β-sitosterol upon formation of coprostanol and 7-dehydroxylation of bile acids in the rat, *Lipids,* 9, 1024, 1974.
47. **Grundy, S. M., Ahrens, E. H., Jr., and Miettinen, T. A.,** Quantitative isolation and gas-liquid chromatographic analysis of total fecal bile acid, *J. Lipid Res.*, 6, 397, 1965.
48. **Cohen, B. I., Raicht, R. F., Salen, G., and Mosbach, E. H.,** An improved method for the isolation, quantitation and identification of bile acids in rat feces, *Anal. Biochem.*, 64, 567, 1975.
49. **Clapp, N. K., Lushbaugh, C. C., Humason, G. L., Gangaware, B. L., and Henke, M. A.,** Natural history and pathology of colon cancer in *Saguinus oedipus oedipus, Digest. Dis. Sci.*, 30, 107S, 1985.
50. **Clapp, N. K., Lushbaugh, C. C., Humason, G. L., Gangaware, B. L., and Henke, M. A.,** The marmoset as a model of ulcerative colitis and colon cancer, in *Colorectal Cancer and Its Precursors,* Ingalls, J. F. and Mastromarino, A., Eds., Alan R. Liss, New York, 1985, 247.
51. **Clapp, N. K., Henke, M. A., Lushbaugh, C. C., Humason, G. L., and Gangaware, B. L.,** Effect of various biological factors on spontaneous marmoset and tamarin colitis: a retrospective histopathological study, *Digest. Dis. Sci.*, 33, 1013, 1988.
52. **Chalifoux, L. V. and Bronson, R. T.,** Colonic adenocarcinoma associated with chronic colitis in cotton-top marmosets, *Saguinus oedipus, Gastroenterology,* 80, 942, 1981.

Chapter 18

A SERUM MARKER FOR COLON CANCER DETECTION: THE USE OF THE COTTON-TOP TAMARIN

Nicholas J. Petrelli, Garth Anderson, Lemuel Herrera, Kenneth Manly, Marsha A. Henke, and Neal K. Clapp

TABLE OF CONTENTS

0-8493-5363-7/93/$0.00 + $.50

I. INTRODUCTION

This chapter will deal with the potential clinical use of tumor markers, specifically carcinoembryonic antigen (CEA) and lactate dehydrogenase-k (LDH_k), in the human and cotton-top tamarin populations. The potential role for tumor markers includes screening asymptomatic individuals for disease, as an aid in establishing the diagnosis in symptomatic individuals, assisting in staging, and in the prognosis of malignancies, and monitoring patients for progression or recurrence of disease.

The definition of a tumor marker can best be described as any means, primarily chemical, that may help to identify the presence of a malignancy as opposed to a benign process. Such markers may be used to develop probes for blood serum tests, tissue *in vitro* testing, or radioimmunodetection. When evaluating a tumor marker one must take into consideration its sensitivity and specificity. Sensitivity (true positive/true positive + false negative) indicates the percentage of patients in a particular population with tumor who test positive for the particular marker. Specificity (true positive/false positive + true negative) refers to the results of the number of negative tests compared with the total number of individuals in a population free of the malignancy being evaluated.

II. CLASSIFICATION OF TUMOR MARKERS

The most widely studied tumor markers include the oncofetal antigens as well as other tumor antigens, hormones, and enzymes. The oncofetal antigens consist of a group of tumor-associated antigens that are also found during fetal growth. They represent a qualitative but not quantitative departure from normal that creates problems with the specificity of the assay.

The development of tumor markers has been made possible in the past three decades by the technology of immunodiffusion in the 1960s, radioimmunoassays in the 1970s, and enzyme-linked immunoassays in the 1980s. Although lactate dehydrogenases exist as multiple isozymes in humans, LDH_k is a protein which is expressed by normal cells exposed to a hypoxic environment. LDH_k will be discussed in detail later in this chapter in both the human and cotton-top tamarin populations.

CEA, originally described by Gold and Freedman,[1] is probably the most widely studied tumor marker. One of the concerns about any tumor marker is whether or not its presence correlates with the extent of disease in a patient. Although CEA does, in part, relate to extent of colorectal disease,[2,3] this is largely a qualitative relationship, e.g., large carcinomas may not produce or release significant levels of CEA and small elevations in CEA can be encountered in patients with small colorectal cancers. Other disease conditions which complicate CEA evaluation are elevated serum levels in benign conditions such as chronic obstructive pulmonary disease, alcoholism, pancreatitis, diabetes mellitus, and hypertension, as well as in patients with a cigarette smoking history.

The more accurately a tumor marker correlates with the stage of cancer, the more useful it becomes as a prognostic tool. Staab et al.[4] and other investigators[5] have found that CEA measurement is predictive statistically and within a given histologic stage of colorectal carcinoma. The consideration of a tumor marker and its relationship to stage of disease and prognostic efficacy will also be discussed with LDH_k.

Because tumor antigens such as CEA and LDH_k may be present in normal tissue and tumor which may be damaged during a surgical procedure, a temporary rise in these tumor markers in serum may be seen immediately following surgery. Also, the half-life of a marker in terms of its clearance from the serum must be considered if it is to be useful as a monitor following curative surgery. Can tumor markers such as CEA and LDH_k allow us to monitor patients with colorectal carcinoma to the patient's advantage? The prospective analysis of LDH_k is presently undergoing evaluation at Roswell Park Cancer Institute (RPCI) in patients following curative surgical resection of a primary colorectal carcinoma. However, monitoring CEA is complicated by the fact that the customary polyclonal antibody to CEA which is usually employed in the assays can have unexplained laboratory variations as well as elevations from the other etiologic benign factors that have been cited. Therefore, a major question that a clinician faces is, how often is the tumor marker successful and how often is it not? Increasing the specificity of a particular marker such as CEA has been attempted by using monoclonal antibodies.[6] Monoclonal antibodies have been identified which are reactive with specific CEA epitopes against 12 or more noncarcinoembryonic antigen substances with cross-reacting epitopes.

Despite the enormous data in the literature dealing with CEA and its role in patients with colorectal carcinoma, a more accurate tumor marker is needed. This fact has led our RPCI group to study LDH_k as a potential marker in patients with colorectal carcinoma. The data collected on human subjects and the cotton-top tamarin will be discussed in the remainder of this chapter.

III. THE PHYSIOLOGY OF LACTATE DEHYDROGENASE-k (LDH_k)

Lactate dehydrogenase-k is a major anoxic stress response protein which is expressed by normal cells subjected to hypoxic conditions. This protein, with a subunit molecular weight of 34 kDa, is also found at very high levels in cells neoplastically transformed by Kirsten murine sarcoma virus and is expressed at high levels in many human cancers. LDH_k is frequently found in human cancer patient sera and appears to have possibilities as a cancer marker.

Lactate dehydrogenases in mammalian systems exist as multiple isozymes. Tetrameric combinations of muscle (M), heart (H), and reproductive

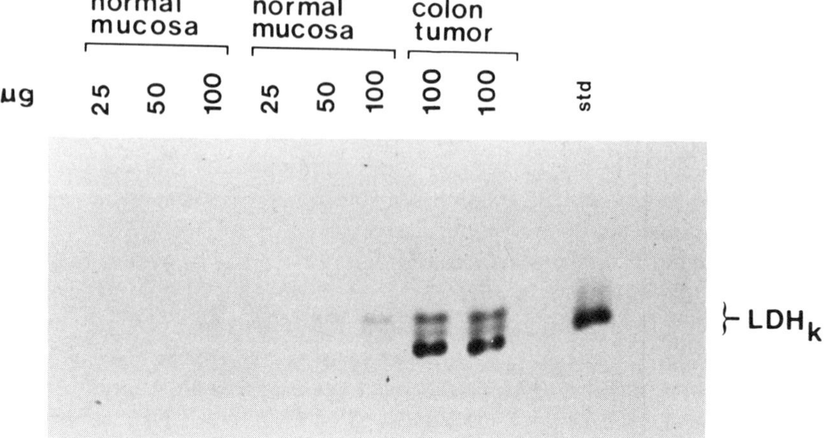

FIGURE 1. LDH_k is expressed at much higher levels in human tumor tissues than in adjoining normal tissues, with qualitative differences also apparent. Extracts of two colonic tumors were compared with adjoining colonic mucosa. LDH_k was detected by nondenaturing gel electrophoresis on imidazole/borate-buffered gels following by activity staining, as described elsewhere.[21] (From left) Lanes 1, 2, 3: 25, 50, and 100 μg of protein extract of one normal colonic mucosa; Lanes 4, 5, 6: 25, 50, and 100 μg of protein of another normal colonic mucosa; Lanes 7, 8: 100 μg of protein from extracts of the two colonic tumors; Lane 9: blank; Lane 10: pure LDH_k standard.

tissue (X) subunits have been known for over 25 years, dating to the studies of Markert and Moller[7] and Kaplan and Ciotti.[8] These lactate dehydrogenases catalyze the interconversion of pyruvate and NADH with lactate and NAD^+. In lower eukaryotes such as yeast, an additional lactate dehydrogenase (cytochrome LDH or cytochrome b_2) exists which transfers electrons directly to cytochrome c.[9,10]

In 1979, we first identified LDH_k as an antigen specific to Kirsten sarcoma virus-transformed cells which was absent from uninfected fibroblasts.[11] This antigen copurified with a lactate dehydrogenase activity. It is electrophorectically separable from conventional LDH isozymes and is designated LDH_k.[12]

Examination of normal and cancerous human tissues has revealed substantial (10- to 500-fold) elevation of LDH_k activity in tumor tissues as compared to normal adjoining tissues, while other isozymes of LDH are elevated only 2- to 5-fold[13,14] (Figure 1).

LDH_k has been found associated with 56,000-, 34,000-, and 21,000 Da subunits[12,15] although it can be purified to yield only the 34,000-Da form. It has not as yet been established that the larger peptide is a precursor of the other two. A recent report by Wu et al. has demonstrated that two 56,000-Da and 35,000-Da polypeptides immunologically related to LDH are translated from tumor mRNA *in vitro,* and mRNA isolation indicates the messages for each are about 15S.[16] The exact nature of the 56,000-Da polypeptide remains unclear.

Significant advances in understanding the normal role of LDH_k occurred with the finding that high levels of a closely related activity were expressed in mammalian retina.[17] In the retina of lower vertebrates, LDH_k activity was much lower, equivalent to that found in brain of mammals and lower vertebrates.[18] This pattern of LDH_k expression in vertebrate retina paralleled the dependency of retina on a metabolism based on aerobic glycolysis. This metabolism, known as the Warburg effect, is observed only in normal retina and in most cancerous tissues.

In 1983, Morin and Hance[19] reported that one attribute of LDH_k, namely oxygen inhibition, was in part an artifact of the imidazole-based gel electrophoresis system. Furthermore, a commercial preparation of LDH-5 had some LDH_k activity, as determined by the standard electrophorectic separation and assay methods. These findings led the authors to suggest that LDH_k may be identical with LDH-5, with the new properties artifactually due to the gel electrophoresis buffer. Subsequent studies that used cuvette assays confirmed that imidazole renders the phenazine/nitroblue tetrazolium coupled assay system oxygen responsive by a factor of two, by transferring electrons from the phenazine oxygen instead of to nitroblue tetrazolium. In addition, a greater part of the oxygen response was an intrinsic property of LDH_k itself, since LDH isolated from the retinas of different species exhibited markedly different oxygen responsiveness even when assayed together on the same gel.[18]

We have since developed affinity chromatography procedures which totally separate LDH_k from LDH-5, verifying that these two isozymes are not identical.[20] FAD (flavin adenine dinucleotide) was found to be a specific inhibitor of LDH_k with no effects on LDH-5 (Figure 2). Further studies have revealed that clear differences exist in peptide composition.

Perucho et al.[21] first described an interaction between lactate dehydrogenase and RNA in 1977. $NADH_2$ could release the RNA and LDH.[22] Recently, Williams et al. demonstrated that a 35-kDa helix-destabilizing protein is also a lactate dehydrogenase which can interact with nucleic acid.[23] Immunofluorescence studies by these authors specifically localized it to the nucleus, unlike LDH-5.[24] Independently, we have determined that nucleic acids bind LDH_k. There is some preference for single-stranded over double-stranded DNA, although binding also occurs to a variety of single- and double-stranded RNAs. A preference exists for binding to A- and T-rich nucleic acids.[20]

LDH_k is noncompetitively inhibited by 5′,5′-dipurine nucleoside tetraphosphates; the K_i value for Gp4G is $2 \times 10^{-5}\ M$ and Ap4A $5 \times 10^{-5}\ M$. Other related compounds such as AP2A, Ap3A, Ap5A, and Gp4 show no inhibitory activity. Other LDH isozymes are not inhibited by Ap4A or Gp4G. This inhibition by Gp4G may be closely linked to functions of LDH_k as an anoxic stress response protein. Ames and colleagues have presented evidence

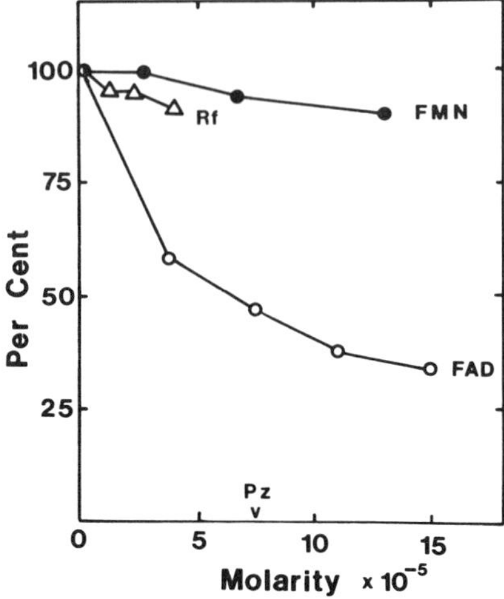

FIGURE 2. Effects of flavin compound on LDH_k activity. LDH_k (0.1 g) was assayed in a cuvette assay in a formazan blue coupled system. Assays were in the presence of FMN (●), FAD (○), or riboflavin (△) at the indicated concentrations.

that these dinucleoside tetraphosphates are cellular alarmones, signal molecules that alert cells to the onset of metabolic stresses.[25,26] Ap4A in particular appears to be synthesized in response to oxidative stress. The regulation of levels of the dinucleoside tetraphosphates is not yet clear. Defining the role and regulation of LDH_k by the class of alarmones may help us understand a key feature of their link to cellular metabolism.

IV. LACTATE DEHYDROGENASE-k (LDH_k) VS. CARCINOEMBRYONIC ANTIGEN (CEA) IN PATIENTS WITH COLORECTAL CARCINOMA

This section will present data that demonstrate an association between metastatic colorectal cancer and the appearance of LDH_k in the serum of patients with this carcinoma. The comparison of serum CEA to serum LDH_k as an indicator of metastatic colorectal carcinoma will also be described. Preliminary data have been published previously by our group.[27,28] The staging of colorectal patients was based upon the Gastrointestinal Tumor Study Group modification of the Dukes system. This is briefly described as follows: Dukes A — tumor not penetrating beyond the mucosa; Dukes B_1 — tumor penetrating the mucosa but not the serosal layer; Dukes B_2 — tumor penetrating into the periserosal fat; Dukes C_1 — one to four lymph nodes involved with metastases; Dukes C_2 — more than four lymph nodes involved with metastases; Dukes D — evidence of distant metastases.

Initially, LDH_k was assayed in the serum of 206 patients with a variety of cancers and in 30 healthy donors.[29] This study showed LDH_k to be expressed

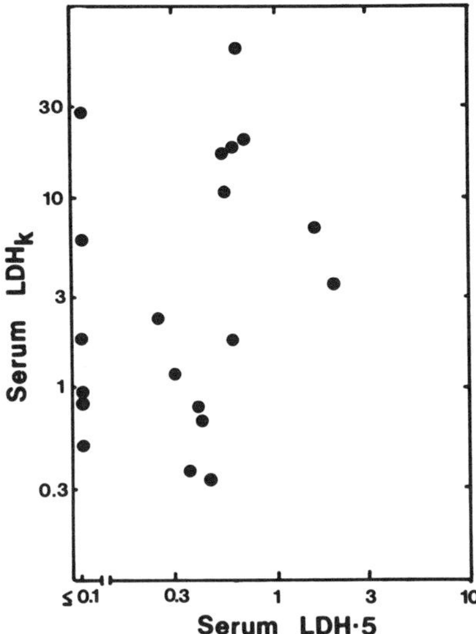

FIGURE 3. Serum expression of LDH_k is independent of other serum lactate dehydrogenase, including LDH-5. The data shown is for human neuroblastoma patients, with LDH_k assayed by nondenaturing gel electrophoresis on imidazole/borate-buffered gels run cathodally, and LDH-5 from tris/glycine-buffered gels run anodally according to procedures reported elsewhere.[21]

in a substantial fraction of the cancer patients but only rarely in the healthy controls. Expression was found to be independent of total serum LDH. Further study of LDH_k in serum has confirmed the specificity of expression of LDH_k, showing no correlation with the most basic conventional isozyme, LDH-5 (Figure 3).

To test the correlation between the presence of metastases from colorectal carcinoma and on elevated serum LDH_k a group of patients with documented distant metastases were selected who could be followed on a serial basis during the course of their treatment. A second group of patients who were admitted to Roswell Park Cancer Institute (RPCI) with a documented primary colorectal cancer were also evaluated for serum levels of LDH_k. In the latter group of patients serum samples were collected prior to surgery, 2 to 3 days following the curative surgical resection, 1 week following the surgical resection, and every 3 months thereafter. CEA data were obtained at the same time as LDH_k.

Following surgery the pathology specimens were examined and patients were staged according to the Dukes classification previously described. Table 1A shows the mean preoperative serum LDH_k and CEA levels as a function of the Dukes stage. The average serum LDH_k is about a sixfold higher level for Dukes D patients than for Dukes B or C patients. The average CEA value was about threefold higher for Dukes D than for Dukes B or C. Thus, the

TABLE 1A
Average Serum LDH_k and Serum CEA Values in Human Patients with Colorectal Adenocarcinoma Prior to Surgery

Dukes (GITSG) Stage	Mean LDH_k level (units)	Mean CEA level (ng/ml)
B (tumor within or through bowel wall)	4.3	13.0
C (lymph nodes positive)	3.5	13.2
D (distant metastases)	26.5	35.1

TABLE 1B
Average Serum Levels on Follow-Up

Patient status	Mean LDH_k (units)	Mean CEA (ng/ml)
No evidence of cancer	1.1	10.4
Metastases documented	35.2	58.3

serum LDH_k seemed to be correlated with the presence of distant metastases from colorectal carcinoma.

Postoperative patients were classified according to the presence of known distant metastases. In this group of patients follow-up serum samples were obtained every 3 months. These samples provided 229 LDH_k values and 132 CEA values, the results of which are presented in Table 1B. There is a 30-fold difference between the average serum LDH_k in patients with documented distant metastases and those without metastases. There is a sixfold difference in average serum CEA between patients with known distant metastases and those without known metastases.

If LDH_k and CEA are both associated with metastases in patients with colorectal carcinoma then it could be expected that both markers may be correlated with each other. This would be true if both markers were controlled by the same mechanism. However, the correlation between serum LDH_k and CEA is low. For preoperative serum samples the LDH_k-CEA correlation coefficient ranges from -0.02 for Dukes C_2 patients to 0.22 for Dukes D patients. For postoperative samples the correlation coefficients were -0.01 for patients with no evidence of distant metastases and 0.16 for those patients with known distant metastases. This lack of correlation suggests that serum LDH_k and CEA are not controlled by a common mechanism.[30]

Therefore, both serum CEA and serum LDH_k are correlated with known distant metastases but they are poorly correlated with each other. Hence, both markers may be able to make independent analysis to an estimate of a patient's disease status and both markers should give a better estimate of a patient's status than either marker alone. In view of this association between LDH_k and metastases from colorectal carcinoma it was decided to evaluate LDH_k

TABLE 2
LDH_k Evaluation in Cotton-Top Tamarins *(S. oedipus)* (LDH_k Values >200 Units)

Animal no.	Species	Sex	Colon cancer (+, −)	Colon sites	LDH_k (units)
1706	*S. oed.*	F	+	Cecum; transverse; rectum	340
1716	*S. oed.*	F	−	NED[a]	300
4561	*S. oed.*	F	−	NED[a]	6560
4585	*S. oed.*	F	−	NED[a]	450
1612	*S. oed.*	M	−	Cecum	330
3941	*S. oed.*	F	−	NED[a]	402
4022	*S. oed.*	M	+	Transverse; descending	483
4180	*S. oed.*	M	−	NED[a]	345

[a] NED, No evidence of disease.

in the cotton-top tamarin model in both susceptible and nonsusceptible animals to colorectal carcinoma.

V. LDH_k EVALUATION IN THE COTTON-TOP TAMARIN MODEL

During the research with LDH_k and CEA in the human population at RPCI, a collaborative research effort was begun with Dr. Neal Clapp, Director of the Marmoset Research Center at Oak Ridge, MARCOR, in Tennessee. The plan was to look at serum levels of LDH_k in the cotton-top tamarin, since this tamarin species is at high risk in 35% of adults for developing colon cancer[31,32] and this animal model would be a unique environment in which to test the efficacy of LDH_k. It was also decided to evaluate CEA and compare it to LDH_k as had been previously reported in this chapter in the human population. However, previous efforts to study CEA had not been fruitful in that CEA was not readily detectable in the tamarin colony.[33] Also, an attempt to look for CEA in tissue specimen blocks was previously unsuccessful with current technology.[34] In view of these technical difficulties with the isolation of CEA it was decided to focus attention on LDH_k analysis alone.

A blinded study was performed and between 1.5 and 2.0 ml of whole blood was drawn from each tamarin; 0.5 ml of serum was shipped frozen to RPCI for analysis of LDH_k. The serum of 11 animals was analyzed. The results of the LDH_k serum analysis is presented in Tables 2 and 3.

Immediately noticeable in Tables 2 and 3 is that the levels of serum LDH_k in the cotton-top tamarin animals with or without colon cancer are at least 100 times the levels seen in the human population. Table 2 lists eight animals along with their history, characteristics, and levels of LDH_k. All of the LDH_k values in Table 2 are greater than 200 units, whereas in Table 3 the animals

TABLE 3
LDH_k Evaluation in Cotton-Top Tamarins, and Other Species (LDH_k Values <200 Units)

Animal no.	Species	Sex	Colon cancer (+, −)	Colon sites	LDH_k (units)
3650	*S. oed.*	M	−	NED[a]	190
4709	*C. jacchus*	M	−	NED[a]	130
1501	*S. oed.*	M	+	Cecum; ascending; descending	90

[a] NED, No evidence of disease.

listed have LDH_k values less than 200 units. In Table 2, six of the eight animals had no evidence of tumor at the time the serum LDH_k was drawn (#1716, #4561, #4585,#3941, #4042, #4180). The two remaining animals (#1706, #1612) had documented colon cancer with serum LDH_k values of 340 units and 330, respectively. Interestingly, animal #4561 had a LDH_k serum level of 6560 units. However, this female animal had no evidence of tumor at autopsy. In this particular animal all LDH isozymes were extremely elevated (H_4, 910 units; M_1H_3, 2180 units; M_2H_2, 2540 units; M_3H_1, 1590 units; M_4, 19,200 units). Table 3 lists three animals whose LDH_k values were less than 200 units. Two animals (#3650, #4709) were from species that are not susceptible to developing spontaneous colon cancer. The third animal (#1501) was a male with documented cancers of the descending colon and cecum whose serum LDH_k value was 90 units.

All tamarins and marmosets that were tested had higher LDH_k values than humans. In addition, a species effect is suggested in that 8/9 cotton-top tamarins had LDH_k values very dramatically higher (up to $100\times$) than those found in humans. The values of noncancer-susceptible species (*Callithrix jacchus* and *Saguinus fuscicollis*) were lower than cotton-top values but were still 5 to 6 times the normal human values. Although the cotton-top tamarin values were generally much higher than in the species not susceptible to colon cancer, the differences between individual cotton-top values did not appear to be affected by either age, colitic state as determined at necropsy or by colonic biopsy, or the presence or absence of colon cancer.

In summary, all cotton-top tamarins (colon cancer-susceptible species) and two animals from noncolon cancer-susceptible species (*C. jacchus* and *S. fuscicollis*) had extremely high levels of LDH_k as compared with values found in the human population. Of 3/4 colon cancer-positive cotton-tops, LDH_k values were >200 units and 1 was <200. Seven animals (including all three species) had no evidence of colon cancer but only three had serum LDH_k values less than 200.

VI. DISCUSSION AND CONCLUSION

The cotton-top tamarin offers a unique animal model to analyze a tumor marker for colorectal carcinoma. Our results in the human population indicate that LDH_k is a useful marker for metastatic colorectal carcinoma, particularly when used with CEA. The extremely high levels of serum LDH_k in both tumor-bearing tamarins and species not susceptible to colon cancer cannot be explained at this time. In a small number of animals no relationship was seen between the disease status of the tamarin and the serum LDH_k level. In fact, in one female tamarin with no evidence of colon cancer at autopsy all LDH isozymes had extremely high levels as compared to the human population. Following new technology it would be imperative to test CEA in the same animal model. The fact that we have demonstrated CEA and LDH_k in the human model being associated with metastases and not correlated with each other emphasizes the need to evaluate CEA in the cotton-top tamarin. Because *S. oedipus* is the colon cancer-susceptible animal species, the testing of a tumor marker can provide a unique environment for serial monitoring of the marker and its correlation with the clinical status of the animal.

Current rapid development of the use of older, well-established techniques and of new tumor markers in the field of colorectal carcinoma will depend upon hybridoma technology and the production of monoclonal antibodies. Perhaps the cotton-top tamarin species can contribute to the future research development of tumor markers in the field of colorectal carcinoma.

REFERENCES

1. **Gold, P. and Freedman, S. O.,** Demonstration of tumor-specific antigens in human colonic carcinomata by immunologic tolerance and absorption techniques, *J. Exp. Med.*, 121, 439, 1985.
2. **Wilking, N., Petrelli, N. J., Herrera, L., Holyoke, E. D., and Mittleman, A.,** Abdominal exploration for suspected recurrent carcinoma of the colon and rectum based upon elevated carcinoembryonic antigen alone or in combination with other diagnostic methods, *Surg. Gynecol. Obstet.*, 162, 465, 1986.
3. **Martin, E. W., Copperman, M., King, G., Rinker, L., Carey, L. C., and Minton, J. P.,** A retrospective and prospective study of serial CEA determinations in the early detection of recurrent colon cancer, *Am. J. Surg.*, 137, 167, 1979.
4. **Staab, H. J., Anderer, F. A. et al.,** Prognostic value of preoperative serum CEA level compared to clinical staging. I. Colorectal carcinoma, *Br. J. Cancer,* 44, 652, 1981.
5. **Holyoke, E. D., Block, G. E., Jensen, E., Sizemore, G. W., Heath, H., Chu, T. M., Murphy, G. P., Mittelman, A., Ruddon, R. W., and Arnott, M. S.,** Biological markers in cancer diagnosis and treatment, *Curr. Probl. Cancer,* 6, 1, 1981.
6. **Hedin, A., Wahren, B., and Hammarstrom, S.,** Tumor localization of CEA containing human tumors in nude mice by means of monoclonal anti-CEA antibodies, *Br. J. Cancer,* 30, 547, 1982.

7. **Markert, C. L. and Moller, F.,** Multiple forms of enzymes: tissue, ontogenetic, and species patterns, *Proc. Natl. Acad. Sci. U.S.A.,* 45, 753, 1959.
8. **Kaplan, N. O. and Ciotti, M. M.,** Evolution and differentiation of dehydrogenases, *Ann. N.Y. Acad. Sci.,* 94, 701, 1961.
9. **Hatefi, T. and Stiggal, D. L.,** Metal containing flavoprotein dehydrogenases, in *The Enzymes,* Boyer, P. D., Ed., Academic Press, 1976, 263.
10. **Ghrir, R., Becam, A. M., and Lederer, E.,** Primary structure of flavocytochrome b_2 from baker's yeast: purification by reverse-phase high-pressure liquid chromatography and sequencing of fragment cyanogen bromide peptides, *Eur. J. Biochem.,* 139, 59, 1984.
11. **Anderson, G. R., Marotti, K. R., and Whitaker-Dowling, P.,** A candidate rate-specific gene product of the Kirsten murine sarcoma virus, *Virology,* 99, 31, 1979.
12. **Anderson, G. R., Kovacik, W. P., and Marotti, K. R.,** LDH_k, a uniquely regulated cryptic lactate dehydrogenase associated with transformation by Kirsten sarcoma virus, *J. Biol. Chem.,* 256, 10583, 1981.
13. **Anderson, G. R., Polonis, V. R., Petell, J. K., Saavedra, R. A., Manly, K. F., and Matovcik, L. J.,** *Isozymes,* Alan R. Liss, New York, 1983.
14. **Anderson, G. R. and Kovacik, W. P.,** LDH_k, an unusual oxygen-sensitive lactate dehydrogenase expressed in human cancer, *Proc. Natl. Acad. Sci. U.S.A.,* 78, 3209, 1981.
15. **Anderson, G. R., Polonis, V. R., Manly, K. F., Saavedra, R. A., Evans, M. J., and Petell, J. K.,** *Oncogenes,* Alan R. Liss, New York, 1982, 185.
16. **Wu, G. J., Lu, S. Y., Lowe, L. L., and Kinkade, J. M.,** Identification of lactate dehydrogenase-M polypeptide translated in vitro from human and mouse tumor cell poly(A)-containing messenger RNA, *Int. J. Biochem.,* 17, 355, 1985.
17. **Saavedra, R. A. and Anderson, G. R.,** A cancer associated lactate dehydrogenase is expressed in normal retina, *Science,* 291, 221, 1983.
18. **Saavedra, R. A., Cordoba, C., and Anderson, G. R.,** LDH_k in the retina of diverse vertebrate species: a possible link to the Warburg effect, *Exp. Eye Res.,* 41, 365, 1985.
19. **Morin, M. E. and Hance, A. J.,** LDH_k, the lactate dehydorgenase associated with transformation by the Kirsten sarcoma virus: a re-evaluation, *J. Biol. Chem.,* 258, 2864, 1983.
20. **Anderson, G. R. and Farkas, B. K.,** The major anoxic stress response protein p34 is a distinct lactate dehydrogenese, *Biochemistry,* 27, 2187, 1988.
21. **Perucho, M., Salas, J., and Salas, M. L.,** Identification of the mammalian DNA-binding protein P8 as glyceraldehyde-3-phosphate dehydrogenase, *Eur. J. Biochem.,* 81, 557, 1977.
22. **Perucho, M., Salas, J., and Salas, M. L.,** Study of the interaction of glyceraldehyde-3-phosphate dehydrogenase with DNA, *Biochim. Biophys. Acta,* 606, 181, 1980.
23. **Williams, K. R., Reddigari, S., and Patel, G. L.,** Idetntification of a nucleic acid helix-destabilizing protein from rat liver as lactate dehydrogenase-5, *Proc. Natl. Acad. Sci. U.S.A.,* 82, 5260, 1985.
24. **Patel, G. J. and Thompson, P. E.,** Immunoreactive helix-destabilizing protein localized in transcriptionally active regions of Drosophila polytene chromosomes, *Proc. Natl. Acad. Sci. U.S.A.,* 77, 6749, 1980.
25. **Lee, P. C., Bochner, B. R., and Ames, B. D.,** ApppppA, heat-shock stress, and cell oxidation, *Proc. Natl. Acad. Sci. U.S.A.,* 90, 7496, 1983.
26. **Bochner, B. R., Lee, P. C., Wilson, S. W., Cutler, C. W., and Ames, B. D.,** ApppppA and related adenylated nucleotides are synthesized as a consequence of oxidation stress, *Cell,* 37, 225, 1984.
27. **Petrelli, N. J., Mittelman, A., Brzykcy, J., Polonis, V. R., and Manly, K. F.,** Anaerobic shock protein/lactate dehydrogenase (ASP/LDH_k) as a marker for human carcinoma. A preliminary report, *Proc. Am. Soc. Clin. Oncol.,* 33, 9, 1983.

28. **Petrelli, N. J., Manly, K. F., Herrera, L., Mittelman, A., and Anderson, G.,** Anaerobic shock protein/lactate dehydrogenase (LDH_k): a tumor marker for colorectal carcioma, *Proc. Am. Assoc. Cancer Res.,* 25, 158, 1984.
29. **Polonis, V. R., Anderson, G. R., Brzykcy, J., Vladutiu, A. O., and Manly, K. F.,** An unusual oxygen-sensitive lactate dehydrogenase isozyme associated with Kirsten murine sarcoma virus in human serum, *Cancer Res.,* 44, 2236, 1984.
30. **Petrelli, N. J., Manly, K. F., Herrera, L., Anderson, G., and Mittelman, A.,** The relationship of anaerobic shock protein/lactate dehydrogenase (LDH_k) and carcinoembryonic antigen (CEA) to Dukes' classification for colorectal carcinoma, *Proc. Am. Assoc. Cancer Res.,* 26, 146, 1985.
31. **Clapp, N. K., Lushbaugh, C. C., Humason, G. L., Gangaware, B. L., and Henke, M. A.,** Natural history and pathology of colon cancer in *Saguinus oedipus oedipus, Digest. Dis. Sci.,* 30, 107S, 1985.
32. **Clapp, N. K., Lushbaugh, C. C., Humason, G. L., Gangaware, B. L., and Henke, M. A.,** The marmoset as a model of ulcerative colitis and colon cancer, in *Colorectal Cancer and its Precursors,* Ingalls, J. F. and Mastromarino, A., Eds., Alan R. Liss, New York, 1985, 247.
33. **Clapp, N. K.,** personal communication.
34. **Thomas, P.,** personal communication (to Dr. Clapp).

Chapter 19

COLONIC GLYCOPROTEIN HETEROGENEITY IN THE COTTON-TOP TAMARIN: GLYCOCONJUGATE MODIFICATIONS ASSOCIATED WITH THE NONHUMAN PRIMATE MODEL OF INFLAMMATORY BOWEL DISEASE AND COLONIC CANCER

C. Richard Boland and Daniel K. Podolsky

TABLE OF CONTENTS

0-8493-5363-7/93/$0.00 + $.50

I. INTRODUCTION

Colonic epithelium expresses a rich variety of glycoconjugates, including cell surface membrane-bound glycoproteins and glycolipids, and several secreted glycoproteins. Heterogeneity among glycoconjugates may be expressed in the core structures, or in the attached oligosaccharide chains, giving rise to a wide range of molecular diversity. A number of observations suggest that many glycoconjugates may be important mediators of cellular behavior and intercellular communication.

The most abundant secretory product of colonic epithelial cells is mucin, the principal glycoprotein substance in the mucus coat which protects all epithelial surfaces. Mucins are high-molecular-weight, carbohydrate-rich glycoproteins that express an extraordinary degree of microheterogeneity. Although very little is known about the primary structure of the apoprotein core of mucin, several studies have provided insight into their oligosaccharide side chains. Because of their complexity, many analytical techniques have been applied to mucins. This chapter reviews information obtained using histochemical and biochemical techniques to analyze mucin structure in the colon, which will provide perspective for an interpretation of data derived from studies in the cotton-top tamarin (CTT).

II. LECTIN HISTOCHEMISTRY

Lectins are carbohydrate-binding probes that can be utilized to identify and localize specific terminal carbohydrate sequences in tissue glycoconjugates. They may be readily conjugated to fluorescein isothiocyanate (FITC) for fluorescence microscopy. Lectin histochemistry was initially found to be valuable in the human colon for the identification of markers of differentiation and malignant transformation.[1-3] Through this technique it has been recognized that terminal galactose (Gal) residues are expressed in goblet cell glycoconjugates in the lower half of the epithelial crypt in the normal human colon. This terminal structure tends not to be expressed in the upper half of the colonic crypt, where *N*-acetylgalactosamine (GalNAc) residues predominate. Since colonic epithelial cells migrate from the lower to the upper portion of the colonic crypt during normal maturation, this suggests that the state of differentiation of the epithelial cell is one determinant of glycoconjugate expression.[1]

In man, the differential expression of glycoconjugates within the colonic crypt has been found to be more pronounced in the proximal than distal colon.[4] In the mouse, differentiation-dependent glycoconjugate expression has also been seen in the proximal but not distal colon. However the structure expressed in the lower half of the proximal mouse colon (in this instance, that bound by peanut agglutinin) is not found anywhere in the normal human colon.[5] Thus, terminal carbohydrate expression is also species dependent.

Comparisons have been made between specimens of normal and malignant human colon. Although a wide variety of terminal carbohydrate structures is expressed in normal goblet cell glycoconjugates (including Gal, GalNAc, *N*-acetylglucosamine, sialic acid, and fucose), the lectin peanut agglutinin (PNA) does not bind to tissue sections from normal human colon.[1] Binding by this lectin requires exposure of the disaccharide linkage Gal-β-1,3-GalNAc.[6] It is therefore of great interest to note that PNA binds to secreted glycoconjugates in most specimens of colonic adenocarcinoma.[1] Furthermore, PNA has been proven to bind to mucin-secreting human colon cancer cell lines when grown as xenografts in nude mice.[7] Thus, a change in glycoconjugate expression also occurs with the process of malignant transformation.

Adenomatous polyps are well-established examples of premalignant epithelium in the human colon. A series of neoplastic colonic polyps has been examined using FITC-PNA, and the percentage of glands labeled with this lectin correlated with the size and pathological grade of the polyp.[8] In order to quantitate the expression of PNA-binding glycoconjugates in the polyps, each lesion was given a score based upon the percentage of glands labeled. Among benign tubular adenomas, a median labeling score of 7% was obtained. The expression of PNA-binding glycoconjugates correlated both with size and histology. Among the polyps ≤7 mm in size (diameter of the fixed tissue specimen on the slide), a median labeling score of 2% was observed and nearly half showed zero labeling. Among the larger lesions (>7 mm), a median labeling score of 24% was found and all showed some degree of labeling. Similarly, 26% of glands were labeled among villoglandular adenomas, and 41% of glands were labeled in polyps containing carcinoma. Thus, the expression of the cancer-related carbohydrate sequence is observed in premalignant colonic lesions during the stepwise evolution of cancer.

Binding of lectins to glycoconjugates has also been examined in a series of rectal biopsies obtained from 18 patients with chronic ulcerative colitis.[9] All the patients had colitis for at least 8 years. None had dysplasia or carcinoma at the time of entry into the study. In the initial samples, 9 of the 18 showed marked reductions in the expression of terminal GalNAc residues (i.e., those bound by the lectins *Dolichos biflorus*, DBA, or soybean agglutinin, SBA). Eleven biopsies showed binding by PNA in the supranuclear cytoplasmic region of the epithelial cells. In one biopsy, all of the goblet cell mucin was labeled by PNA.

Annual colonoscopies were performed on the 18 patients over a 4-year period, with biopsies taken at 10-cm intervals from cecum to rectum at the time of each examination. During the follow-up period, six patients developed dysplasia; of these six patients, five were from the group of eleven that had exhibited PNA-binding glycoconjugates in their initial rectal biopsy. The single exception was a patient who developed high-grade dysplasia in the cecum. This patient underwent colectomy (because of the dysplasia), at which time no other evidence of carcinoma or dysplasia was found. A cancer was detected 2 years after entry into the study in the only patient whose rectal goblet cell mucin had been labeled initially by FITC-PNA. In addition, extensive labeling of intracellular glycoconjugates by FITC-PNA was present in those samples that demonstrated moderate or severe dysplasia. Thus, patients with ulcerative colitis expressing PNA-binding glycoconjugates in colonic mucosa appear to be at high risk for the subsequent development of neoplasia.

The expression of a cancer-associated glycoconjugate structure has also been demonstrated in CF-1 mice treated with the chemical carcinogen 1,2-dimethylhydrazine.[10] The CF-1 mouse has been a valuable experimental model for two reasons: the pathological features resemble those found in human disease, and alterations in mucin are similar to those in the human model. PNA-binding glycoconjugates are expressed in control animals, but only in the lower half of the colonic crypts of the proximal colon. After the administration of the carcinogen, colonic neoplasms develop in the distal, but not proximal, colon. In this model, PNA binds to glycoconjugates in both benign and malignant neoplastic lesions (i.e., adenomas and carcinomas). In addition, PNA-binding glycoconjugates emerge throughout the normal-appearing distal colon, although no changes are seen in the proximal colon of carcinogen-treated animals nor in controls. Thus, the carbohydrate structure (i.e., the Thomsen-Friedenreich antigen) which is preferentially expressed in neoplastic lesions of human colon is also found in premalignant epithelium in a nonhuman primate species. The latter findings are consistent with the concept that colonic epithelium undergoes substantial changes in cell kinetics[11] and glycoprotein synthesis[12,13] after exposure to carcinogen.

Small New World monkeys are especially valuable for the study of certain aspects of inflammatory bowel disease. While in captivity, some of these primates develop a disease that resembles chronic colitis in humans. Moreover, approximately 35% of the adults of one species, the cotton-top tamarin (CTT), spontaneously develop carcinoma of the colon in a manner similar to that seen in man. (The CTT is formally named *Saguinus oedipus,* which has been abbreviated S.O. in portions of the text and figures to correspond with previously published material.) Two closely related species of New World monkey, *Saguinus fuscicollis illigeri* (SF) or the white-lipped tamarin, and *Callithrix jacchus* (CJ) or the common marmoset, develop colitis while in captivity but do not develop colonic cancer.

In view of the apparent association of some cancer-associated glycoconjugates with an increased risk for development of dysplasia in humans with ulcerative colitis, colonic tissue was obtained from New World monkeys for an analogous study using FITC-PNA.[14] These samples came from four groups of ten animals each, as follows: S.O. with cancer, S.O. without cancer, CJ, and SF. A full-thickness specimen of non-neoplastic colon was obtained at necropsy and imbedded in paraffin. The samples were sectioned, rehydrated, and stained as previously described.[1,4,8,9] The specimens were first evaluated pathologically and scored for inflammatory infiltrate. Inflammation was cat-

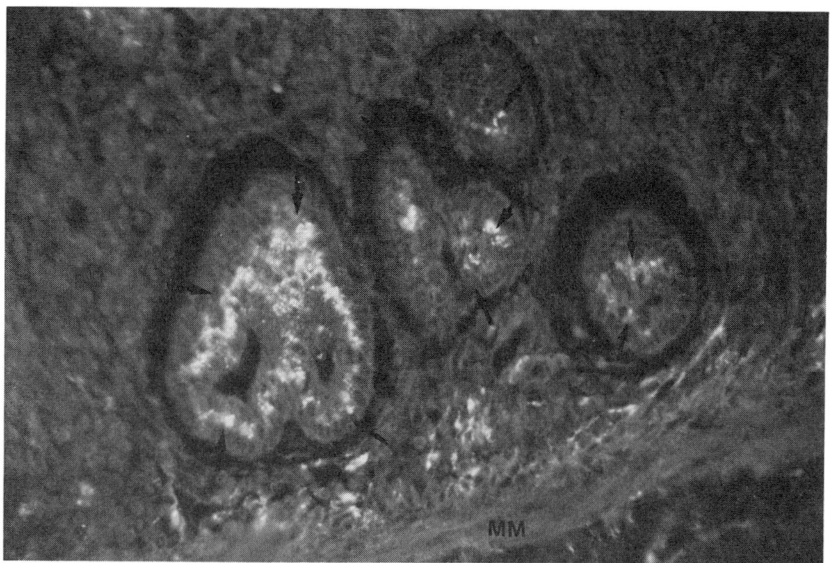

FIGURE 1. Photomicrograph of FITC-PNA labeled marmoset colon, demonstrating four glands (arrows) labeled by FITC-PNA. The lectin labels the supranuclear region of the colonic epithelial cells in the four glands, but there is neither diffuse cytoplasmic labeling nor labeling of secreted mucins in the section. This degree of labeling is similar to that seen in some human rectal biopsies of patients with chronic ulcerative colitis. This type of labeling was grade II; absent or barely perceptible labeling was called grade I, and extensive labeling of the epithelium scored grade III. MM, Muscularis mucosae. (Magnification × 500.)

egorized as chronic in 34, acute in 7, and subacute in 8.[14] The labeling of glycoconjugates in the colonic epithelium was categorized on the basis of our prior experience using the human colon.[9] Grade I labeling indicated trace or absent labeling in the specimen, as previously observed in normal human colons. Grade II indicated labeling of the supranuclear cytoplasm of the colonic epithelial cell, as illustrated in Figure 1. Goblet cell mucin or secreted mucus was not labeled. Grade II labeling resembles that found in rectal biopsies of humans with ulcerative colitis.[9] Grade III labeling indicated diffuse fluorescence throughout the cytoplasm of the epithelial cell or the labeling of secreted mucus. This last degree of labeling is similar to that observed in human colon cancers,[1] adenomatous polyps,[8] and dysplasia in the setting of ulcerative colitis.[9]

When all members of S.O. (CTT), the only species at risk for cancer, were compared with animals from CJ and SF (both develop colitis, but no cancer), there was a significant increase in grade III labeling ($p < .01$) and grades II or III labeling ($p < .01$), as indicated in Figure 2. Indeed, these findings were much more marked than that observed in man. Epithelial cell glycoconjugates in the normal human colon are minimally labeled by FITC-

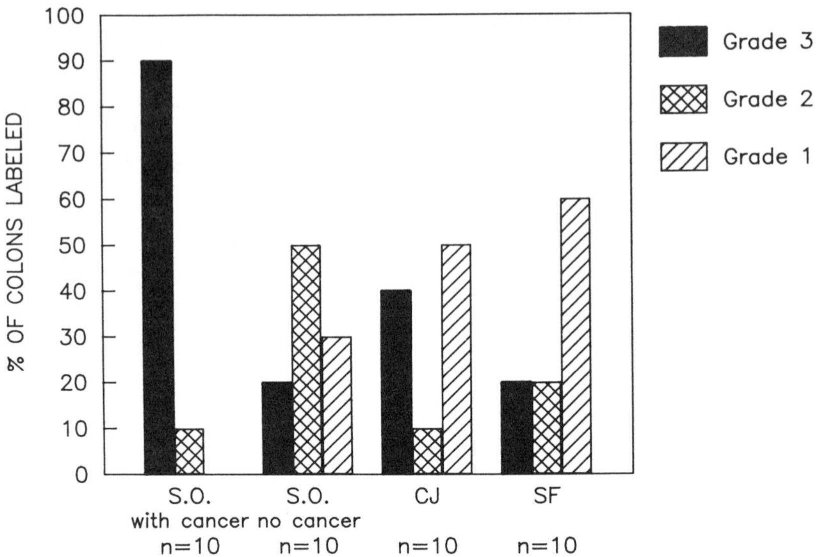

FIGURE 2. FITC-PNA labeling of marmoset and tamarin colons, by species. The grades of labeling of colonic tissues by FITC-PNA are expressed by species. S.O. with cancer = labeling in the non-neoplastic colonic epithelium of CTTs that also had colonic cancer. No animal in this group had grade 1 labeling. S.O. no cancer = labeling in colonic epithelium of CTTs that did not develop cancer. CJ, *Callithrix jacchus* (common marmoset); SF, *Saguinus fuscicollis illigeri* (white-lipped tamarin). CJ and SF all had colitis, but none had carcinoma.

PNA and increases in expression of PNA-binding glycoconjugates are relatively subtle in the rectal biopsies of patients with chronic ulcerative colitis. In contrast nearly two thirds of New World monkey colons demonstrated grade II or greater labeling and 43% of the group showed grade III labeling. Interestingly, 55% of the colons from CJ and SF showed grade I labeling, whereas 90% of the S.O. animals that developed cancer showed grade III labeling. Therefore, although PNA-binding glycoconjugates were broadly expressed in these colons, there was a significant correlation between the presence of PNA staining in non-neoplastic mucosa and the concurrent presence of cancer elsewhere in the colon. Together with the data accumulated previously, these findings suggest that the glycoconjugate structure bound by PNA is a marker of an increased risk for cancer in the colon. However, expression of this glycoconjugate marker in inflamed colonic epithelium of animals that do not develop cancer indicates that other factors may result in its production.

Seven of the 50 specimens of colon examined demonstrated acute (as well as chronic) inflammatory changes. Six of these samples were derived from animals with cancer. Of interest, all seven of the colonic specimens with acute inflammatory activity had grade III labeling with FITC-PNA, as demonstrated in Figure 3. There is currently no direct evidence to link acute

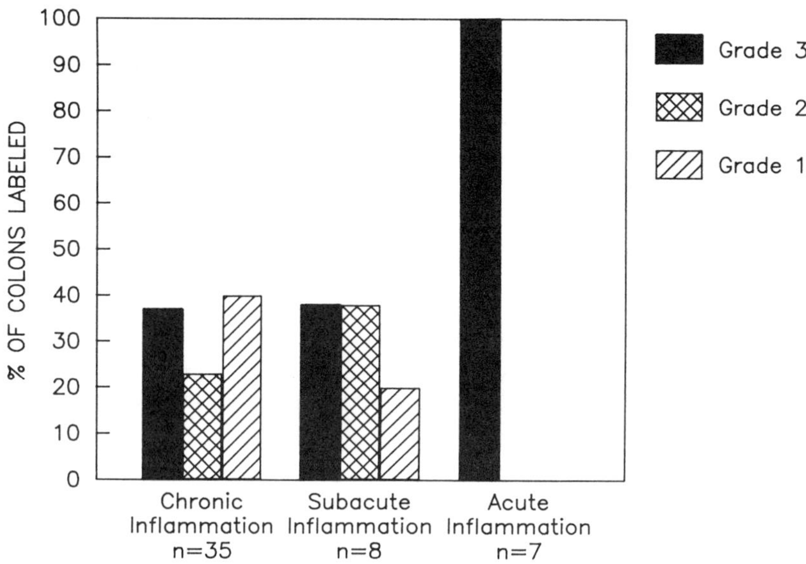

FIGURE 3. FITC-PNA labeling according to degrees of inflammation: the results of FITC-PNA labeling of tamarin and marmoset colons are expressed according to degrees of inflammation. None of the animals with acute inflammation had grades 1 or 2 labeling.

inflammation with the pathogenesis of cancer in this animal model. However, since all acutely inflamed epithelium demonstrated grade III labeling, and 6/8 of subacutely inflamed specimens showed grades II or III labeling, it is possible that inflammation may independently affect glycoconjugate synthesis in the primate colon.

III. BIOCHEMICAL ANALYSIS OF MUCINS FROM NONHUMAN PRIMATE COLONS

As indicated above, some important insights into the nature of glycoconjugates in human and tamarin colonic mucosa have been achieved through the use of fluoresceinated lectin probes and histochemical staining techniques. Studies using these techniques demonstrate the presence of regional variation in glycoconjugate determinants. Insights into the spectrum of glycoprotein structures present in normal human mucosa have also been obtained through direct compositional and structural analysis of isolated glycoproteins.[15-19] These studies have provided a reference for understanding alterations associated with disease states as well as a foundation for comparative studies in CTT and related primates.

While mucin glycoproteins are comprised of 40 to 85% carbohydrate by weight, the actual pattern of oligosaccharide substitution remains unknown. Despite these limitations, considerable information has been learned about the oligosaccharide structures. Slomiany and co-workers first defined structures of colonic mucin glycoprotein oligosaccharides using material isolated from the rat.[20] They identified and characterized eight structures ranging from two to eight carbohydrate residues in length. Composition was typical of O-glycosidically linked oligosaccharides with a preponderance of hexosamines, the uniform presence of galactosaminitol (indicative of the participation of galactosamine in the peptide-oligosaccharide linkage), and the absence of mannose. Several oligosaccharides possessed carbohydrate residues which would confer various blood group-related reactivities.

An even more extensive variety of oligosaccharides has been isolated from human colonic mucins.[21,22] Human colonic mucin appears to include at least 26 discrete oligosaccharides which range in size from 2 to 12 residues. Their compositional characteristics are similar to those found in the rat-derived oligosaccharides. Generally, they appear to represent fundamental linear or biantennary branched structures in varying degrees of completion. Many structures contain residues at nonreducing terminal and other positions of substitution which could confer reactivity with lectins and other probes.

As yet, the structures of oligosaccharide chains of CTT colonic mucin glycoproteins have not been directly defined. It may be reasonably supposed that they are closely similar to those found in man. This assumption is supported by the similarity in the lectin-staining patterns described above, the observation of analogous chromatographic behavior of intact CTT colonic glycoproteins, and the extensive cross-recognition of CTT goblet cells by monoclonal antibodies prepared against human colonic glycoproteins (see below). By the same criteria it must also be assumed that CTT colonic mucin glycoproteins are not identical to those present in man and other mammalian species. While extensive cross-reactivity has been observed, a number of anti-human colonic mucin glycoprotein monoclonal antibodies fail to recognize CTT glycoproteins.[23,24] Conversely, a number of monoclonal antibodies prepared against CTT colonic mucosa do not bind to colons of even closely related primate species.[31]

Ultimately, definition of the fine structure of the oligosaccharides present on CTT colonic glycoproteins may be useful in facilitating understanding of the transition from normal to malignant mucosa in this primate and its relevance to comparable processes in man. The potential value of this information is suggested by the accumulating evidence of the presence of aberrant oligosaccharide structures in human colonic carcinoma tissue, some of which are described above. While a variety of different structural alterations have been described, there is an emerging recognition that some oligosaccharides of colonic carcinoma cells are more extended than their normal counterparts and may acquire additional blood group-related specificities in association with these alterations.[14,25,26] It will certainly be important to determine whether comparable alterations develop in the colonic mucosa of the CTT and the relationship of their appearance to the duration of colitis.

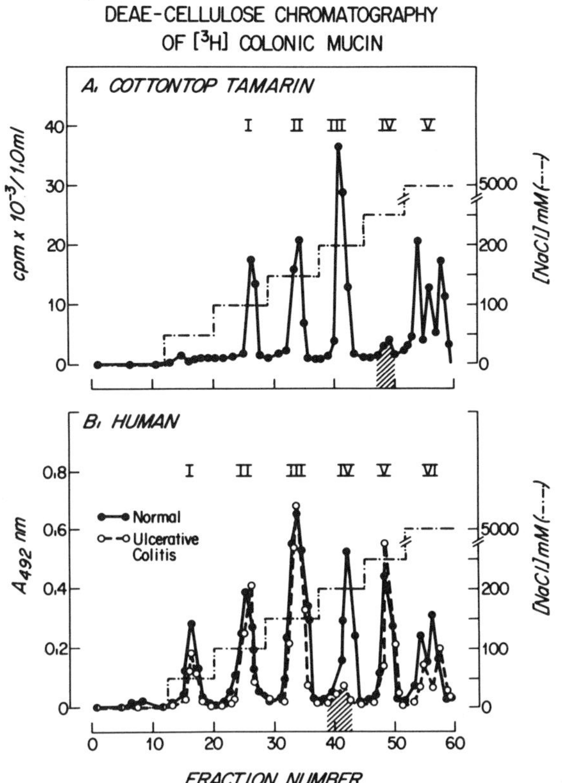

FIGURE 4. Separation of tamarin and human colonic mucin species on DEAE-cellulose. Glycoproteins in colonic mucosal biopsies were radiolabeled and separated from other components by Sepharose 4B chromatography. Mucin glycoproteins were then chromatographed on DEAE-cellulose as previously described.[28] (A) Cotton-top tamarin; (B) human from normal or ulcerative colitic colon. Shading emphasizes reduction in species IV in CTT and ulcerative colitis tissues.

Although the primary structure of the colonic mucin glycoprotein peptide backbones remain undetermined, it has been possible to define chromatographic heterogeneity of intact glycoproteins. Observations using material from a number of experimental animals suggest that colonic mucosa may contain different populations of mucin glycoproteins. Thus, it has been possible to further dissociate purified mucin glycoprotein from rabbit, rat, and sheep into discrete fractions by various chromatographic procedures.[15,17]

Analysis of colonic mucin glycoproteins isolated from normal human mucosa has also suggested the consistent presence of several "species" of glycoproteins.[27] Indeed, at least six distinct peaks of mucin glycoprotein (designated species I to VI) are recovered following chromatography of purified material on DEAE-cellulose (Figure 4B). None of the peptide cores of these individual populations has yet been isolated, precluding confirmation that these chromatographically defined components represent the products of a comparable number of discrete genes. Alternatively, these entities could represent variably modified products of a smaller number of genes. Nonetheless, a number of observations support the suggestion that a multiplicity of structurally distinct mucin glycoproteins exist in colonic mucosa and may well reflect the ultimate result of separate mucin peptide-encoding genes.

Each of the chromatographically defined species exhibits a unique carbohydrate and amino acid composition. It should also be noted that each of the mucin species has been found to contain a distinctive spectrum of oligosaccharide side chains and, in most instances, perhaps unique oligosaccharides. However, the latter findings probably do not represent the fundamental basis for the separation of these populations and could result from differences in the relative efficiency of the formation of the various structures on the different mucin glycoproteins. The latter conclusion follows from the recognition that the various oligosaccharides probably reflect the products of similar or identical combinations of glycosyltransferases.

The presence of structurally distinct populations of mucin glycoproteins has been further supported through the use of monoclonal antibodies prepared against mucin glycoprotein.[23] While binding assays demonstrated the presence of shared structural determinants common to all of the separated mucin glycoprotein species, some monoclonal antibodies were found to bind to individual mucin glycoprotein fractions or various subsets of the six species. These latter observations suggest that the chromatographically defined populations possess distinctive structural features. Furthermore, these anti-mucin monoclonal antibodies have made it possible to define the distribution of mucin species I to VI within human colonic mucosa using indirect immunofluorescence.[24] These latter studies have indicated that mucin glycoprotein species may be relatively segregated within different subpopulations of goblet cells. While individual goblet cells invariably contain more than one type of mucin species, certain glycoproteins exist in mutually exclusive populations of goblet cells. Thus, the spectrum of mucin glycoproteins may reflect the products of goblet cell heterogeneity. While these observations raise the possibility for differential response to a range of specific stimuli, the factors regulating mucin synthesis and secretion in the colon remain unknown.

Although the role of each glycoprotein species remains obscure, a selective deficiency of one species (IV) has been found in specific association with ulcerative colitis in man.[27,28] Reduction in the content of mucin species IV has been observed in mucosa of patients with ulcerative colitis, both in association with the inflammatory process itself, as well as independently. Similar reduction in species IV has been observed in the proximal colon of patients with disease confined to the left colon. In addition, the reduction of species IV in areas of disease involvement persists even after resolution of the acute inflammatory process. These findings indicate that the observed reduction in this glycoprotein constituent may be related to the disease process primarily rather than reflect a nonspecific response to inflammation. This impression is supported by the failure to observe comparable alterations in other inflammatory conditions, including Crohn's colitis, radiation injury, ischemic colitis, or a variety of infectious disorders of the large intestine. However, insofar as assessment of colonic glycoprotein heterogeneity has only been determined after the onset of the clinical disorder, the existence of the reduction of mucin species IV preceding the development of ulcerative colitis in man has not been demonstrated.

Similar approaches to the examination of colonic glycoprotein heterogeneity have been used to evaluate the CTT.[29] Studies have been limited due to the small quantities of colonic tissue which may be obtained from these diminutive primates. Therefore, it has not been possible to undertake detailed compositional and structural characterization of the CTT-derived material. Despite these limitations, it has been possible to assess heterogeneity by radiolabeling the nonreducing termini of oligosaccharide side chains which permits analysis of minute quantities of material solubilized from mucosal biopsies.[28]

The results of the latter studies indicate the presence of multiple mucin glycoproteins in the CTT colon which are partly analogous to those found earlier in the human colon (Figure 4). However, some consistent differences were observed. Although six distinct peaks are recovered from human mucosa, only five were found when CTT colonic glycoproteins were studied. Moreover, the first peak of CTT glycoprotein is not recovered until a salt concentration equivalent to that sufficient to elute the second human species is achieved. The chromatographic profiles suggest that CTT colonic mucin glycoproteins differ from their human counterparts in a consistent fashion. However, the existence of a systematic structural modification or feature leading to consistent displacement of all six tamarin mucin species in their chromatographic elution profile remains unproven in the absence of specific compositional and structural analysis of the CTT material.

Mucin from CTT had a very small amount of the mucin fraction designated primate species IV in a manner similar to that observed in patients with ulcerative colitis. It should be noted that primate mucin IV actually corresponds in its elution properties to human mucin V and not human mucin IV, and their structural similarity remains presumptive. Nonetheless, it is notable that CTT mucin species IV encompasses less than 6% of total colonic mucin glycoprotein content.

Interpretation of the relationship of low levels of the primate mucin species IV and the coexistent chronic colitis is clouded by the high prevalence of colitis in this population. The presence of substantial amounts of mucin eluting at the same position as CTT mucin IV in colonic glycoproteins solubilized from other New World and Old World primates indicates that the observed paucity of this constituent in the CTT is not simply a feature distinguishing

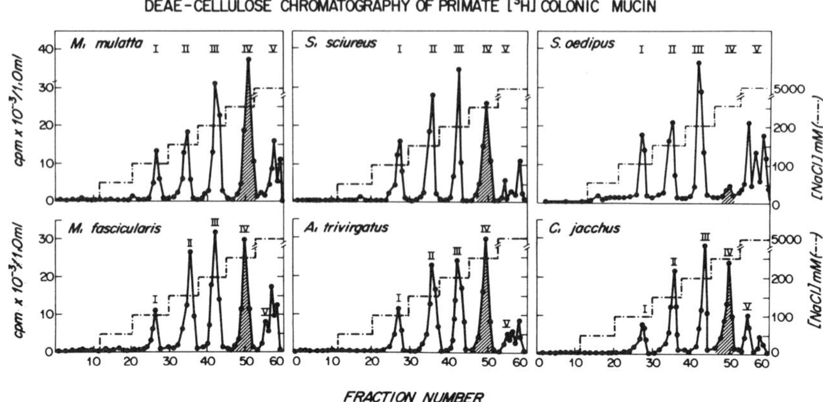

FIGURE 5. Colonic mucin heterogeneity in various primates: shading emphasizes relative differences in nonhuman primate mucin species IV.

lower primates from man (Figure 5). It is interesting to note that the common marmoset (*Callithrix jacchus*), a tamarin closely related to the CTT which experiences a mild chronic colitis without any apparent predisposition to carcinoma, was observed to have an intermediate concentration of the primate species IV. Furthermore, the recovery of primate mucin species IV from the CTT could not be related to the activity of the colitis per se, but remained constant despite histological resolution of acute activity in response to treatment with sulfasalazine.[30] The persistence of the apparent deficit of primate mucin species mirrors a comparable analysis in man.

In addition to the uniformly low content of the primate species IV, CTT colonic mucosa is remarkable for increased content of primate species III. However, in contrast to the low recovery of species IV, the enhanced representation of species III is present only in association with acute inflammatory activity and recedes with resolution of the acute colitis. It appears that this alteration may be directly related to mucosal injury rather than being an inherent feature of CTT mucosa associated with the potential for chronic colitis.

The basis of the observed apparent deficit of primate mucin species IV remains unknown and its relationship to the predisposition to colitis and colon cancer in the CTT is unclear. This primate offers the opportunity to evaluate the extent of species IV reduction or depletion prior to the onset of colitis. Limitations of methodology have precluded analysis in the live infant CTT in the past but should be feasible in the future. While it is not yet known whether the failure to observe a significant primate species IV peak in the CTT is the result of a biosynthetic deficit reflecting an underlying genetic disorder, or an aberration of degradation, it may be possible to gain insight into these processes through organ culture or establishment of cell lines from CTT colonic mucosa.

Ultimately it will be important to define the similarity of the colon mucin glycoproteins of the CTT to those of man. As suggested above, preliminary studies using monoclonal antibodies prepared against human colonic glycoproteins show extensive cross-reactivity with CTT. Fourteen of 17 anti-human colonic mucin antibodies efficiently stained CTT colonic mucosa using indirect immunofluorescent techniques.[24] The availability of these reagents with defined specificity toward separate human colonic mucin glycoprotein species permits clarification of the relatedness of the primate species to their human counterparts. Despite the many limitations in our current knowledge, available information indicates that the CTT possesses a complex but distinct array of colonic glycoproteins which has an important relationship to its development of a chronic colitis with predisposition to cancer. Conversely, the results of studies using both lectin probes and biochemical characterization provide further credence to the notion of the relevance of the CTT disorder to human disease.

IV. SUMMARY

In summary, colonic epithelial glycoconjugates are highly heterogeneous, and a variety of techniques have been utilized to understand their structural complexities. Lectin histochemistry can be used to identify and localize terminal glycosylation patterns on fixed specimens of tissue. A cancer-associated structure has been identified in the human colon by its ability to bind the lectin PNA. Studies of the CTT and related New World monkeys indicate a high degree of correlation between PNA-binding glycoconjugates in non-neoplastic tissue and the presence of carcinoma, suggesting a diffuse mucosal abnormality in those colons that develop cancer. In addition, it was found that acutely inflamed colons show a marked degree of labeling with PNA. The relationship between acute inflammation and carcinogenesis in this model has not been studied, but it appears that factors other than neoplasia can produce modification in glycoconjugate structures.

Studies using ion-exchange chromatography have permitted a more precise molecular definition of the mucin glycoproteins. A selective deficiency of mucin species IV has been found in human colons with ulcerative colitis which appears to be independent of acute inflammatory activity. The recent production of monoclonal antibodies against the mucin species by ion-exchange chromatography and the identification of the carbohydrate epitopes to which these antibodies are directed will make it possible to study the factors that regulate the expression of different mucin species in normal and diseased colons. Selective deficiency of an analogous colonic mucin species has been observed in the CTT and, to a lesser extent, in *C. jacchus*.

Further study of colonic mucin heterogeneity may provide insight into the unique susceptibility of these primates to chronic colitis and cancer, and the role of selective glycoprotein alterations in the pathophysiology of these diseases.

REFERENCES

1. **Boland, C. R., Montgomery, C. K., and Kim, Y. S.,** Alterations in colonic mucin structure in differentiation and malignant transformation, *Proc. Natl. Acad. Sci. U.S.A.,* 79, 2051, 1982.
2. **Boland, C. R. and Kim, Y. S.,** Lectin markers of differentiation and malignancy, in *Progress in Cancer Research and Therapy,* Vol. 29, Wohlman, S. and Mastromarino, A. J., Eds., Raven Press, New York, 1984, 1987.
3. **Boland, C. R.,** Mucin histochemistry in colonic polyps and cancer, *Semin. Surg. Oncol.,* 3, 183, 1987.
4. **Bresalier, R. S., Boland, C. R., and Kim, Y. S.,** Regional differences in normal and cancer-associated glycoconjugates of the human colon, *J. Natl. Cancer Inst.,* 75, 249, 1985.
5. **Boland, C. R. and Ahnen, D. J.,** The binding of lectins to goblet cell mucin in premalignant colonic epithelium of the CF-1 mouse, *Gastroenterology,* 89, 127, 1985.
6. **Lotan, R., Skutelsky, E., Danon, D., and Sharon, N.,** The purification, composition and specificity of the anti-T lectin from peanut (Arachis hypogaea), *J. Biol. Chem.,* 254, 8518, 1975.
7. **Boland, C. R., Roberts, J. A., Siddiqui, B., Byrd, J., and Kim, Y. S.,** Cancer-associated colonic mucin in cultured human tumor cells and athymic (nude) mouse xenografts, *Cancer Res.,* 46, 5724, 1986.
8. **Boland, C. R., Montgomery, C. K., and Kim, Y. S.,** Cancer-associated mucin alterations in benign colonic polyps, *Gastroenterology,* 82, 664, 1982.
9. **Boland, C. R., Lance, P., Levin, B., Riddell, R. H., and Kim, Y. S.,** Abnormal goblet cell glycoconjugates in rectal biopsies associated with an increased risk of neoplasia in patients with ulcerative colitis: early results of a prospective study, *Gut,* 25, 1364, 1984.
10. **Boland, C. R. and Ahnen, D. J.,** Binding of lectins to goblet cell mucin in malignant and premalignant colonic epithelium in the CF-1 mouse, *Gastroenterology,* 89, 127, 1985.
11. **Wargovich, M. J., Medline, A., and Bruce, W. R.,** Early histopathologic events to evolution of colon cancer in C57BL/6 and CFI mice treated with 1,2-dimethylhydrazine, *J. Natl. Cancer Inst.,* 71, 125, 1983.
12. **Filipe, M. I.,** Mucous secretions in rat colonic mucosa during carcinogenesis induced by dimethylhydrazine. A morphological and histochemical study, *Br. J. Cancer,* 32, 60, 1975.
13. **Decaens, C., Bara, J., Rosan, B., Daher, N., and Burtin, P.,** Early oncofetal antigenic modifications during rat colonic carcinogenesis, *Cancer Res.,* 43, 355, 1983.
14. **Boland, C. R. and Clapp, N.,** Glycoconjugates in the colons of New World monkeys with spontaneous colitis, *Gastroenterology,* 92, 625, 1987.
15. **Neutra, M. R. and Forstner, J. F.,** Gastrointestinal mucus: synthesis, secretion, and function, in *Physiology of the Gastrointestinal Tract,* Johnson, L. R., Ed., Raven Press, New York, 1987, chap. 34.
16. **Allen, A., Bell, A., Mantle, M., and Pearson, J. P.,** The structure and physiology of gastrointestinal mucus, *Adv. Exp. Med. Biol.,* 144, 115, 1982.
17. **Marshall, T. and Allen, A.,** Isolation and characterization of the high-molecular weight glycoprotein from pig colonic mucus, *Biochemistry,* 173, 569, 1978.
18. **Gold, D. V., Shochat, D., and Miller, E.,** Protease digestion of colonic mucin, *J. Biol. Chem.,* 255, 6354, 1981.
19. **Murty, V. L. N., Downs, F. J., and Pigman, W.,** Rat colonic mucus glycoprotein, *Carbohydr. Res.,* 61, 139, 1978.
20. **Slomiany, B. L., Murty, V. L. N., and Slomiany, A.,** Isolation and characterization of oligosaccharides from rat colonic mucus glycoprotein, *J. Biol. Chem.,* 255, 9719, 1980.

21. **Podolsky, D. K.,** Oligosaccharide structures of human colonic mucin, *J. Biol. Chem.,* 260, 8262, 1985.
22. **Podolsky, D. K.,** Oligosaccharide structures of isolated human colonic mucin, *J. Biol. Chem.,* 260, 15510, 1985.
23. **Podolsky, D. K., Fournier, D. A., and Lynch, K. E.,** Development of anti-human colonic mucin monoclonal antibodies: characterization of multiple colonic mucin species, *J. Clin. Invest.,* 77, 1251, 1986.
24. **Podolsky, D. K., Fournier, D. A., and Lynch, K. E.,** Human colonic goblet cell. Demonstration of distinct subpopulations defined by mucin specific monoclonal antibodies, *J. Clin. Invest.,* 77, 1263, 1986.
25. **Itzkowitz, S. H., Yuan, M., Ferrell, L. D., Palekar, A., and Kim, Y. S.,** Cancer-associated alterations of blood group antigen expression in human colorectal polyps, *Cancer Res.,* 46, 5976, 1986.
26. **Feizi, T. and Childs, R. A.,** Carbohydrates as antigenic determinants of glycoproteins, *Biochem. J.,* 245, 1, 1987.
27. **Podolsky, D. K. and Isselbacher, K. J.,** Composition of human colonic mucin. Alterations in inflammatory bowel disease, *J. Clin. Invest.,* 72, 142, 1983.
28. **Podolsky, D. K. and Isselbacher, K. J.,** Glycoprotein composition of colonic mucosa: specific alterations in ulcerative colitis, *Gastroenterology,* 87, 991, 1984.
29. **Podolsky, D. K., Madara, J. L., King, N., Sehgal, P., Moore, R., and Winter, H. S.,** Colonic mucin composition in primates: selective alterations associated with spontaneous colitis in cotton-top tamarins, *Gastroenterology,* 88, 20, 1985.
30. **Madara, J., Podolsky, D. K., King, N. W., Sehgal, P. K., Moore, R., and Winter, H. B.,** Characterization of spontaneous colitis in cotton top tamarins (Saguinus oedipus) and its response to sulfasalazine, *Gastroenterology,* 88, 13, 1985.
31. **Podolsky, D. K.,** unpublished observations.

Chapter 20

POLYAMINE METABOLISM IN COLONIC DISEASES

Gordon D. Luk

TABLE OF CONTENTS

0-8493-5363-7/93/$0.00 + $.50

I. INTRODUCTION

The naturally occurring polyamines (putrescine, spermidine, and spermine) and the first and often rate-limiting enzyme regulating their synthesis, ornithine decarboxylase (ODC), are important for cell and tissue growth, particularly in small intestinal and colonic mucosa. Mucosal ODC and polyamines are also increased during chemical colonic carcinogenesis in rodents. Difluoromethylornithine (DFMO), a specific inhibitor of ODC, suppresses the increases in mucosal ODC and polyamines and blocks normal mucosal growth and carcinogenesis. The growth of human colon cancer cells is also inhibited by DFMO. This growth inhibition of colon cancer cells is enhanced by 5-fluorouracil and *cis*-platinum in some *in vitro* models. DFMO also suppresses the growth of human colon cancer xenografts in nude mice. Increased ODC levels appear to be markers for colorectal polyps and cancers, and possibly also for the hereditary risk of developing adenomatous polyposis coli. Preliminary evidence shows that ODC and the polyamines are increased in dysplastic lesions in colitis, in humans and in the cotton-top tamarin. In conclusion, the available evidence suggests that ODC and the polyamines are important for the growth of normal and neoplastic colon mucosal cells, may serve as markers for colorectal polyps and cancer, and may be potential targets for chemotherapy of colorectal cancer. Studies of ODC and polyamines in the cotton-top tamarin model may help clarify their potential role in colitis, dysplasia, and colon cancer.

II. ORNITHINE DECARBOXYLASE AND POLYAMINE METABOLISM

The amino acid ornithine is unique in that it is not used to synthesize protein, not represented by any triplet codon in the genetic code, and is not recognized by any specific tRNA. However, ornithine does participate in three metabolic pathways. It can enter the Krebs cycle through the action of ornithine transaminase. Ornithine also participates in the urea cycle, being converted by ornithine transcarbamylase to citrulline, which is then converted in sequence to arginosuccinate, arginine, and urea. The third metabolic pathway for ornithine, and the subject of this chapter, is polyamine biosynthesis.[1,2]

Ornithine is the precursor for the biosynthesis of the three naturally occurring polyamines, putrescine, spermidine, and spermine. It is decarboxylated by ornithine decarboxylase (ODC) to form putrescine, and this reaction appears to be the first and often rate-limiting step in polyamine biosynthesis. The second critical enzyme is *S*-adenosylmethionine decarboxylase (SAM-DC), which catalyzes the decarboxylation of *S*-adenosylmethionine to decarboxylated *S*-adenosylmethionine, which provides the aminopropyl groups for the subsequent biosynthesis of spermidine and spermine via spermidine and spermine synthase, respectively.[1-5]

The structures of the polyamines are as follows:

Putrescine	$NH_2(CH_2)_4NH_2$
Spermidine	$NH_2(CH_2)_4NH(CH_2)_3NH_2$
Spermine	$NH_2(CH_2)_3NH(CH_2)_4NH(CH_2)_3NH_2$

The polyamines are ubiquitous, low-molecular-weight, polycationic compounds found in all nucleated prokaryotic and eukaryotic cells studied. They form noncovalent complexes with many organic molecules, including nucleic acids, and have been shown, *in vitro,* to facilitate nearly all aspects of DNA, RNA, and protein synthesis. They are also known growth factors for many prokaryotic and eukaryotic cells.[4,5] The basal activity of ODC is low in quiescent tissues. However, marked increases in enzyme activity and rapid accumulation of tissue polyamines are characteristically associated with rapid cell and tissue growth, including embryonic growth, tumor growth, and increased secretory activity of endocrine glands. This increase in ODC activity is one of the earliest events that occur during the transition of cells from quiescence to active proliferation.[4,5]

ODC has one of the shortest half-lives known for a mammalian enzyme, ranging from 7 to 15 minutes from different studies. In the rat hepatectomy model, increased ODC activity and increased RNA synthesis occur almost simultaneously. The early increase in ODC activity in the initial phases of cell proliferation may be a trigger mechanism for critical processes in cell proliferation and protein synthesis.[1,4,5]

Studies using blockade of polyamine synthesis have provided important information about the potential role of polyamine metabolism. Particularly important in this regard is the specific enzyme-activated, irreversible ODC inhibitor, difluoromethyl ornithine (DFMO, MDL 71,782), synthesized at the Merrell-Dow Research Institute.[6,7] DFMO administration leads to the sustained depletion of polyamines and has helped document the critical role of polyamine metabolism in many biologic processes.[8,9] DFMO's only documented pharmacologic activity appears to be the selective inhibition of ODC, and it is virtually nontoxic in normal mice and rats at doses sufficient for *in vivo* inhibition of tissue ODC activity.[8,9]

In vitro, DFMO suppresses the early increase in ODC activity during the onset of proliferation of several cell types.[8] This inhibition of ODC retards the growth of many cell types in culture, including rat hepatoma cells,[8] mouse mammary EMT6 sarcoma cells,[10] mouse L1210 leukemia cells,[8] human leukemia cells,[11] and human small cell lung carcinoma cells.[12,13] *In vivo,* DFMO suppresses increases in tissue ODC activity and results in growth inhibition of many organ systems.[14-16] DFMO suppresses the increases in uterine ODC activity associated with early embryogenesis and arrests embryonic development.[17] DFMO also inhibits the growth of tumor cells in rodent models.[16,18-21] These results suggest that increases in ODC activity and polyamine biosynthesis are essential in mammalian growth processes.

III. ORNITHINE DECARBOXYLASE AND INTESTINAL AND COLONIC MUCOSAL GROWTH

Increases in ODC activity and polyamine content in the intestinal mucosa are associated with cell growth and hyperplasia. In the rat intestinal tract, increased ODC activity and polyamine content occur during maturation in neonatal small intestine,[16] mucosal regeneration after cytotoxic injury,[16] intestinal adaptation post-jejunectomy,[22] and intestinal adaptation during lactation.[23] Upon treatment with the specific ODC inhibitor, DFMO, intestinal mucosal growth in all these models is suppressed.[16,23,24] In addition, we demonstrated that this intestinal growth inhibition is due to a suppression of crypt cell DNA synthesis and proliferation.[24] Similar results have subsequently been found using a pancreatico-biliary diversion model of intestinal adaptation.[25]

During adaptive hyperplastic growth of the small intestine in response to jejunectomy and to starvation-refeeding, there is an associated increase, although to a lesser degree, in colonic mucosal growth. This increase in colonic mucosal growth is also associated with increases in ODC and polyamines. With DFMO administration, ODC activity and polyamine content are suppressed, and colonic mucosal cell growth is abrogated.[24]

IV. ORNITHINE DECARBOXYLASE AND CHEMICAL COLONIC CARCINOGENESIS

Induction of ODC has been associated with carcinogenesis in animal models.[26] Studies in the mouse skin tumor promotion model have shown a strong relationship between induction of ODC activity and the tumor-promoting ability of a variety of substances.[26] Tumor promoters also induce ODC activity in other carcinogenesis models in their respective target tissues.[26] ODC is induced during chemical colonic carcinogenesis in the rodent model.[27-29] Early carcinogenesis studies found increased ODC levels in the rat colon before the appearance of tumors.[27] We have subsequently found, in the rat colon carcinogenesis model, distinct and prolonged increases in ODC activity occurring within 4 hours of a single injection of the carcinogen azoxymethane, and persisting for at least 14 days. With serial weekly injections, there were persistent and prolonged increases in ODC. With the administration of ten serial weekly injections of carcinogen, the increase in ODC activity was distinctly biphasic, higher at week 2 and again during weeks 11 through 13, and occurring before the appearance of colonic tumors.[29] A progressive increase in ODC activity in the course of colonic tumor evolution was also noted. ODC activity was higher in normal appearing colonic mucosa from carcinogen-treated rats compared to normal colonic mucosa in untreated rats, but was highest in the colonic tumors.[29]

These increases in colonic mucosal ODC activity were shown to be critical for colonic carcinogenesis. DFMO reduced the incidence of dimethylhydrazine-induced colonic tumors in mice.[30] DFMO also reduced the increases in colonic mucosal ODC activities and suppressed the induction of colonic tumors by azoxymethane in rats.[28,31,32] These data suggest that DFMO, or other polyamine biosynthesis inhibitors, may have potential in the chemoprevention of colorectal cancer.

V. ORNITHINE DECARBOXYLASE AND HUMAN COLON CANCER CELL GROWTH

The proliferation of human colonic carcinoma cells in culture, similar to other *in vitro* cell culture systems, is associated with increases in ODC activity and polyamine content.[33,34] In several human colon cancer cells, we found marked transient increases in ODC activity and polyamines during their rapid logarithmic growth phase. When DFMO was added to the culture medium at a concentration that is achievable in human serum in clinical trials, ODC activity was suppressed and cell growth and plating efficiency were inhibited.[33,34]

DFMO also enhanced the human colon cancer cell growth-inhibitory effects of other antineoplastic agents, including 5-fluorouracil[35] and flavone acetic acid.[34] Since human colon cancer is poorly responsive to currently available chemotherapy, DFMO alone or in combination might be a potentially useful regimen. Furthermore, DFMO works by a different mechanism of action than currently available chemotherapeutic agents, and has nonoverlapping toxicities with most agents.[36] These preliminary data in culture systems are undergoing further clinical investigation.

VI. POLYAMINES AND HUMAN COLON CANCER XENOGRAFTS

Using an established nude mouse xenograft model,[16,20,21] we tested the *in vivo* therapeutic efficacy of DFMO against human colon cancer cells. The administration of DFMO prior to tumor inoculation completely prevented the development of colonic tumors. When DFMO was given after the tumor xenografts had become palpable (3 to 5 mm diameter nodules), the growth of the tumor implants was inhibited beginning approximately 4 weeks after continuous DFMO administration.[37] Using a cyclic regimen of DFMO administration that was previously shown to have decreased host toxicities, we were able to show persistent antitumor effects of DFMO.[37] These results helped in the implementation of phase I and phase II clinical trials of DFMO.[36,38] Although the efficacy of DFMO has not been established for colon cancer, the results suggest that the efficacy of DFMO might be tested in chemoprevention or consolidation studies.

VII. POLYAMINES AS MARKERS OF COLON NEOPLASIA

The hyperproliferative state of colorectal polyps and cancers, normal-appearing colonic mucosa adjacent to colonic tumors, and normal-appearing colonic mucosa in the hereditary polyposis syndromes has been well established.[39] The association of increased ODC activity with increased colonic mucosal growth and with chemical colonic carcinogenesis suggests that ODC activity may be useful as a biological marker for colorectal neoplasia.

We first tested ODC as a marker for colon neoplasia in adenomatous polyposis coli (familial polyposis), the autosomal dominant hereditary disorder in which virtually all of the affected subjects develop multiple adenomatous polyps and eventually colon cancers. ODC activity in macroscopically normal-appearing areas of colonic mucosa from patients affected with familial polyposis was 3- to 4-fold higher than ODC levels in normal colonic mucosa from unaffected controls.[40] In patients affected with adenomatous polyposis coli, mucosal ODC activity progressively increased, from normal-appearing flat mucosa to polyps, and to polyps with severe dysplasia. In addition, ODC activity was highest in colonic carcinomas.[28] This suggested that increased colonic mucosal ODC activity may reflect the abnormal proliferative status of the mucosa associated with polyposis and colonic neoplasia.[40] In colonic mucosa from clinically unaffected, first-degree relatives of patients with adenomatous polyposis coli (who have a 50% theoretical risk of inheriting the polyposis genotype), there was a bimodal distribution of ODC activity, with one peak at the mean of normal controls, and the other at the mean for normal-appearing flat mucosa from affected patients. These results suggest that increased ODC activity may identify clinically normal family members who carry the genotype.[40] The potential usefulness of ODC as a marker for the genotype for polyposis syndromes await further follow-up studies.

In addition to serving as a marker for adenomatous polyposis coli, mucosal ODC activity may be helpful in nonhereditary colon neoplasia. ODC activity increased progressively from normal-appearing mucosa to adenoma to adenocarcinoma.[28] The polyamines themselves were also found to be elevated in colon cancers. Spermidine was threefold higher and spermine fourfold higher in colon cancers than in adjacent, apparently uninvolved, resection margins. There was no correlation of polyamine levels with histologic grade, tumor size, Dukes stage, or presence of palpable metastases.[41] In another study, ODC activity and polyamine content were increased in colon polyps and cancers compared to normal colonic mucosa.[42] Other investigators have also found that ODC (and SAM-DC) activities were progressively increased from normal colonic mucosa to polyps and to adenocarcinomas.[43]

We have found that rectal mucosal ODC may serve as a marker for the existence of more proximal colonic neoplasia. ODC activity in normal-appearing flat rectal mucosa was markedly higher in patients with adenomatous

TABLE 1
Rectal Mucosal ODC Activity in Patients with Distant Colonic Neoplasia

	ODC (pmol/mg/h)	
	Men	Women
No neoplasia	117 ± 47[a]	125 ± 46[b]
Distant adenoma	182 ± 63[c]	212 ± 58[d]
Distant carcinoma	345 ± 149[e]	427 ± 171[f]

[a] n = 29
[b] n = 23
[c] n = 18
[d] n = 13
[e] n = 4
[f] n = 3

polyps, and even higher in patients with colon cancer, when compared to patients who have no colonic neoplasia. In these patients with nonhereditary colon cancer, ODC activity was higher in women than in men. High ODC activity was positively correlated with coexistence of colonic neoplasia at some distance away from the rectal mucosal biopsy (Table 1).

These results suggest that a diffuse hyperproliferative colonic mucosa exists in patients with colonic neoplasia. The findings are compatible with previous results showing hyperproliferation of rectal mucosa in both human colonic neoplasia[44] and in rodent chemical carcinogenesis models.[45] Not only would increased ODC activity provide a useful marker for long-term surveillance of patients at high risk for colorectal polyps and cancer, it may provide a target for chemotherapy and chemoprevention because of the availability of specific inhibitors of ODC, such as DFMO. In addition, ODC activity may provide a useful intermediate assay for testing the effectiveness of chemopreventive agents. With the development of newer and more potent ODC and polyamine synthesis inhibitors, such as polyamine analogs,[46,47] the potential usefulness of ODC as a therapeutic target deserves further investigation.

VIII. POLYAMINES AND COLITIS IN THE COTTON-TOP TAMARIN

Chronic idiopathic ulcerative colitis in man may be characterized histologically by marked mucosal inflammation, injury, and regeneration. One of the most serious complications of ulcerative colitis is the development of colon cancer, often taking place over a period of 10 years or more. There are often precursor lesions, represented by dysplasia of varying degree, ranging from minimal dysplasia to "precancer" to carcinoma *in situ*. The

TABLE 2
Colonic Mucosal ODC Activity in Inactive Ulcerative Colitis

	ODC (pmol/mg/h)
Negative for dysplasia	318 ± 112[a]
Low-grade dysplasia	792 ± 316[b]
High-grade dysplasia	1374 ± 498[c]

[a] n = 6
[b] n = 7
[c] n = 4

TABLE 3
Colonic Mucosal ODC Activity in the Tamarin

	ODC (pmol/mg/h)
Negative for cancer	543 ± 285[a]
Cancer in adjacent segment	718 ± 492[b]
Cancer	1357 ± 974[a]

[a] n = 2
[b] n = 3

progression from inflammation and regeneration to dysplasia and cancer has prompted measurements of ODC activity and polyamines in ulcerative colitis. In one study, urinary polyamine levels were elevated in patients with colitis, and the increases were similar to those found in patients with colon cancer.[48] In patients with clinically and histologically inactive ulcerative colitis, we have found that colonic mucosal ODC activity was increased in or adjacent to dysplastic lesions, compared to areas without dysplasia (Table 2).

In recent years an animal model for ulcerative colitis and its evolution to colon cancer has received increasing recognition.[49] Studies have shown that cotton-top tamarins (*Saguinus oedipus,* also called marmosets) develop a disease with many features resembling ulcerative colitis, including acute and chronic inflammation and colon carcinoma. This model has been used successfully for studies of colonic mucin,[50] and lectin histochemistry.[51] An oncofetal glycoconjugate, identified by peanut lectin binding and described in human colonic mucosa with malignant, premalignant, and inflammatory diseases, is expressed in the colons of 65% of the tamarins. Expression of this glycoconjugate is highly correlated with the development of colon cancer and with acute inflammatory activity in these animals.[51] We have found an association of increased ODC activity with the coexistence of colon cancer (Table 3). The biology and biochemistry of the natural progression of ulcerative colitis to colon cancer can be studied extensively in the cotton-top tamarin, and such studies are ongoing in many laboratories.

IX. CONCLUSION

Polyamine metabolism, and in particular ODC activity, appears critical for cell and tissue proliferation in general, and colonic mucosal proliferation and neoplastic evolution in particular. In addition, suppression of ODC activity with the specific inhibitor, DFMO, results in inhibition of normal and neoplastic growth processes of the colonic mucosa. This includes inhibition of growth of human colon cancer cells in culture, and in an *in vivo* nude mouse xenograft model. Furthermore, increased ODC activity is a promising biological marker for the presence and/or development of colorectal polyps and cancer. Preliminary evidence shows that ODC and the polyamines are increased in dysplastic lesions in colitis in humans and in cotton-top tamarins. Polyamine metabolism warrants further investigation as a biological tool to understanding the neoplastic process, and as a potential therapeutic target for colorectal malignancy. Studies of polyamine metabolism in colitis, dysplasia, and neoplasia in the cotton-top tamarin may be applicable to human disease.

ACKNOWLEDGMENTS

We thank Dr. Vainutis K. Vaitkevicius, for encouragement, advice, and support; and William Theiss for technical assistance.

The studies were supported in part by grants R01-CA43280, RO1-CA45831, and U01-CA50399 from the National Institutes of Health and by the Department of Veterans Affairs Research Service. GDL was a recipient of a faculty research award from the American Cancer Society and the American Gastroenterological Association/Robbins Research Scholar Award.

REFERENCES

1. **Williams-Ashman, H. G. and Canellakis, Z. N.,** Polyamines in mammalian biology and medicine, *Perspect. Biol. Med.*, 22, 421, 1979.
2. **Luk, G. D. and Casero, R. A.,** Polyamines in normal and cancer cells, *Adv. Enzyme Regul.*, 26, 91, 1987.
3. **Janne, J., Poso, H., and Raina, A.,** Polyamines in rapid growth and cancer, *Biochim. Biophys. Acta,* 473, 241, 1978.
4. **Pegg, A. E. and McCann, P. P.,** Polyamine metabolism and function, *Am. J. Physiol.*, 243, C212, 1982.
5. **Tabor, C. W. and Tabor, H.,** Polyamines, *Annu. Rev. Biochem.*, 53, 749, 1984.
6. **Bey, P.,** Substrate-induced irreversible inhibition of alpha-aminoacid decarboxylase. Application to glutamate; aromatic-L-alpha-aminoacid and ornithine decarboxylases, in *Enzyme-Activated Irreversible Inhibitors,* Seiler, N., Jung, M. J., and Koch-Weser, J., Eds., Elsevier/North Holland, New York, 1978, 27.
7. **Metcalf, B. W., Bey, P., Danzin, C., Jung, M. J., Casara, P., and Vevert, J. P.,** Catalytic irreversible inhibition of mammalian ornithine decarboxylase (E.C.4.1.1.17) by substrate and product analogues, *J. Am. Chem. Soc.*, 100, 2551, 1978.

8. **Mamont, P. S., Duchesne, M.-C., Grove, J., and Bey, P.,** Anti-proliferative properties of DL-alpha-difluoromethyl-ornithine in cultured cells. A consequence of the irreversible inhibition of ODC, *Biochem. Biophys. Res. Commun.*, 81, 58, 1978.
9. **Seiler, N., Danzin, C., Prakash, N. J., and Koch-Weser, J.,** Effects of ornithine decarboxylase inhibitors *in vivo,* in *Enzyme-Activated Irreversible Inhibitors,* Seiler, N., Jung, M. J., and Koch-Weser, J., Eds., Elsevier/North Holland, New York, 1978, 55.
10. **Prakash, N. J., Schechter, P. J., Mamont, P. S., Grove, J., Koch-Weser, J., and Sjoerdsma, A.,** Inhibition of EMT6 tumor growth by interference with polyamine biosynthesis; effects of alpha-difluoromethylornithine, an irreversible inhibitor of ornithine decarboxylase, *Life Sci.*, 26, 181, 1980.
11. **Luk, G. D., Civin, C. I., Weissman, R. M., and Baylin, S. B.,** Ornithine decarboxylase: essential in proliferation but not differentiation of human promyelocytic leukemia cells, *Science,* 216, 75, 1982.
12. **Luk, G. D., Goodwin, G., Marton, L. J., and Baylin, S. B.,** Polyamines are necessary for the survival of human small-cell lung carcinoma in culture, *Proc. Natl. Acad. Sci. U.S.A.*, 78, 2355, 1980.
13. **Luk, G. D., Goodwin, G., Gazdar, A. F., and Baylin, S. B.,** Growth-inhibitory effects of DL-alpha-difluoromethylornithine in the spectrum of human lung carcinoma cells in culture, *Cancer Res.*, 42, 3070, 1982.
14. **Bartolome, J., Huguenard, J., and Slotkin, T. A.,** Role of ornithine decarboxylase in cardiac growth and hypertrophy, *Science,* 210, 793, 1980.
15. **Danzin, C., Claverie, N., Wagner, J., Grove, J., and Koch-Weser, J.,** Effect on prostatic growth of alpha-difluoromethylornithine, an effective inhibitor of ornithine decarboxylase, *Biochem. J.*, 202, 175, 1982.
16. **Luk, G. D., Marton, L. J., and Baylin, S. B.,** Ornithine decarboxylase is important in intestinal mucosal maturation and recovery from injury in rats, *Science,* 210, 195, 1980.
17. **Fozard, J. R., Part, M.-L., Prakash, N. J., Grove, J., Schechter, P. J., Sjoerdsma, A., and Koch-Weser, J.,** L-Ornithine decarboxylase: an essential role in early mammalian embryogenesis, *Science,* 208, 505, 1980.
18. **Marton, L. J., Levin, V. A., Hervatin, S. J., Koch-Weser, J., McCann, P. P., and Sjoerdsma, A.,** Potentiation of the antitumor therapeutic effects of 1,3-bis(2-chloroethyl)-1-nitrosourea by alpha-difluoro-methylornithine, an ornithine decarboxylase inhibitor, *Can. Res.*, 41, 4436, 1981.
19. **Bartholeyns, J. and Koch-Weser, J.,** Effects of alpha-difluoromethyl-ornithine alone and combined with adriamycin or vindesine on L1210 leukemia in mice, EMT6 solid tumors in mice, and solid tumors induced by injection of hepatoma tissue culture cells in rats, *Cancer Res.*, 41, 5158, 1981.
20. **Luk, G. D., Abeloff, M. D., Griffin, C. A., and Baylin, S. B.,** Successful treatment with DL-alpha-difluoromethylornithine in established human small cell variant lung carcinoma implants in athymic mice, *Cancer Res.*, 43, 4239, 1983.
21. **Luk, G. D., Abeloff, M. D., McCann, P. P., Sjoerdsma, A., and Baylin, S. B.,** Long-term maintenance therapy of established human small cell variant lung carcinoma implants in athymic mice with a cyclic regimen of difluoromethylornithine, *Cancer Res.*, 46, 1849, 1986.
22. **Luk, G. D. and Baylin, S. B.,** Polyamines and intestinal growth-increased polyamine biosynthesis after jejunectomy, *Am. J. Physiol.*, 245, G656, 1983.
23. **Yang, P., Baylin, S. B., and Luk, G. D.,** Polyamines and intestinal growth: absolute requirement for ODC activity in adaptation during lactation, *Am. J. Physiol.*, 247, G553, 1984.
24. **Luk, G. D. and Baylin, S. B.,** Inhibition of intestinal epithelial DNA synthesis and adaptive hyperplasia after jejunectomy in the rat by suppression of polyamine biosynthesis, *J. Clin. Invest.*, 74, 698, 1984.

25. **Dowling, R. H., Hosomi, M., Stace, N. H., Lirussi, F., Miazza, B., Levan, H., and Murphy, G. M.,** Hormones and polyamines in intestinal and pancreatic adaptation, *Scand. J. Gastroenterol.*, 20 (Suppl. 112), 84, 1985.
26. **Boutwell, R. K.,** Biochemical mechanism of tumor promotion, *Carcinogenesis,* 2, 49, 1978.
27. **Ball, W. J., Salser, J. S., and Balis, M. E.,** Biochemical changes in preneoplastic rodent intestines, *Cancer Res.*, 36, 2686, 1976.
28. **Rozhin, J., Wilson, P. S., Bull, A. W., and Nigro, N. D.,** Ornithine decarboxylase activity in the rat and human colon, *Cancer Res.*, 44, 3226, 1984.
29. **Luk, G. D., Hamilton, S. R., Yang, P., Smith, J. A., O'Ceallaigh, D., McAvinchey, D., and Hyland, J.,** Kinetic changes in mucosal ornithine decarboxylase activity during azoxymethane-induced colonic carcinogenesis in the rat, *Cancer Res.*, 46, 4449, 1986.
30. **Kingsnorth, A. N., King, W. W. K., Diekema, K. A., McCann, P. P., Ross, J. S., and Malt, R. A.,** Inhibition of ornithine decarboxylase with alpha-difluoromethylornithine reduced incidence of dimethylhydrazine-induced colon tumors in mice, *Cancer Res.*, 43, 2545, 1983.
31. **Nigro, N. D., Bull, A. W., and Boyd, M. E.,** Importance of the duration of inhibition on intestinal carcinogenesis by difluoromethylornithine in rats, *Cancer Lett.*, 35, 153, 1987.
32. **Luk, G. D., Zhang, S. Z., and Hamilton, S. R.,** Effects of timing of administration and dose of difluoromethylornithine on rat colonic carcinogenesis, *J. Natl. Cancer Inst.*, 81, 421, 1989.
33. **Silverman, A. L., Parikh, N., Gesell, M. S., Maliakkal, B. J., and Luk, G. D.,** Prolonged exposure to difluoromethyl ornithine is cytotoxic to anchorage dependent human colon cancer cell lines, *Proc. Am. Assoc. Cancer Res.*, 31, 419, 1990.
34. **Neelam, S. S., Bernabei, A., Freedland, C., Thompson, R., Corbett, T., and Luk, G. D.,** Combination of flavone acetic acid with adriamycin, cis-platinum, and difluoromethyl ornithine in vitro against human colon cancer cells, *Invest. New Drugs,* 8, 263, 1990.
35. **Kingsnorth, A. N., Russell, W. E., McCann, P. P., Diekema, K. A., and Malt, R. A.,** Effects of difluoromethylornithine and 5-fluorouracil on the proliferation of a human colon adenocarcinoma cell line, *Cancer Res.*, 43, 4035, 1983.
36. **Abeloff, M. D., Slavik, M., Luk, G. D., Griffin, C. A., Hermann, J., Blanc, O., Sjoerdsma, A., and Baylin, S. B.,** Phase I trial and pharmacokinetic studies of alpha-difluoromethyl ornithine — an inhibitor of polyamine biosynthesis, *J. Clin. Oncol.*, 2, 124, 1984.
37. **Luk, G. D.,** Successful treatment with difluoromethylornithine in established human colon carcinoma implants in athymic mice, *Gastroenterology,* 92, 1511, 1987.
38. **Abeloff, M. D., Rosen, S. T., Luk, G. D., Baylin, S. B., Zeltzman, M., and Sjoerdsma, A.,** Phase II trials of alpha-difluoromethyl-ornithine, an inhibitor of polyamine synthesis, in advanced small cell lung cancer and colon cancer, *Cancer Treat. Rep.*, 70, 843, 1986.
39. **Deschner, E. E.,** Cell proliferation as a biological marker in human colorectal neoplasia, in *Colorectal Cancer: Prevention, Epidemiology and Screening,* Winawer, S. J., Schottenfeld, P., and Sherlock, P., Eds., Raven Press, New York, 1980, 133.
40. **Luk, G. D. and Baylin, S. B.,** Ornithine decarboxylase as a biologic marker in familial colonic polyposis, *N. Engl. J. Med.*, 311, 80, 1984.
41. **Kingsnorth, A. N., Lumsden, A. B., and Wallace, H. M.,** Polyamines in colorectal cancer, *Br. J. Surg.*, 71, 791, 1984.
42. **Lamuraglia, G. M., Lacaine, F., and Malt, R. A.,** High ornithine decarboxylase activity and polyamine levels in human colorectal neoplasia, *Ann. Surg.*, 204, 89, 1986.
43. **Porter, C. W., Herrera-Ornelas, L., Clark, J., Pera, P., Petrelli, N. J., and Mittleman, A.,** Polyamine biosynthetic activity in normal and neoplastic human colorectal tissues, *Cancer,* 60, 1275, 1987.

44. **Shamsuddin, A. K. M., Weiss, L., Phelps, P. C., and Trump, B. F.,** Colon epithelium. IV. Human colon carcinogenesis. Changes in human colon mucosa adjacent to and remote from carcinoma of the colon, *J. Natl. Cancer Inst.,* 66, 413, 1981.
45. **Pan, Q., Hamilton, S. R., Hyland, J. and Biotnott, J. K.,** Effects of carcinogen dosage on experimental colonic carcinogenesis by azoxymethane: an ultrastructural study of grossly normal colonic mucosa, *J. Natl. Cancer Inst.,* 74, 689, 1985.
46. **Sjoerdsma, A.,** Suicide enzyme inhibitors as potential drugs, *Clin. Pharmacol. Ther.,* 30, 3, 1981.
47. **Sjoerdsma, A. and Schechter, P.,** Chemotherapeutic implications of polyamine biosynthesis inhibition, *Clin. Pharmacol. Ther.,* 35, 287, 1984.
48. **Thompson, J. S., Edney, J. A., and Laughlin, K. I.,** Urinary polyamines in colorectal cancer, *Dis. Colon Rectum,* 29, 873, 1986.
49. **Clapp, N. K., Lushbaugh, C. C., Humason, G. L., Gangaware, B. L., Henke, M. A., and McArthur, A. H.,** The marmoset as a model of ulcerative colitis and colon cancer, *Prog. Clin. Biol. Res.,* 1986, 247, 1985.
50. **Podolsky, D. K., Madara, J. L., King, N., Sehgal, P., Moore, R., and Winter, H. S.,** Colonic mucin composition in primates, *Gastroenterology,* 88, 20, 1985.
51. **Boland, C. R. and Clapp, N. K.,** Glycoconjugates in the colons of New World monkeys with spontaneous colitis, *Gastroenterology,* 92, 625, 1987.

Chapter 21

IMMUNOBIOLOGY OF THE COTTON-TOP TAMARIN

David I. Watkins and Norman L. Letvin

TABLE OF CONTENTS

0-8493-5363-7/93/$0.00 + $.50

I. INTRODUCTION

The cotton-top tamarin (*Saguinus oedipus*) has been widely used as a model in biomedical research to study the pathogenesis of certain human diseases.[1] The reason for using this particular species stems, in part, from its extreme susceptibility to a variety of viruses. *S. oedipus* develops fatal lymphoproliferative syndromes following infections with Epstein-Barr virus (EBV)[2] and *Herpesvirus saimiri*.[3] The cotton-top tamarin also appears to be far more susceptible to retrovirus-induced sarcomas and fatal measle virus infections than other species.[4,5] Additionally, as many as 60% of captive *S. oedipus* spontaneously develop ulcerative colitis and 15% develop adenocarcinoma of the colon.[6]

Cotton-top tamarins are usually born as dizygotic twins and, due to anastomosing placental circulations, they are bone marrow-chimeric.[7] Since these primates are naturally occurring "A" + "B" → "A" bone marrow chimeras, it has been suggested by some investigators that the need to maintain tolerance between the genetically distinct "A" and "B" lymphocyte populations in these chimeras results in a depression in the function of the cotton-top tamarin's immune system. It has been proposed that such an immune depression accounts for the cotton-top tamarin's increased susceptibility to tumors and virally induced diseases.[8]

To explore the unusual susceptibility of the cotton-top tamarin to a number of viral infections, we have examined various aspects of the immune system involved in host defense against viruses. Virus-specific CD8+ cytotoxic T lymphocytes (CTLs) constitute an important host response to viral infection. These CTLs recognize viral antigens expressed on the membrane of infected cells in association with class I allelic products of the major histocompatibility complex (MHC). Infected cells are then lysed by these CTLs, thereby preventing fulminant viral infections.[9] Codominant expression of MHC class I alleles and an extraordinary degree of polymorphism in these gene products is felt to confer a survival advantage to individuals and the species through facilitating the immune system's ability to interact with a variety of viral antigens.[9]

In this review, we demonstrate that a number of important functional parameters of the immune system of the cotton-top tamarin appear to be normal. We show, however, that the immune system of the cotton-top tamarin differs from that of other primate species in that its MHC class I loci exhibit an extremely limited degree of variation and polymorphism. We explore the ramifications of this limited MHC class I diversity on the immune system of the species.

II. FUNCTIONAL IMMUNE STATUS OF *S. oedipus*

The functional immune status of the peripheral blood lymphocytes (PBLs) of these animals was assessed by ^{3}H-thymidine incorporation following

TABLE 1
Proliferation of *S. oedipus* PBLs in Response to Lectin Stimulation

PHA (μg/ml)	Hours of culture 48	72	96
None	190 ± 33[a]	260 ± 31	1030 ± 370
0.6	4560 ± 270 (24[b])	16800 ± 680 (64)	34700 ± 270 (34)
1.3	3910 ± 270 (21)	12100 ± 700 (46)	26300 ± 870 (26)

Note: PBLs were isolated from whole blood on a Ficoll-Diatrozoate gradient and cultured in round-bottomed microtiter plates at 5×10^4 cells/well in RPMI containing 10% FBS and various concentrations of PHA; 16 h before harvesting each well was pulsed with 1 μCi ^{3}H-thymidine.

[a] Data are expressed as mean ± SD of triplicate wells.
[b] Value represents stimulation index: experimental counts divided by counts in similar wells without PHA.

stimulation by the lectin phytohemagglutinin (PHA). The results of one such experiment are shown in Table 1. After 96 h in culture using 50,000 PBLs per well and 0.6 μg/ml of PHA, a peak response of 34,700 counts per minute (cpm) as a stimulation index of 34 was generated. These results are in the expected range for lectin-stimulated proliferation of primate PBLs.[10]

A more sensitive test of immune function is the proliferative response of lymphocytes to antigen stimulation. We examined the response of *S. oedipus* PBLs to allogeneic stimulation in the mixed lymphocyte culture (MLC) assay. The allogeneic stimulator cells were derived from cotton-top tamarins in the colony that were unrelated to the animals from which cells were used as a responder population. Representative data shown in Table 2 indicate that cpm of above 30,000 with a stimulation index over 10 are commonly generated. Again, these responses in alloantigen-driven proliferation assays are comparable to those seen with lymphocytes from other primate species.[11]

Trinitophenyl (TNP)-specific CTL have also been generated in tamarins.[12] As targets, B cells from tamarins were cloned after transforming by coculturing with supernatants derived from the EBV-producing tamarin B cell line B95-8. They were grown up, cloned in soft agar, and their genetic homogeneity was confirmed by karyotypic analysis. These clones were then used as genetically homogeneous stimulator and target cell populations in the generation and assaying of CTL function to confirm that these EBV-transformed clones, when haptenated, could serve to stimulate the generation of hapten-specific CTL and act as targets in the assay of that function. Killer cells were generated in a population of unprimed PBL from a chimeric *S. oedipus* which kill TNP-conjugated but not unconjugated cells when assayed on EBV-transformed B cell clones. It was then established that primary alloantigen-specific and TNP-specific CTL can be generated under conditions of limiting dilution. Alloantigen-specific target cell lysis can be measured after a primary *in vitro*

TABLE 2
Proliferation of *S. oedipus* PBLs in Response to Allogeneic Cells

Responder cells[a]	Stimulator cells	cpm (E/C)[b] Exp. 1			Exp. 2	
		144 h	**168 h**	**192 h**	**168 h**	**192 h**
10^5	10^5	NT[c]	11200 (4.1)	11500 (4.5)	47700 (12.1)	26000 (6.1)
	5×10^4	9690 (4.4)	4600 (2.2)	4970 (2.6)	28700 (11.6)	20000 (7.0)
5×10^4	5×10^4	1980 (2.4)	14600 (2.9)	2500 (2.9)	35000 (6.8)	NT

[a] PBLs were incubated with mitomycin-C-treated stimulator cells in round-bottomed microtiter wells, then pulsed with ^{3}H-thymidine and harvested for counting.
[b] Value represents E/C where E is mean ^{3}H-thymidine incorporation in triplication wells containing allogeneic stimulators and C is the incorporation in wells containing an equal number of syngeneic stimulator cells.
[c] Not tested.

TABLE 3
Proliferative Response of a TNP-Specific Tamarin T Cell Clone[a]

	cpm[b]	
Clone	**Self**	**TNP-self**
1.8	2,399	15,849

[a] Phenotype of clone 1.8 was as follows: 92% T4, 22% T8, 90% T11, 0% NKH1, and 0% B1.

[b] Responder cells were incubated with mitomycin-treated stimulator cells and interleukin-2 pulsed with ^{3}H-thymidine at 72 h and harvested at 88 h.

TABLE 4
Cytotoxic Responses of TNP-Specific Tamarin T Cell Clones[a]

	% Specific ^{51}Cr release[b]	
Clone	**Self**	**TNP-self**
1.7	0	17
1.8	0	2

[a] Cytotoxicity was measured during 6-h ^{51}Cr-release assay with 10^4 targets and E:T of 20:1.

[b] Phenotype of clone 1.8 was as described in Table 3. Phenotype of 1.7 was as follows: 0% T4, 95% T8, 97% T11, 0% NKH1, 0% B1.

education of progressively smaller numbers of naive *S. oedipus* PBL. Experiments of this type indicate that this tamarin alloantigen-specific CTL precursor frequency under these conditions is 1:490. Similarly, TNP-coupled target cell lysis can be generated under these conditions. The TNP-specific CTL precursor frequency as determined under these conditions is 1:2600. Finally, we have generated CTLs in bulk culture and cloned them. Several different clones resulted. Of these, two were selected for further study. One of these was CD4+ CD8− and responded in a proliferative assay to TNPlated self (Table 3). The other clone was CD8+ CD4− and killed TNPlated self (Table 4). Thus, long-term culture of TNP-specific CTLs and helper cell clones can be generated in the cotton-top tamarin.

III. CHARACTERIZATION OF THE MHC MOLECULES OF *S. oedipus*

We studied animals from six different colonies, a population which should be representative of 30,000 to 40,000 *S. oedipus* that have been exported from Colombia for use in medical research.[13] Lectin-stimulated PBLs of 20 wild-caught and 6 colony-born, unrelated *S. oedipus* were metabolically labeled, MHC class I molecules were immunoprecipitated with the monoclonal

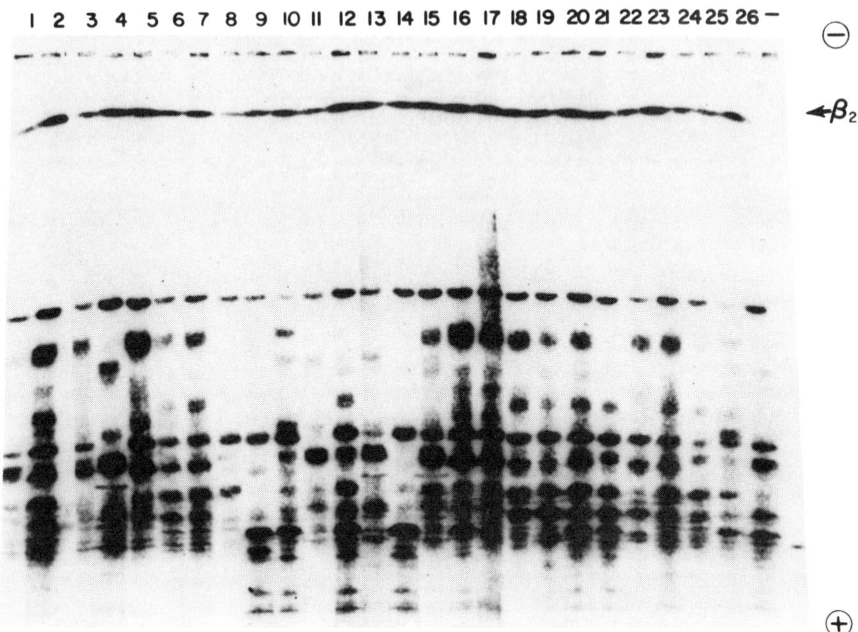

FIGURE 1. One of the *S. oedipus* MHC class I molecules is expressed by the lymphocytes of all cotton-top tamarins tested. 1-D IEF of class I molecules from the PBLs of 26 unrelated *S. oedipus*. PBLs were PHA-stimulated, ^{35}S-labeled, MHC class I molecules were immunoprecipitated with a mouse anti-human MHC class I monoclonal antibody and subjected to 1-D IEF. PBLs studied from *S. oedipus* originally housed in the following colonies: New England Regional Primate Research Center (1 to 5), Bristol (6 to 9), Oak Ridge (10 to 12 and 20 to 26), Miami (13, 14), Wayne State (15 to 17), and Yale (18, 19). The lysate prepared from the PBLs of animal 26 was precipitated with a monoclonal antibody with an irrelevant specificity (–). The position of β-2 microglobulin is indicated (β-2).

anti-class I antibody BB7.7[14] and analyzed by one-dimensional isoelectric focusing (1-D IEF) (Figure 1).[15] Strikingly, a single MHC class I molecule was common to all animals tested. Moreover, a second product was shared by 24 of the 26 animals. Considerable heterogeneity was observed in the other 11 class I glycoproteins expressed by the PBLs of these animals. This degree of heterogeneity was, however, less than might have been predicted when one considers that there are more than 97 alleles at the class I human leukocyte antigen *(HLA)-A* and *-B* loci.[16] Additionally, we have recently analyzed the MHC class I molecules of a group of wild cotton-top tamarins. These animals expressed MHC class I molecules that were indistinguishable from those expressed by captive tamarins, supporting the notion that the captive animals are representative of those in the wild (data not shown).

The polymorphism evident in the nonidentical *S. oedipus* class I molecules suggested that a founder effect or a genetic bottleneck was probably not

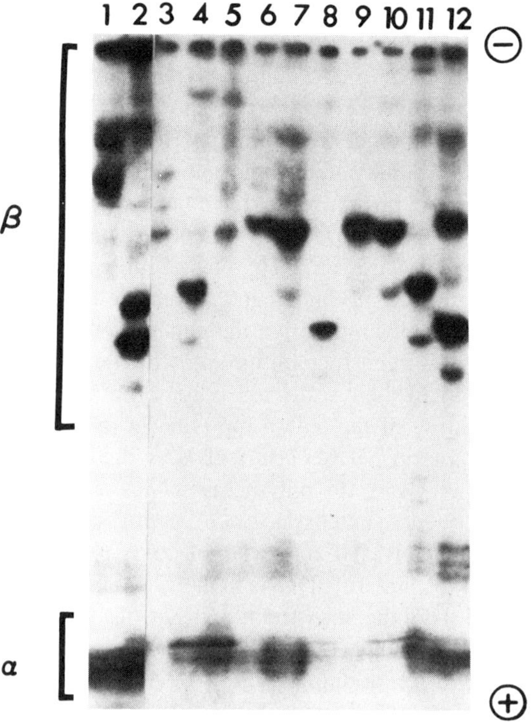

FIGURE 2. *S. oedipus* MHC class II glycoproteins are polymorphic. 1-D IEF of class II molecules immunoprecipitated with a mixture of two mouse anti-human class II monoclonal antibodies. MHC class II glycoproteins from 12 unrelated animals were iodinated, immunoprecipitated, and analyzed by 1-D IEF. PBLs studied were from *S. oedipus* originally housed in the following colonies: New England Regional Primate Research Center (1 to 5), Oak Ridge (6, 7, and 11, 12), Bristol (8), Miami (9), and Yale (10). The positions of the alpha (α) and beta (β) chains are shown.

responsible for this remarkable conservation of two alleles at the MHC class I loci of this species. We nevertheless pursued such possibilities further by similarly analyzing MHC class II-encoded gene products in the cotton-top tamarin. Analysis of ^{125}I surface-labeled lectin-stimulated PBLs from 12 *S. oedipus* showed that MHC class II alpha gene products, which exhibit little heterogeneity in all species previously studied, are also relatively nonpolymorphic in these animals. However, extensive polymorphism was seen in the MHC class II beta gene products (Figure 2). At least eight different beta-chain allelic products are clearly expressed by the lymphocytes of the cotton-top tamarin population studied. This finding provides further evidence that a founder effect or genetic bottleneck is unlikely to account for the strikingly high frequency of certain alleles at the MHC class I loci in *S. oedipus*.

To investigate whether the structure of the tamarin MHC class I molecule was related to the extraordinary susceptibility of the species to pathogens, we then cloned and sequenced three tamarin MHC class I molecules.[17] These tamarin MHC class I cDNAs coded for amino acid substitutions not found in any of the 39 previously sequenced human MHC class I alleles.[18] Moreover, the majority of these unique amino acid substitutions were located in the antigen recognition site at positions that have been shown to be critical in the presentation of viral peptides to T cells in mice and humans. These data suggest that selective pressures on MHC class I molecules preferentially act on the antigen recognition site and that the peptide-binding or -presenting functions of these molecules may drive the generation of MHC class I polymorphism. The novel antigen recognition sites of the tamarin MHC class I molecules, in addition to their restricted polymorphism, might account for the unusual susceptibility of the cotton-top tamarin to human pathogens.

The expressed tamarin MHC class I cDNAs displayed little nucleotide sequence variation.[19,20] Using the polymerase chain reaction (PCR) we were then able to clone, sequence, and express cDNAs encoding all of the tamarins' electrophoretically defined MHC class I molecules. Comparison of the nucleotide sequences of the tamarin cDNAs to their human counterparts indicates that they are derived from the ancestral homologs of the human nonclassical, nonpolymorphic *HLA-G* locus (Figure 3). A deletion of the *HLA-A, -B,* and *-C* locus homologs and recent duplication of *HLA-G* locus homolog accounts for the limited variation and polymorphism of the tamarin MHC class I loci. The expression of *HLA-G*-related, relatively nonpolymorphic MHC class I molecules in the tamarin may limit the variety of viral and tumor antigens which can be presented to tamarin T cells and may thus increase the susceptibility of this species to these pathogens. Moreover, utilization of *HLA-G*-related, nonpolymorphic MHC class I molecules may be important in the establishment of tolerance in these bone marrow chimeras. In fact, these findings, and the observation that the human fetal trophoblast expresses high levels of *HLA-G* products,[21,22] suggest that expression of nonpolymorphic MHC class I gene products may facilitate maintenance of allotolerance.

IV. THE MHC CLASS I GENES OF THE COTTON-TOP TAMARIN ARE UNIQUE

To determine whether the cotton-top tamarin's MHC class I genes are unique when compared to the MHC class I genes of other primates, we and others have cloned, sequenced, and expressed MHC class I cDNAs from nine other primate species[23-27] (and data not shown). MHC class I cDNAs from Old World and great ape species were all related to the human *HLA-A, -B,* and *-C* loci. We then cloned cDNAs from several species of New World primates. These cDNAs were all found to be related to *HLA-G* (data not shown). However, the cotton-top tamarin's MHC class I genes clustered separately from those of the common marmoset and from those of all other

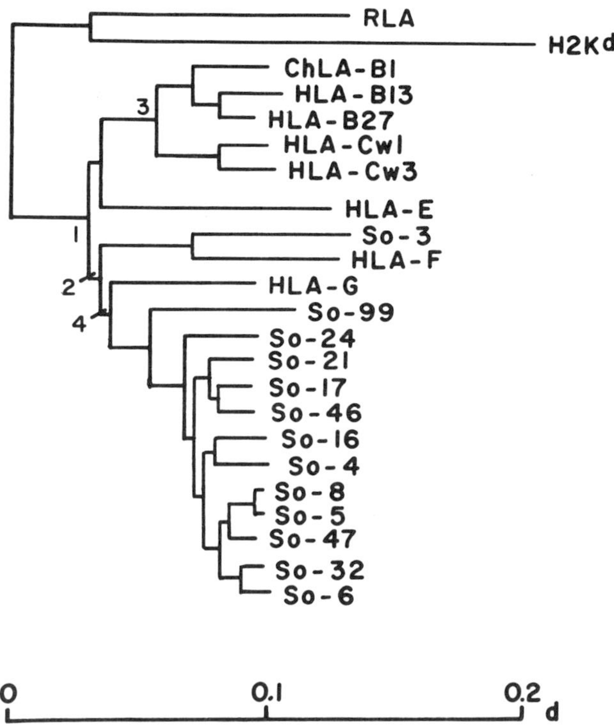

FIGURE 3. The tamarin MHC class I loci are related to the *HLA-G* and *-F* nonclassical loci. Phylogenetic trees based on nucleotide substitutions per side (d) among cotton-top tamarin and other primate MHC class I genes: tree for 1005 aligned nucleotides from exons 1–7. Rabbit (*RLA*) and mouse (*H2K^d*) MHC class I alleles are used as outgroups to establish the root of the tree. The internal branch length d_{1-2} (between the cluster containing the tamarin genes plus *HLA-G* and *-F* and the cluster of human and chimpanzee classical genes) = 0.042 ± 0.007 ($P < .001$); and the internal branch length d_{34} (between the *HLA-F*/3 cluster and the cluster including *HLA-G*, 99, and the tamarin classical cDNAs) = 0.027 ± 0.005 ($P < .001$).

New World primate species. This indicates that the cotton-top tamarin MHC class I genes probably have independent evolutionary origins. Additionally, several of the unique substitutions found in the antigen recognition sites of the MHC class I molecules of the cotton-top tamarin were not found in the antigen recognition site of any of the other primate species examined. Thus, it appears that the cotton-top tamarin's MHC class I genes are indeed unique among other primates.

V. RAMIFICATIONS OF LIMITED MHC CLASS I VARIATION AND POLYMORPHISM IN *S. oedipus*

We have reviewed the data suggesting that a number of parameters of the immune function of *S. oedipus* appear to be normal. A significant difference, however, does exist between the cotton-top tamarin and other primate species thus far studied. The MHC class I genes of the cotton-top tamarin appear to be very limited in their variation and polymorphism when compared to the MHC class I genes of other species. This limited MHC class I polymorphism does not appear to be the result of a founder effect, since MHC class II molecules of these animals are polymorphic.

The relatively low level of MHC class I polymorphism detected using biochemical techniques is consistent with previously established functional data. Extensive studies of skin graft rejection, a largely MHC class I-mediated response, have been performed with *S. oedipus*. While the cotton-top tamarin will reject skin grafts from other species of tamarins in 12 to 20 days, they tolerate allogeneic grafts for greater than 70 days.[28] Studies of mixed lymphocyte reactions,[12] an MHC class II-mediated phenomenon, are consistent with the biochemically defined MHC class II polymorphism in this species.

It has been proposed that a few other species may lack MHC class I gene polymorphism. Grafts exchanged between unrelated cheetahs are accepted indefinitely.[29] Since a number of their serum enzymes are virtually nonpolymorphic, it has been suggested that this species has been through at least one genetic bottleneck.[30] Cheetah MHC-encoded gene products, however, have never been biochemically characterized. Studies have also suggested that the Syrian hamster has polymorphic MHC class II gene products, but may be monomorphic at its class I loci. An analysis of the Syrian hamster's MHC class I gene products revealed that all animals tested expressed monomorphic MHC class I allelic products.[31] Studies of their class II molecules demonstrated that the three strains tested shared identical $\alpha 2$ and $\beta 2$ molecules, and that only two of these three hamster strains differed at their $\alpha 1$ and $\beta 1$ allelic products.[32] Since the available inbred lines of Syrian hamsters are derived from the offspring of only a few animals caught in Syria, the genotypes of these captive animals may not be representative of those in the wild. Additionally, recent data suggest that electrophoretic variation can be detected among the MHC class I molecules expressed by different Syrian hamsters.[33] Interestingly, both the cheetah and the Syrian hamster are highly susceptible to a number of viral infections.[29,34]

The MHC haplotype of an individual has been shown clearly to correlate with the susceptibility of that individual to a variety of pathogenic processes. In chickens, resistance to a fatal infection by Marek's Disease Virus cosegregates with the B21 haplotype,[35] and humans with the HLA-B27 allele have a markedly increased susceptibility to ankylosing spondylitis.[36] The recent demonstration that the human HLA-B27 gene (present in over 80% of individuals with ankylosing spondylitis) causes ulcerative colitis in HLA-B27-transgenic rats suggests that a particular MHC class I allele may predispose an individual to autoimmune disease.[37] It may well be that one of the two conserved MHC class I molecules expressed by all tamarins may be similar to HLA-B27 in its ability to predispose tamarins to ulcerative colitis. Although

MHC class I polymorphism is not essential for the survival of isolated populations,[38] the absence of such a polymorphism may have a negative impact on host defenses when species or individuals encounter new pathogens that are not normally present in their environment. An extreme selective pressure in its natural environment for a limited number of MHC class I alleles may have left the cotton-top tamarin susceptible to a variety of pathogens that it does not encounter in its native habitat. This may explain its striking susceptibility to a variety of human viruses, ulcerative colitis, and adenocarcinoma of the colon.

VI. SUMMARY

The New World primate *Saguinus oedipus* (the cotton-top tamarin) has an extremely high incidence of ulcerative colitis and adenocarcinoma of the colon and is unusually susceptible to lethal infection with a variety of viruses. Cotton-top tamarins are also unusual in that their cells express relatively nonpolymorphic, nonvariable, *HLA-G*-related MHC class I molecules. The limited MHC class I diversity of the cotton-top tamarin may predispose these primates to various pathogenic processes.

ACKNOWLEDGMENTS

We thank A. Petto for his assistance in genealogical analysis of *S. oedipus* from the New England colony, N. Clapp for sending blood samples from the Oak Ridge Colony, D. Brosseau and S. Kotlikoff for preparation of this manuscript. This work was supported by grants RR00168, DK43351, and AI32426 from the National Institutes of Health. Dr. Letvin is a recipient of an American Cancer Society Faculty Research Award.

REFERENCES

1. **Wolfe, L. G. and Deinhardt, F.,** Overview of viral oncology studies in Saguinus and Callithrix species, in *Primate Medicine,* Vol. 10, Goldsmith, E. I. and Moor-Jankowski, J., Eds., S. Karger, Basel, 1978, 96.
2. **Miller, G., Shope, T., Coope, D., Waters, L., Pagano, J., Bornkamm, G. W., and Henle, W.,** Lymphoma in cotton-topped marmosets after inoculation with Epstein-Barr virus: tumor incidence, histologic spectrum, antibody responses, demonstration of viral DNA and characterization of viruses, *J. Exp. Med.,* 145, 948, 1977.
3. **Fleckenstein, B. and Desrosiers, R. C.,** Herpesvirus saimiri and Herpesvirus ateles, in *The Herpesviruses,* Vol. 1, Roizman, B., Ed., Plenum Press, New York, 1982, 253.
4. **Deinhardt, F., Wolfe, L., Northrop, R., Marczynska, B., Ogden, J., McDonald, R., Falk, L., Shramek, G., Smith, R., and Deinhardt, J.,** Induction of neoplasms by viruses in marmoset monkeys, *J. Med. Primatol.,* 1, 29, 1972.

5. **Albrecht, P., Lorenz, D., Klutch, M. J., Vickers, J. H., and Ennis, F. A.,** Fatal measles infection in marmosets, pathogenesis and prophylaxis, *Infect. Immun.*, 27, 969, 1980.
6. **Chalifoux, L. V. and Bronson, R. T.,** Colonic adenocarcinoma associated with chronic colitis in cotton marmosets, *Saguinus oedipus, Gastroenterology,* 80, 942, 1982.
7. **Benirschke, K., Anderson, J. M., and Brownhill, L. E.,** Marrow chimerism in marmosets, *Science,* 128, 513, 1962.
8. **Nickerson, D. A. and Gengozian, N.,** Functional capabilities of marmoset T and B lymphocytes *in vitro* antibody formation, *Cell. Immunol.*, 57, 408, 1981.
9. **Zinkernagel, R. and Doherty, P.,** Restriction of *in vitro* T cell mediated cytotoxicity in lymphocytic choriomeningitis within a syngeneic or allogeneic system, *Nature,* 248, 701, 1974.
10. **Humber, D. P. and Hetherington, C. M.,** A micro-method for the evaluation of PHA-responsive T cells in *Callithrix jacchus* and *Macaca fascicularis, J. Med. Primatol.*, 10, 170, 1981.
11. **Steele, R. W., Eichberg, J. W., Heberling, R. L., Kalter, S. S., and Kniker, W. T.,** Correlation and mixed lymphocyte reactivity and skin graft rejection in non-human primates, *J. Med. Primatol.*, 6, 119, 1977.
12. **Picus, J., Aldrich, W. R., and Letvin, N. L.,** A naturally occurring bone-marrow-chimeric primate, *Transplantation,* 39, 297, 1985.
13. **Hernandez-Camacho, J. and Cooper, R. W.,** The nonhuman primates of Columbia, in *Neotropical Primates: Field Studies and Conservation,* Thorington, R. W., Ed., National Academy of Sciences, Washington, D.C., 1976, 35.
14. **Brodsky, F. J., Parham, P., Barnstable, C. J., Crumpton, M V., and Bodmer, W. F.,** Monoclonal antibodies for analysis of the HLA system, *Immunol. Rev.*, 47, 3, 1979.
15. **Neefjes, J. J., Breur-Breisendorp, B. S., van Seveneter, G. A., Ivanyi, P., and Ploegh, H. L.,** An improved biochemical method for the analysis of HLA-class I antigens. Definition of new HLA-class I subsets, *Hum. Immunol.*, 16, 169, 1986.
16. **Yang, S. Y.,** Population analysis of class I antigens by one-dimensional isoelectric focusing gel electrophoresis, Workshop Summary Report, in *Histocompatibility Testing,* Dupont, B., Ed., Springer-Verlag, New York, 1989, 309.
17. **Watkins, D. I., Letvin, N. L., Hughes, A. L., and Tedder, T. F.,** Molecular cloning of cDNAs that encode MHC class I molecules from a New World primate (*Saguinus oedipus:*) natural selection acts at positions that may affect peptide presentation to T cells, *J. Immunol.*, 146, 1136, 1990.
18. **Parham, P., Lomen, C. E., Lawlor, D. A., Ways, J. P., Holmes, N., Coppin, H. L., Salter, R. D., Wan, A. M., and Ennis, P. D.,** Nature of polymorphism in HLA-A, -B, and -C molecules, *Proc. Natl. Acad. Sci. U.S.A.*, 85, 4004, 1988.
19. **Watkins, D. I., Chen, Z. W., Hughes, A. L., Evans, M. G., Tedder, T. F., and Letvin, N. L.,** Evolution of the MHC class I gene of a New World primate from ancestral homologues of human non-classical genes, *Nature,* 346, 60, 1990.
20. **Watkins, D. I., Chen, Z. W., Toukatly, G., Hughes, A. L., and Letvin, N. L.,** Unusually limited nucleotide sequence variation of the expressed major histocompatibility complex class I genes for a New World primate species *(Saguinus oedipus), Immunogenetics,* 33, 79, 1991.
21. **Ellis, S. A., Palmer, M. S., and McMichael, A. J.,** Human trophoblast and the choriocarcinoma cell line BEWO express a truncated HLA class I molecule, *J. Immunol.*, 144, 731, 1990.
22. **Kovats, S., Main, E. K., Librach, C., Stubblebine, M., Fisher, S. J., and DeMars, R.,** A class I antigen, HLA-G, expressed by human trophoblasts, *Science,* 248, 220, 1990.

23. **Lawlor, D. A., Ward, F. E., Ennis, P. D., Jackson, A. P., and Parham, P.,** HLA-A and B polymorphism predate the divergence of humans and chimpanzees, *Nature,* 335, 268, 1988.
24. **Mayer, W. E., Jonker, M., Klein, D., Ivanyi, P., van Seventer, G., and Klein, J.,** Nucleotide sequences of chimpanzee MHC class I alleles: evidence for trans-species mode of evolution, *EMBO J.,* 7, 2765, 1988.
25. **Watkins, D. I., Chen, Z. W., Garber, T. L., Hughes, A. L., and Letvin, N. L.,** Segmental exchange between MHC class I genes in a higher primate. Recombination in the gorilla between the ancestor of a human non-functional gene and an A locus gene, *Immunogenetics,* 34, 185, 1991.
26. **Lawlor, D. A., Warren, E., Taylor, P., and Parham, P.,** Gorilla class I alleles: comparison to human and chimpanzee class I, *J. Exp. Med.,* in press.
27. **Lawlor, D. A., Warren, E., Ward, F. E., and Parham, P.,** Comparison of class I MHC alleles in humans and apes, *Immunol. Rev.,* 113, 147, 1990.
28. **Gengozian, N. and Porter, R. P.,** Transplantation immunology in the marmoset, in *Medical Primatology,* S. Karger, Basel, 1971, 165.
29. **O'Brien, S. J., Roelke, M. E., Marker, L., Newman, A., Winkler, C. A., Meltzer, D., Colly, L., Evermann, J. F., Bush, M., and Wildt, D. E.,** Genetic basis for species vulnerability in the cheetah, *Science,* 227, 1428, 1985.
30. **O'Brien, S. J., Wildt, D. E., Bush, M., Caro, T. M., FitzGibbon, C., Aggundey, I., and Leady, R. E.,** East African cheetahs: evidence for two population bottlenecks?, *Proc. Natl. Acad. Sci. U.S.A.,* 84, 508, 1987.
31. **Darden, A. G. and Streilein, J. W.,** Syrian hamsters express two monomorphic class I major histocompatibility complex molecules, *Immunogenetics,* 20, 603, 1984.
32. **Sung, E., Duncan, W. R., Streilein, J. W., and Jones, P. O.,** Detection of two distinct class I $\alpha:\beta;I_i$ complexes in the syrian hamster, *Immunogenetics,* 16, 425, 1982.
33. **Watkins, D. I., Chen, Z. W., Hughes, A. L., Lagos, A., Lewis, A. M., Jr., Shadduck, J. A., and Letvin, N. L.,** Syrian hamsters express diverse MHC class I gene products, *J. Immunol.,* 145, 3483, 1990.
34. **Toolan, H. W.,** Susceptibility of the syrian hamster to virus infection, *Fed. Proc.,* 37, 2065, 1978.
35. **Briles, W. E., Stone, H. A., and Cole, R. K.,** Marek's disease: effects of B histocompatibility alloalleles in resistant and susceptible chicken lines, *Science,* 195, 193, 1977.
36. **Schlosstein, L., Terasaki, P. I., Bluestone, R., and Pearson, C. M.,** High association of an HLA antigen, w27 with ankylosing spondylitis, *N. Engl. J. Med.,* 288, 700, 1973.
37. **Hammer, R. E., Maika, S. D., Richardson, J. A., Tang, J. P., and Taurog, J. D.,** Spontaneous inflammatory disease in transgenic rats expressing HLA-B27 and human β-2 microglobulin: an animal model of HLA-B27-associated human disorders, *Cell,* 65, 1099, 1990.
38. **Figueroa, F., Tichy, H., Berry, K. J., and Klein, J.,** MHC polymorphism in island populations of mice, *J. Curr. Top. Microbiol. Immunol.,* 127, 100, 1986.

Chapter 22

SCINTIGRAPHIC IMAGING OF TAMARIN COLORECTAL CARCINOMA WITH RADIOLABELED MONOCLONAL ANTIBODIES

James E. Crook and Neal K. Clapp

TABLE OF CONTENTS

0-8493-5363-7/93/$0.00 + $.50

I. INTRODUCTION

Colon carcinoma persistently remains one of the leading causes of death in the U.S., despite significant technological advances in diagnosis and improved treatment. Colon cancer is the second most common malignant tumor in the U.S., with a death rate second to lung cancer.[1]

The first introduction to the possibilities that the cotton-top tamarin (CTT) could offer in the arena of radiopharmaceutical research began in 1987 with an attempt to identify areas of the tamarin colon involved with colitis in animals that had been diagnosed with acute colitis. Identification of the disease was thought to be important since less than 5% of all cotton-top tamarins in the MARCOR facility have colons unaffected with colitis, albeit present in a chronic, inactive stage. Since colitis is an inflammatory process, increased numbers of leukocytes are generally present when there is an exacerbation of the disease such as that occurring in acute colitis. Colon cancer in the cotton-top tamarin is associated with acute colitis and identifying areas of acutely affected bowel using radiolabeled leukocytes would have been of interest.

Utilizing methodology previously described for indium-111 labeling of white blood cells,[2] seven cotton-top tamarins with varying stages of colitis underwent this procedure. The selected tamarins were reinjected intravenously with autologous leukocytes that had been previously radiolabeled *in vitro* with indium-111 by a commercial radiopharmacy. Scintigraphic imaging of the tamarins was relatively straightforward as their size is amenable to obtaining whole body and torso-only images with a standard gamma camera equipped with various collimators, i.e., medium energy, fine focus, and pin hole. To our knowledge, this was the first successful attempt at producing images of the cotton-top tamarin with its associated colitic diseases. Although the scintigraphic images revealed regions of increased activity throughout the colon, it was not possible by visible inspection to demonstrate discrete foci of increased uptake of the radiolabeled leukocytes.[3] This may have resulted, in part, from the limited number of leukocytes available for radiolabeling. Although leukocyte counts performed prior to radiolabeling experiments were in the normal reference range, the total amount of blood that could be withdrawn for leukocyte radiolabeling was limited to approximately 2.0 ml. However, we were encouraged by these early experimental imaging attempts.

II. BACKGROUND

The preclinical and clinical radiopharmaceutical development program at Oak Ridge Associated Universities (ORAU) had a long and abiding interest in the development of radiolabeled monoclonal antibodies developed primarily for radioimmunotherapy with a strongly associated area of endeavor in radioimmunodetection of cancer, especially colon cancer. However, the great majority of investigative effort was focused on a specific monoclonal antibody identified as CO17-1A, isotype IgG2a, and its associated specificity for gastrointestinal tumors, especially colonic adenocarcinoma. Radiolabeling of

CO17-1A with yttrium-90 was shown to be efficacious in producing a marked regression of subcutaneously xenografted human carcinomas in nude mice.[4,5] It thus seemed a natural extension of this endeavor to include and apply this area of expertise toward another of ORAU's valuable resources, viz., the cotton-top tamarin model of colon cancer.[6]

Early assessment of the immunological status of the spontaneously occurring CTT carcinoma began with a determination of whether there was production and shedding into the systemic circulation of common fetal associated antigens such as carcinoembryonic antigen (CEA). The potential presence or absence of this antigen would influence the choice of monoclonal antibodies intended for the early determination of colon cancer *in situ* in the cotton-top tamarin model of colon cancer; some investigators reported the use of anti-CEA antibodies for the scintigraphic demonstration of gastrointestinal neoplasms.[7] To determine the CEA status of cotton-top tamarins with a known clinical condition, i.e., presence or absence of acute or chronic colitis with or without colonic carcinoma,[8,9] six tamarins were selected to undergo testing by an external laboratory that routinely performed this test. Sera were collected from this group of tamarins which included three who had biopsy-proven colon cancer and three who had no colon cancer but had colitis present in various stages — one acute and two chronic. All six tamarins had serum concentrations of CEA which were below the levels of detection of the immunoassay used, e.g., less than 0.5 ng/ml.[10] These results effectively eliminated the possibility of using a radiolabeled anti-CEA monoclonal antibody in scintigraphic studies.

III. METHODOLOGY

A. SELECTION OF MONOCLONAL ANTIBODY

The initial foray into the area of scintigraphic imaging of CTT colon cancer was thus directed toward obtaining a suitable monoclonal antibody, i.e., one with activity against tumor-associated antigens that could then be successfully conjugated and radiolabeled with an appropriate radionuclide. The half-life and energy characteristics should be such that the early identification of the CTT colon cancer would be possible with images obtained with instrumentation readily available to a majority of investigators. The monoclonal antibody BR55-2, specific for human colorectal carcinoma with activity toward the tamarin tumor, was initially selected for radiolabeling studies.[11] BR55-2, isotype 2a, at a concentration of 5.9 mg/ml, was coupled with diethylenetriaminepentaacetic acid (DTPA) using the cyclic DTPA anhydride technique.[12] An anhydride-to-antibody molar ratio of 2:1 was employed to assure that an adequate number of DTPA groups were present for radiolabeling with the gamma emitter indium-111 ($T_{1/2}$ = 2.8 days). In this and all subsequent experiments, a demonstrated requirement for purification by high-performance liquid chromatography (HPLC) was carried out.[4] All scintigraphic imaging studies also included the coadministration of unlabeled monoclonal antibody in order to achieve maximum tumor specificity which in turn translates into maximum tumor uptake.[13] Early investigations with five different tamarins, two of which were noncancer-bearing controls, were performed to serve two purposes: (1) to evaluate the cotton-top tamarin as a suitable animal model employing the technique of radiolabeled monoclonal antibodies and (2) to determine whether or not monoclonal antibodies labeled with radionuclides possessed the specificity and sensitivity needed to demonstrate the presence of an early colorectal carcinoma, especially on a background of chronic/acute colitis. These were all cogent points that could limit the CTT's usefulness.

The tamarin's small size, approximately 400 g, makes it ideal for performing studies with agents only available in limited amounts and often early in their development. However, vascular access, either arterial or venous, is essentially restricted to percutaneous puncture of the femoral artery or vein. Normally, as part of the routine preliminary animal investigation with radioactively labeled monoclonal antibodies, biodistribution studies of the labeled protein throughout a variety of organs and tissues, in addition to the tumor, are conducted. This very important terminal maneuver is not possible when using the cotton-top tamarin, which is an endangered species. As a result, parallel studies were performed in the more classical athymic nude mouse model with extrapolation of the results to the nonhuman primate.

These caveats aside, femoral venous injections of ^{111}In-labeled BR55-2 were carried out using doses ranging from 100 to 200 μCi. Serial scintigraphic images were obtained at 4, 24, 48, and 72 h, using a standard gamma camera. Taking into consideration the weak affinity of the monoclonal antibody, the colon, spleen, and liver could be satisfactorily evaluated.[14]

Based on the encouraging results of these preliminary investigations, additional efforts were directed toward establishing the tamarin adenocarcinoma cell line (TAC-1) as an *in vitro* culture. This task was successfully completed and the TAC-1 cell line was then exposed to a panel of 13 monoclonal antibodies including a positive control for all human cells.[15] The results of the suspension radioimmunoassay revealed that the only positive monoclonal antibody was WGHS22-2 which was also highly specific for human colorectal cancer.[11]

B. TISSUE DISTRIBUTION STUDIES

Accordingly, a standardized protocol was initiated by subcutaneously injecting 10 million cells of TAC-1 into young, female nude mice. These xenografted mice were utilized in tissue distribution studies when the xenografts had attained a usable size generally measuring 2 to 5 mm in diameter; the maximal diameter occurred approximately 3 months following inoculation. Other investigators have described radiolabeling monoclonal antibodies against tumor-associated antigens with either iodine or indium as a means for detecting by gamma scintigraphy the presence of tumors in experimental animals or man.[16] The monoclonal antibody WGHS22-2 was radiolabeled with iodine-123 ($T_{1/2}$ = 13.1 h) by the chloramine-T method typically producing yields with greater than 40% radiolabeling.[17] Labeled and unlabeled monoclonal antibody was separated by size exclusion HPLC. Radiolabeled ^{123}I-WGHS22-2 of greater than 90% purity, with specific activity in the range of 3 to 6 mCi/mg protein, was produced and approximately 1 mCi of activity was used for scintigraphic studies.

Unlike the previous study, which used the monoclonal antibody BR55-2 conjugated by a different method, WGHS22-2 was conjugated using 1(2)-methyl-4-(*p*-isothiocyanatobenzyl) DTPA, (SCN-Bz-Mx-DTPA), a gift from Drs. O. A. Gansow and M. W. Brechbiel, National Cancer Institute, Maryland. By this method, the indium-111-labeled WGHS22-2 used in the imaging studies had a greater than 99% purity and the activity of the injected solution contained 0.3 mCi/ml. As previously alluded to, the first set of investigations was focused on tissue distribution. Using ^{90}Y-WGHS22-2, produced by reacting yttrium-90 chloride with WGHS22-2 previously conjugated with SCN-Bz-Mx-DTPA, nude mice bearing xenografted TAC-1 tamarin colorectal carcinoma tumors received intravenously coadministered injections of the radiolabeled and nonradiolabeled WGHS22-2. A total of 13 organs and tissues, including bone and bone marrow, were assayed for the percent uptake of the administered dose per gram of tissue present at 72 h post-injection. The radiolabeled monoclonal antibody was present in all tissues examined. Significantly, the data indicated a marked affinity for the xenografted tumor which contained concentrations that were orders of magnitude greater than the liver, which demonstrated the second highest concentration of activity. Calculations of tumor-to-tissue ratios disclosed a wide range of values which were maximal when tumor uptake was compared to muscle. At a ratio approximating 2, tumor-to-liver uptake was the closest to unity — the normalized ratio for tumor. Important for consideration in terms of evaluating either the iodine- or indium-radiolabeled monoclonal antibody was the tumor-to-large bowel ratio with uptake in the tumor approximately 13 times greater than bowel uptake. A ratio of this order is preferable and predicts that the background normal bowel uptake of the radiolabeled monoclonal antibody should not interfere with scintigraphic imaging of the *in situ* colon carcinoma. Thus, the tissue distribution data gave credence to plans to determine the utility of WGHS22-2 radiolabeled with either of the two gamma-emitting radionuclides, iodine and indium.

C. IMAGING TECHNIQUES

Nine cotton-top tamarins were anesthetized and placed supine on a small Mylar restraint board and prepared for femoral intravenous injection of either ^{123}I- or ^{111}In-radiolabeled WGHS22-2 following a protocol approved by ORAU's Animal Care Standard Committee.[18] To prevent thyroidal uptake, tamarins scheduled to receive the iodinated monoclonal antibody were administered NaI orally 24 h before and immediately prior to injection. Serial images were obtained with a Searle Pho-Gamma V gamma camera equipped with a low-energy, all-purpose collimator at time intervals of 6, 24, 48, and 72 h. Of the nine tamarins studied, two were controls, three were classified as cancer suspects (radiographic evidence of colonic stricture without histological confirmation of cancer), and four demonstrated histological evidence of cancer.

IV. DISCUSSION

All nine tamarins received the I-123 derivative;[19] only three tamarins, one from each of the three groups also received the indium-111-labeled monoclonal antibody. Results of the scintigraphic studies using In-111 and I-123 demonstrated the three colon and one rectal cancers known to be present in this group of tamarins. Irrespective of the radionuclide used for radiolabeling, the two controls and the three cancer suspects all yielded negative scintigraphic images. The prognostic value is suggested by the circumstances surrounding positive scans obtained from two of the tamarins. Although radiographically classified as cancer suspects, imaging studies for these CTTs were clearly positive. Subsequently, at necropsy, colon carcinomas were diagnosed and confirmed histologically. The scintigraphic images obtained from the cancer-positive tamarins revealed good correlation with radiographs obtained by barium enema double air contrast pneumoperitoneography. The timed study which collected 100,000 counts at different periods of time indicated that optimal images were obtained at 24 h when either radionuclide was used as the radiolabeling agent. However, the overall quality of the images was substantially better with the I-123 radiolabeled monoclonal antibody. This may be due to the high liver uptake associated with In-111-labeled monoclonal antibodies. The exaggerated liver uptake presents substantial difficulties because of the proximity of the liver to the transverse and ascending colon which are frequent sites of occurrence of CTT colon cancer.

V. SUMMARY

In summary, scintigraphic studies of colorectal carcinomas in the cotton-top tamarin indicate that it is feasible and technically possible to image *in situ* carcinomas in this model of colon cancer which arises spontaneously and without chemical inducement. As a unique nonhuman primate model of a frequently occurring cancer in man, it offers a number of opportunities for future investigation.

ACKNOWLEDGMENTS

The authors gratefully acknowledge the contributions of B. L. Byrd, M. Henke, E. C. Holloway, Y. C. C. Lee, Z. Steplewski, T. T. H. Sun, and L. C. Washburn. This article, in part, is based on work supported by contract

No. DE-AC05-76OR00033 between the U.S. Department of Energy and Oak Ridge Associated Universities and by the National Cancer Institute under grant No. CA 39706.

REFERENCES

1. **Beart, R. W., Jr.,** Colorectal cancer, in *Textbook of Clinical Oncology,* Holleb, A. I., Fink, D. J., and Murphy, G. P., Eds., American Cancer Society, Atlanta, GA, 1991, 213.
2. **McAfee, J. G. and Thakur, M. L.,** Survey of radioactive agents for in vitro labeling of phagocytic leukocytes. I. Soluble agents, *J. Nucl. Med.,* 17, 480, 1976.
3. **Crook, J. E.,** unpublished data, 1987.
4. **Washburn, L. C., Lee, Y. C. C., Sun, T. T. H., Byrd, B. L., Crook, J. E., Stabin, M. G., and Steplewski, Z.,** Preclinical assessment of ^{90}Y-labeled monoclonal antibody CO17-1A, a potential agent for radioimmunotherapy of colorectal carcinoma, *Nucl. Med. Biol.,* 15, 707, 1988.
5. **Lee, Y. C. C., Washburn, L. C., Sun, T. T. H., Byrd, B. L., Crook, J. E., Holloway, E. C., and Steplewski, Z.,** Radioimmunotherapy of human colorectal carcinoma xenografts using ^{90}Y-labeled monoclonal antibody CO17-1A prepared by two bifunctional chelate techniques, *Cancer Res.,* 50, 4546, 1990.
6. **Clapp, N. K., Lushbaugh, C. C., Humason, G. L., Gangaware, B. L., and Henke, M. A.,** Natural history and pathology of colon cancer in Saguinus oedipus, *Digest. Dis. Sci.,* 30, 107S, 1985.
7. **Hine, K. R., Bradwell, A. R., and Reeder, T. A.,** Radioimmunodetection of gastrointestinal neoplasms with antibodies to carcinoembryonic antigen, *Cancer Res.,* 40, 2993, 1980.
8. **Clapp, N. K., Lushbaugh, C. C., Humason, G. I., Gangaware, B. L., and Henke, M. A.,** The marmoset as a model of ulcerative colitis and colon cancer, in *Colorectal Cancer and its Precursors,* Ingalls, J. F. and Mastromarino, A., Eds., Alan R. Liss, New York, 1985, 247.
9. **Clapp, N. K., Henke, M. A., Holloway, E. C., and Tankersley, W. G.,** Carcinoma of the colon in the cotton top tamarin: a radiographic study, *J. Am. Vet. Med. Assoc.,* 183, 1328, 1983.
10. **Crook, J. E.,** unpublished data.
11. **Steplewski, Z.,** personal communication.
12. **Hnatowich, D. J., Layne, W. W., Childs, R. L., Lanteigne, D., and Davis, M. A.,** Radioactive labeling of antibody: a simple and efficient method, *Science,* 220, 613, 1983.
13. **Crook, J. E., Lee, Y. C. C., Washburn, L. C., Sun, T. T. H., Byrd, B. L., Holloway, E. C., and Steplewski, Z.,** Effect of co-administration of IgG isotypes on biodistribution of Y-90 labeled monoclonal antibodies (MAB), *Antibiot. Immunoconjug. Radiopharm.,* 4, 14, 1991.
14. **Crook, J. E., Washburn, L. C., Lee, Y. C. C., Sun, T. T., Byrd, B. L., Holloway, E. C., Clapp, N. K., and Steplewski, Z.,** Imaging and radiolabeling studies of tamarin anticolon carcinoma monoclonal antibody BR55-2 with indium-111, in *Proc. Fourth Asia and Oceania Congress of Nuclear Medicine,* Taipei, Taiwan, 1988, 260.
15. **Littlefield, G. and Colyer, S.,** personal communication.
16. **Larson, S. M. and Carrasquillo, J. A.,** Advantages of radioiodine over radioindium labeled monoclonal antibodies for imaging solid tumors, *Nucl. Med. Biol.,* 15, 231, 1988.

17. **Greenwood, F. C., Hunt, W. M., and Clover, J. S.,** The preparation of ^{131}I-labelled human growth hormone of high specific radioactivity, *Biochem. J.*, 89, 114, 1963.
18. **Holloway, E. C., Crook, J. E., Lee, Y. C. C., Washburn, L. C., Sun, T. T. H., Henke, M., Clapp, N., and Steplewski, Z.,** Imaging techniques for radiolabeled monoclonal antibodies in the tamarin, *J. Nucl. Med. Technol.*, 18, 155, 1990.
19. **Lee, Y. C. C., Crook, J. E., Washburn, L. C., Holloway, E. C., Sun, T. T. H., Henke, M., Clapp, N., and Steplewski, Z.,** Imaging of colorectal cancer in tamarins using I-123-labeled monoclonal antibody, in *Proc. 5th Congress — World Federation of Nuclear Medicine and Biology,* Montreal, Canada, 1990.

E. Summary

Chapter 23

FUTURE DIRECTIONS FOR COLON DISEASE RESEARCH USING COTTON-TOP TAMARINS

Neal K. Clapp, Ronald V. Nardi, and Martin Tobi

TABLE OF CONTENTS

0-8493-5363-7/93/$0.00 + $.50

I. INTRODUCTION

In light of this effort reporting the current status of research on the cotton-top tamarin (CTT), some suggestions of where we have been, where we are, and where we may go in the study of colonic diseases seems appropriate. The answers to these questions may well appear different to individuals from varied perspectives. Consequently, three investigators from different backgrounds and expertise assisted in the assessment of this problem. One of us (Neal Clapp) is an experimental pathologist and a research investigator working in hands-on experiments with the cotton-top tamarins. This involves study of pathogenesis of tamarin colonic diseases, as well as performing the colonoscopy procedures, administering anesthesia, etc., plus the production and care of the animals, working with animal care and use committees, etc. Another (Ron Nardi) is from the private sector, specifically the pharmaceutical industry, which develops new drugs for improving human and animal health. His research interests include mechanisms in disease pathogenesis and intervention in these processes. Finally, Martin Tobi is a gastroenterologist who daily diagnoses colonic afflictions in human patients and seeks to alleviate their suffering. Since we are all concerned with pathogenesis and intervention, we have combined our efforts to evaluate both the successes of the past and present and the needs for the future and how we might address them.

As has been mentioned elsewhere in this volume, an international workshop was convened at Oak Ridge Associated Universities (ORAU) in 1984 to address the question, "Is the Marmoset an Experimental Model for the Study of Gastrointestinal Disease?" Dr. Conrad Richter, who spent some 5 years at ORAU addressing several husbandry and pathological issues, summarized the CTT colon cancer status as follows, "The cotton-top tamarin is an interesting and perhaps phenomenal opportunity to investigate the biology of a neoplastic disease occurring very regularly in a nonhuman primate. If we cannot learn something from this that is important to cancer biology, then we will be accused of being devoid of imagination." Since that time, considerable effort has been expended to better understand the CTT colon cancer as a model, and new arenas have been visited regarding CTT idiopathic colitis as another model with relevance to human disease. Some questions have been answered, many more have been asked, and certainly many more remain undiscovered.

II. COLITIS RESEARCH

Recognition of the inflammatory disease that precedes and is intercurrent with the development of colonic carcinoma has expanded the potential importance of the cotton-top tamarin in biomedical research. Just as the prevalence of colonic carcinoma has been recognized in most CTT colonies worldwide,[1] so has colitis been diagnosed where colonic specimens have been histologically examined. The presence of colitis appears to be independent of the environment in which the CTTs are housed, i.e., zoo population or research colony, individual or family-type caging, type of food provided, or continent (Europe or the U.S.). In feral CTTs of South America, as well as those in captivity, colitis has been observed.[2] It appears that the prevalence is approximately the same in colonies where prospective studies or colonic surveys have been performed by colonoscopy and mucosal biopsy.[3,4] The lower incidence reported in the feral setting may have more to do with numbers sampled and/or predators of sick animals than with actual disease incidence.

The 6-year serial examination in the longitudinal colitis study at ORAU and the colony survey conducted at New England Regional Primate Research Center offer information about the pathogenesis of the disease that may not even be available in humans.[3,4] Human information is obtained largely from clinical observations and reports, and little is known about the asymptomatic and subclinical aspects of the disease which have now been reported in cotton-tops.[3] Admittedly, we have only scratched the surface in studying the pathogenesis of these diseases, but we have a better understanding of their development than that which was evident 8 years ago.

In light of the variety of circumstances and locations in which CTT colitis is observed, a single infectious etiology, e.g., *Staphylococcus, Camplylobacter, Escherichia, Pseudomonas,* etc., seems unlikely. Several organisms have been suggested as etiological agents, and the role of coronaviruses is still under investigation.[5] Thus, in unidentified etiology, the CTT condition closely resembles the idiopathic nature of the disease as seen in humans.[6]

Similarities and dissimilarities between the disease in humans and in the cotton-top tamarin are still being discussed. Most pathologists that have examined both CTT tissues and human lesions agree that the human disease reaches more severe proportions; in particular, the hemorrhagic episodes that are common in man are infrequent in these primates. To date, the possible dissimilarities between colitis in CTTs and humans include the lack of some human extracolonic manifestations, e.g., arthropathies, skin lesions (which may be more difficult to recognize in fur-covered skin), and oral lesions, but hepatic lesions now reported in CTTs may well approximate those found in humans.[7] Admittedly, the total numbers of cotton-top tamarins that have been examined are relatively few (only a few thousand at best) in comparison to the millions of human idiopathic colitis cases from all backgrounds and environments that have been examined over hundreds of years.

Use of the colonoscopic and mucosal biopsy procedures that have been developed appears to be relatively safe as experimental protocols and produce little or no risk to these precious animals.[8] In itself, this is encouraging and avoids some potential conflicts between the biomedical research community and others who might question the justification of using these endangered animals in biomedical research. *The benefit derived is helpful for the afflicted animal species as well as for the anticipated value of data extrapolation to the human problem.* Development of the cotton-top tamarin model for evaluating anti-inflammatory efficacy has been a positive step in exploiting this animal model to more closely predict anticipated pharmacological activity in humans.[9] In addition, this procedure could prove to be financially valuable as a screening technique. Judicious selection of the animals to be used is most important if reasonable interpretation is to be made of the results. Identifying physiological differences in pharmacodynamics between results in rodents,[9] nonhuman primates, and humans encourages the cotton-top tamarin investigator, because these are the specific kinds of results that would make use of this primate model especially attractive. Some of the limitations facing the investigator are the lack of availability of CTTs, the numbers of animals that are needed as a critical mass to provide adequate afflicted CTTs, and the costs involved in producing and using primates in general. Some of these limitations may be resolved as more information becomes available and cost-benefit evaluations better elucidate the role of this model for selected usage.

III. COLORECTAL CARCINOMA

The prevalence of colorectal carcinoma in cotton-top tamarins has been established in almost every captive environment and location in the world. The evasive and, as yet, undetermined aspect of this disease is, why? As in the development of human colon cancer, genetic factors would appear important in species susceptibility as well as apparent species resistance. The fact that no colon cancers have been diagnosed in either common marmosets or saddle-back tamarins in >2500 necropsies of these species housed in an identical environment (at ORAU) supports both species susceptibility (CTTs) and resistance.[10] The familial contribution may also be important, but remains to be proven.[11,12] With larger colonies and more known generations of CTTs to be studied in greater detail, this answer may soon be obtained.

Investigators in several colonies have produced data that incriminate the colitic episodes as predisposing the CTT colon to the neoplastic process in the CTT.[1,3,4] In man, colorectal carcinoma is also more prevalent among individuals with chronic colitis. Whether colitis is a "true promoter" of carcinogenesis may be the focus of some new studies that could elucidate the role of biochemical changes (inflammatory mediators, cytokines, growth factors, etc.) in this process. Study of changes in ploidy may also offer insight into the strong susceptibility of CTTs to colorectal carcinoma.

The study of death rates associated with certain diseases is quite interesting, but a difficult problem is posed in that we have no reliable methods to accurately predict the age of imported CTTs. A previously conservative, admittedly nonscientific "guesstimate" had been simply to assume that the CTT adults on arrival in captivity were at least two years of age (physically mature). This would likely result in underestimation rather than a reliable determination of age. On the other hand, the calculated estimate of age from assuming continuing and identical death rates may also need application of some new evolving techniques that may provide more accurate estimates.

While important differences between tamarin and human cancer exist, the association with colitis in tamarins and man suggests that a common mechanism in carcinogenesis may be operative. The cotton-top tamarin may therefore be an invaluable model in the elucidation of (1) mechanisms of carcinogenesis, (2) cancer diagnosis, surveillance, and screening techniques, and (3) cancer therapy, all of which in the human setting engender considerable controversy.

IV. PHYSIOLOGICAL PARAMETERS

Changes in physiological and pathophysiological parameters continue to offer hope but no pathognomonic perturbation exists for either inflammatory bowel disease or colon cancer. Perhaps some of the frustrating results from these types of studies are due, in part, to the fact that currently available techniques are unable to identify the specific biochemical compounds or changes that could accurately predict the disease state. In a recent abstract, carcinoembryonic antigen-like compounds were identified in cotton-top tamarins that had not previously been recognized.[13] Changes in mucin production and lymphocyte cell numbers may well add insight into the pathogenesis of these diseases as well as their value as markers for the disease occurrence. Further studies in these areas are clearly indicated.

V. CONCLUSIONS

Some progress has been made in better understanding the colonic diseases that occur in the cotton-top tamarin; obviously, many questions remain. Does the cotton-top develop colon cancer in the wild? First, we do not know because not enough animals have been examined to identify even one positive cancer or to be certain that the disease does not occur in the wild; the effect of predators on a wild population and survival behavioral characteristics also enter this picture. Second, it is conceivable that sick animals simply do not survive long enough to develop cancer. They may die during the colitic episodes that were recently recognized in the feral state, albeit these were described as somewhat less severe. However, the observation of feral CTT colon cancer, of itself, is not required for the animal model to be of value to biomedical researchers; it is present in captive colonies. Certainly, the cotton-top tamarin colonic carcinoma needs to be understood in light of the elegant work of Vogelstein[14] and others. If this animal model proves comparable to humans in at least part of its pathogenic mechanisms, much advancement in knowledge could accrue rapidly because of the contracted time frame for colon cancer development in these animals (a few years) as opposed to the decades of latency in humans.

Use of the CTT colitis model may be currently increasing at a more rapid rate than study of the CTT colon cancer because some immediate needs have been met. Information has been obtained regarding pathogenesis as well as mechanisms that have made the animal extremely attractive as a nonhuman primate model. This is also an important area for new pharmaceutical products where much effort needs to be invested. A scientific approach to understanding the basic mechanisms of pathogenesis is essential to develop targeted therapeutic agents in the eradication of this debilitating disease.

Our research opportunities using cotton-top tamarins to study colonic diseases are truly only limited by our ingenuity.

REFERENCES

1. **Clapp, N. K.,** Prevalence of colonic carcinoma in cotton-top tamarin colonies through the world, This volume, Chapter 13.
2. **Wood, J. D. and Peck, O. C.,** Idiopathic colitis and colon cancer in the cotton-top tamarin, in *Effects of Immuno Cells and Inflammation on Smooth Muscle and Enteric Nerves,* Snape, W. J. and Collins, S., Eds., CRC Press, Boca Raton, FL, 1990.
3. **Clapp, N. K., Henke, M. A., Hansard, R. M., Carson, R. L., Adams, L. J., and Nardi, R. V.,** Natural history, time course, and pathogenesis of idiopathic colitis in cotton-top tamarins *(Saguinus oedipus),* This volume, Chapter 4.
4. **King, N. W., Johnson, L. D., Sehgal, P. K., and Ringler, D. J.,** The prevalence of idiopathic colitis in the New England Regional Primate Research Center cotton-top tamarin *(Saguinus oedipus)* colony, This volume, Chapter 5.
5. **Brian, D. A. and Shockley, L. J.,** Coronaviruses in tamarin and marmoset colitis, This volume, Chapter 9.
6. **Goulston, S. J. M. and McGovern, V. J.,** *Fundamentals of Colitis,* Pergamon Press, New York, 1981.
7. **Warren, B. F., Henke, M. A., and Clapp, N.,** Extraintestinal manifestations of cotton-top tamarin colitis, This volume, Chapter 7.
8. **Clapp, N. K., Henke, M. A., Hansard, R. M., Carson, R. L., and Nardi, R. V.,** Do repeated colonic mucosal biopsies impact mortality in cotton-top tamarins?, This volume, Chapter 10.
9. **Clapp, N. K., Henke, R. M., Hansard, R. M., and Carson, R. L.,** A protocol to evaluate the efficacy of anticolitic agents against ulcerative colitis in cotton-top tamarins, This volume, Chapter 8.
10. **Clapp, N. K. and Henke, M. A.,** Spontaneous colonic carcinoma observations in the Oak Ridge Associated Universities' 26-year-old cotton-top tamarin *(Saguinus oedipus)* colony, This volume, Chapter 11.
11. **Petersen, G. M. and Roth, M.-P.,** Genetic epidemiology of colon cancer, This volume, Chapter 12.
12. **Cheverud, J. M., Tardif, S., Henke, M. A., and Clapp, N. K.,** Is colon cancer heritable in the cotton-top tamarin *(Saguinus oedipus)?, Am. J. Phys. Anthropol.,* S14, 59, 1992.
13. **Tobi, M., Chintalapani, S., Kaila, V., Kithier, K., Henke, M., and Clapp, N.,** The cotton-top tamarin (*Saguinus oedipus*) as a model for human inflammatory bowel disease: an antigenic profile, *Gastroenterology,* submitted.
14. **Vogelstein, B., Fearon, E. R., Hamilton, S. R., Preisinger, A. C., Leppert, M., Nakamura, Y., White, R., Smits, A. M. M., and Bos, J. L.,** Genetic alterations during colorectal tumor development, *N. Engl. J. Med.,* 319, 525, 1988.

Index

INDEX

A

B

C

D

E

F

G

H

I

J

K

L

N

O

P

Q

R

T

U

V

W

X

Y

Z